HERPESVIRIDAE

Edited by **József Ongrádi**

Herpesviridae
http://dx.doi.org/10.5772/61923
Edited by József Ongrádi

Contributors
Pablo Alberto Gonzalez, Susan Bueno, Eduardo Tognarelli, Angello Retamal, Alexis Kalergis, Pierre Busson, Gurpreet Kaur, Mudit Chandra, Yukio Kato, Mo Chen, Li-Yi Cai, Takako Kato, Miroslav Andric, Aleksandar Jakovljevic, Aleksandra Knezevic, Katarina Beljic-Ivanovic, Maja Miletic, Tanja Jovanovic, Ljiljana Kesic, Jelena Milašin, Clinton Jones, Carola Otth, Francisca Acuña-Hinrichsen, Luis Leyton, Margarita Concha, Carolina Martin, Julius Rajčáni, Vladimira Ďurmanová, Marian Adamkov, Joseph Ongrádi

Published by InTech
Janeza Trdine 9, 51000 Rijeka, Croatia

Publishing Process Manager Andrea Koric
Technical Editor SPi Global
Cover InTech Design team

First published September, 2016
Printed in Croatia

Additional hard copies can be obtained from orders@intechopen.com

Herpesviridae, Edited by József Ongrádi
p. cm.
Print ISBN 978-953-51-2610-2
Online ISBN 978-953-51-2611-9

For EU product safety concerns:
IN TECH d.o.o., Prolaz Marije Krucifikse Kozulić 3, 51000 Rijeka, Croatia,
info@intechopen.com or visit our website at intechopen.com.

Meet the editor

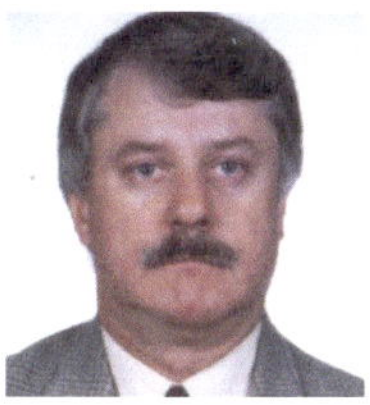

Joseph Ongrádi graduated as MD at the Semmelweis University of Medicine, Budapest, Hungary, in 1976. At this university, he obtained his PhD at the Institute of Microbiology. He is a board-certified medical microbiologist and clinical biologist and has habilitation in medical microbiology. Between 1998 and 2005, he was the Head of Microbiology Laboratory, Department of Dermato-Venereology; between 2005 and 2010, he was the head of the Immunovirology Laboratory, Department of Public Health, and he returned to the Department of Medical Microbiology in 2011. His interests include latency, reactivation, interaction of herpesviruses, adenoviruses, and retroviruses. He described the role of Roseoloviruses in skin diseases, multiple sclerosis and AIDS, and two bacterium species as sexually transmitted infections and isolated the first Adenovirus from Felidae in the feline AIDS model.

Contents

Preface

Herpesviruses possess a complex self-regulatory mechanism and an extremely sophisticated machinery to invade, persist for life in the organism's virome, and cause several forms of, even lethal, acute or chronic debilitating diseases depending on both the virus and host species. Lately, sensitive molecular and immunological methods have shown that herpesviruses evade the immune defense mimicking host functions; furthermore, through altering the normal interleukin pattern and dispersing their components with regulatory potential to remote organs, they modulate the complete physiology of the organism. Several herpesvirus species transactivate heterologous viruses to promote progression of non–herpesvirus-associated diseases. The lack of appropriate animal models due to very intimate host-parasite relationship has long hindered studies on the simultaneous pathological events in vivo.

Novelties regarding the molecular biology and unconventional pathology of *Herpesviridae* will profoundly alter our way of thinking in near future. This book covers more hot topics of contemporary human and veterinary fields of the herpesvirus literature. The "Introduction" shortly raises questions and gives some answers why herpesviruses are somewhat unique among viral parasites. In the first part of this book, more chapters are intended to give an overview on typical clinical syndromes, in which herpesviruses are unambiguously involved through their partial gene expression and inapparent virus production. The first chapter written by Otth and coworkers summarizes up-to-date knowledge on the pathomechanism of herpes simplex virus (HSV)-1 infection in the central nervous system. This is one of the hottest topics in the transplantation setting due to the sharp increase in the number of individuals at risk: immunocompromised patients who suffer from acute encephalitis or its lifelong debilitating sequelae and, furthermore and elderly persons suffering from chronic devastating disorders with unknown etiology. A possible connection of Alzheimer's disease with HSV-1 reactivation is discussed. The second chapter prepared by Jakovljevic and coworkers contains a meta-analysis of four cross-sectional studies on an old topic. It has been suspected for several decades that different viruses from all *Herpesviridae* subfamilies can contribute to periodontal diseases, but no appropriate technology has been available to investigate their effects. Genetic polymorphism of both herpesviruses (especially CMV and the Epstein-Barr virus (EBV)) and the host might sensitize individuals to periapical diseases leading to tooth loss. In the third chapter prepared by Chen et al., we learn how HSV-1 could contribute to male infertility. Herpesviruses cannot infect germ cells; therefore, an unconventional way must exist in this clinical problem. In transgenic rats expressing the open reading frame of HSV-1 thymidine kinase, consequent altered cellular gene expression along with severe morphological alterations in postmeiotic spermatids could be the reason for infertility. From this very well-focused small animal model, the results are extrapolated to human conditions.

The second part of this book is devoted to the recent forefront of virology: immune evasion. Retamaz-Díaz and coworkers classify the modes and how herpes simplex viruses can negatively modulate host immune functions. Modulation of signaling pathways, interference with proper pathogen recognition, hampered innate and adaptive immunity, and all aspects of immune cell damages are thoroughly discussed. Very clearly constructed tables help the reader orientate in the jungle of viral actions and host counteractions.

The third part is devoted to discuss novel therapeutic and prevention strategies in herpesvirus-associated disorders. Oker and coworkers describe a promising way recently that has been applied in onco-virology: viral oncolysis. In contrast to other attempts to infect tumor cells using virus vectors, in the Epstein-Barr virus-associated nasopharyngeal and other carcinomas, pharmacological activation of this virus from latency to lytic infection could destroy tumor cells. Advantages of the potential, activating chemical compounds over conventional chemotherapy are discussed. Several professional tables and figures illustrate the complicated molecular switch from partial gene expression to cell lysis by replicating virus. The following review written by Durmanová and coworkers returns to an old but, in spite of huge efforts, still unresolved problem: vaccination against HSV-1 and HSV-2. Prevention and immunotherapeutic use would bear a significant impact, especially in immunocompromised patients. From analyzing previously unsuccessful attempts, authors draw the conclusion that boosting activity of cytotoxic CD8+ cells using lipopeptides and new adjuvants could lead to clinical application.

The last chapter on bovine herpesvirus infection deals with a severe economical impact in animal husbandry. The general review by Kaur and Chandra describes the complete characteristics and clinical aspects of these viruses, laying emphasis on diagnostic procedures. The accompanying paper from C. Jones focuses on the establishment of neuronal latency and its reactivation, especially after using corticosteroid hormones. This aspect raises the idea that studies on bovine herpesvirus infection could be a valuable, large animal model for its human counterpart.

To conclude, one can say that ongoing herpesvirus research is not exclusively academic. Several data have served as a base for sensitive diagnostic procedures or targets for conventional chemotherapy. Well beyond these aspects, immense amount of knowledge is accumulating about both the alternative, unconventional ways in regulating herpesvirus infections and their contribution to the broad range of clinical disorders with unresolved etiology. These open novel strategies to prevent and treat human and animal herpesvirus infections. The chapters collected in the book are intended to read not only for those who are specialist in the field of *Herpesviridae* but also for other virologists, microbiologists, and medical and veterinary professionals.

The Editor is very thankful to Ms. Andrea Koric (Publishing Process Manager, InTech Editorial Office, Rijeka, Croatia), for her kind technical guidance throughout the preparation of this book, and to Ms. Valéria Kövesdi (Chief Technician, Institute of Medical Microbiology, Semmelweis University, Budapest, Hungary), for her very accurate clerical help in handling manuscripts.

József Ongrádi, MD, PhD, med. habil.
Institute of Medical Microbiology
Semmelweis University
Budapest, Hungary

Section 1

Introduction

Chapter 1

Introductory Chapter: Unconventional Philosophy of Herpesvirus Infections

Joseph Ongrádi

Additional information is available at the end of the chapter

http://dx.doi.org/10.5772/64818

The course of herpesvirus infection in human and animals is not so simple as it has been presumed on the analogy of other microbes at the beginning of virology era. Classification into acute and chronic infections, simple distinction of complete clinical and virological recovery or perishing of the host organism belong to the conventional views on the course and outcome of virus infections. But several other forms of existence of herpesviruses (HHVs) in the host are possible. Many diverse interactions between the macro-organism and herpesviruses have been discovered gradually. In spite of these new data, conventionally, the idea about one organism causing one well-characterized disease has remained in the mind of the majority of both many medical, veterinary professionals and the public. Nowadays we believe that we understand the pathomechanism of herpesviral diseases. Simply saying, this is not true, because, frequently we encounter new experimental evidence that cause surprise and continuously modify dogmas. The conventional way of our thinking on host-viral interaction is somewhat static, but the life-long flow of events between invading herpesviruses and the defensive organism is dynamic: several alternative ways on both sides might influence outcome. Furthermore, their bilateral interplay is modified by many intrinsic and extrinsic factors, consequently it is rather multilateral. This moment there are delicate methods to follow post-infection events at the molecular level. Beside structural polypeptides, herpesviruses encode a large number of proteins with enzymatic or regulatory functions. The exact way of regulating their activities by post-translational modifications, e.g. glycosylation or phosphorylation, is hardly explored. Events at sub-molecular level and energy flow during assembly of their structural components are almost unknown. Basic physics, not conventional virology could help supply knowledge in these matters. Data processing by computers analyses tens of thousands of data obtained in one model experiment or clinical cohorts including large number of patients, but in future we have to extrapolate their pathophysiological meaning to clinical relevance. It is surprising at the first glance, that the same herpesvirus species can contribute to both acute clinical picture exhibiting characteristic symptoms (vesicles, rash, fever, etc.), and chronic, debilitating diseases without apparent virus production (tumours, autoimmune diseases, etc.). Similarly, related herpesviruses could induce the same clinical symptoms, as herpes simplex virus (HSV) 1 and 2, or cytomegalovirus (CMV) and Epstein-Barr virus (EBV), or HHV-6B and HHV-7. These suggest that our detecting systems are not fine enough to distinguish only superficially identical processes. We are on a good path to reveal the importance of genetic background, namely, polymorphism of both the virus and its host in the course of pathogenesis. Latency, persistence can be regarded as a balanced state between herpesviruses and animals. Instead of complete gene expression and virion production, partial gene expression evolved through phylogenesis and co-evolution by the host and its herpesviruses. Even maintenance of episomal latency of herpesviruses is not a passive process, it requires active viral gene expression as it has been shown in the case of Epstein-Barr virus and herpes simplex virus. Partial gene expression was described in EBV-associated or Kaposi sarcoma herpesvirus (KSHV)-associated tumours several decades ago. Both life-long latency without activation and malignant transformation of cells and consequent contribution to tumour induction and progression are a dead end for the virus along with the perishing host instead of replication and spreading to the environment to find new hosts. Another unusual aspect of herpesvirus pathogenicity is that in 0.2–0.85% of the human population HHV-6A and HHV-6B are integrated in the telomeric region of human chromosomes, and transmitted vertically by standard Mendelian inheritance or by any cell donation [1]. The time and mode of integration in our ancestors are unknown. Some of the carrier persons suffer from neurological symptoms for several years with remittances and relapses [2]. At this moment it is not known whether the life span is modified by HHV-6 species. In combatting defence mechanisms of the organism, different herpesviruses developed cascade mechanisms to mimic several molecular events hijacked from their host. Among alternative infection strategies these are regarded as parts of immune evasion. Can we introduce similar or other human host genes into herpesvirus vaccines to improve their efficacy? Can we introduce genes of animal origin into a human or animal herpesvirus vaccine? Would it be dangerous or unethical? How to select a human gene donor? There are attempts to use HHV-7 as a vector to treat genetic disorders, because this virus has been regarded as ubiquitous and harmless. But lately several clinical reports have shown that it reactivates in the recipients after solid organ transplantation and aggravates CMV disease. In bone marrow or stem cell transplant recipients, usually in small children with leukemias, it also reactivates, and can elicit a very severe, frequently lethal encephalitis. Delayed primary HHV-7 infection in adults might result in a generalized infection, tetraplegia and encephalitis [3]. Conventional common belief about HHV-7 has been turned to the opposite direction in a few years of time.

To find new host cells, cell-to-cell spread is a convenient way. Some herpesviruses are regarded as cell associated, but the exact molecular cascade in this process has not been elucidated yet. So far, we have known that alteration of the function of neighbouring cells or distant cells is mediated by soluble mediators, cytokines and chemokines. Discovery of micro-vesicles and exosomes that can contain fragments of viral nucleic acid, mRNAs and microRNAs with regulatory potential will change our ideas about the regulation of the whole body of a macro-organism by viruses. These vesicles are released from infected cells to the microenvironment or

http://dx.doi.org/10.5772/64818

the circulation, and are taken up by another cells in the vicinity or very far in the body, subsequently they induce further pathological changes that have not directly been credited with virus infections so far. Accumulating evidence suggests that this mechanism is widely used by human herpesvirus species. Exosomes released from HSV-1-infected cells can contain viral polypeptides (gH, gD). Interestingly, they contain modified tegument and envelope proteins that usually originate from the light particles of HSV. Tegument proteins outside the nucleocapsid exert very important regulatory functions. Such content of exosomes promote spread and latency by HSVs. CMV-infected cells release exosomes with cellular molecules that are necessary for virus uptake. These might contribute to allograft rejection in transplant recipients. Exosomes released from HHV-6-infected cells transfer MHC I molecules in addition to complete viral particles. This latter is an absolute viral journey in disguise throughout the whole body, even crossing the blood-brain barrier. Furthermore, growth factors that are very important in EBV pathogenesis can be shuttled into exosomes. Viral antigens in the absence of apparent EBV replication can be transferred to other cells, consequently they can induce autoimmune or other diseases. Exosomes produced by KSHV-infected cells can carry both cellular and viral mRNAs promoting sarcoma metastases. All these phenomena contribute to the transient infection, a newly recognized form of viral existence in the body (see references in [4]).

The structure of herpesviruses comprising the nucleocapsid, tegument and envelope resembles the cellular nucleus, cytoplasm and cell membrane, respectively [5]. The regular belief is that the effect of viruses on cells starts when virus genes are expressed in the cells. Really, this effect starts much earlier, when virions attach to receptors and co-receptors instructing them to send fake messages to reprogram cellular machinery.

Asymptomatic virus shedding is very common in all herpesvirus infections. At the population level, it can be difficult to establish the source and time of infection, e.g. in contract tracing, to find and prove the possible donor in certain cases, even in the court, decades later, or to describe viral epidemiology. Simultaneous herpesvirus infections, or in the presence of one species in the body, a super-infection by another herpesvirus species might occur. In such events, direct interaction in the same host cells or indirect interaction between different cells infected by distinct viruses can take place, resulting in intracellular or trans-cellular transactivation between two competent viruses. Interactions among herpesviruses promote reactivation from latency, profoundly modify innate immunity and T-cell activity, only a few facts to mention [6]. Interaction of herpesviruses with other viruses has gained clinical importance lately, especially in AIDS patients. All human herpesvirus species are involved in the one way or mutual transactivation with HIV facilitating AIDS progression. Especially β- and γ-herpesviruses are able to transactivate other unrelated viruses, bacteria and parasites [7]. The net effect of transactivation is neither additive nor synergistic; new formulas have to be created for their mathematical modelling. It is conceivable that formulas will depend on actual virus pairs. These phenomena listed above could be regarded as crossroads of epidemiology: the unknown source and time of infection by the participating viruses pose a nightmare to classical epidemiologists.

The simplest question is: do animals including human contain a normal virus flora similarly to the normal bacterial flora? Latency, persistence of herpesviruses with asymptomatic shedding but without apparent harm to the host might suggest an answer: yes [6]. But appearance of clinical symptoms, tumours, even causing acute lethal complications by the same reactivated viruses imply no. No sharp distinction, a clear answer can be made regarding our virome. It is important for human to undergo several bacterial infections during the early period of our life cycle: some microbes establish the normal flora and all of them induce some form of immunity (e.g. systemic, mucosal). Their presence in the body and wide range effects significantly exceeds these simple facts. It seems that it is also important to acquire herpesvirus infections in early childhood. These infections are usually asymptomatic or mild conferring protection against super-infection. Delayed primary herpesvirus infections of seronegative individuals usually are accompanied by severe clinical manifestations. The order of sequential primary infections could be regulated. A simple example is shown by HSV-1 infection in infants, HSV-2 infection in adolescents or HHV-6B infection around 6 months of age, HHV-7 infection around 3 or 4 years of age in spite of the same, salivary route of transmission. The exact mode of regulation is absolutely unknown. Unfortunately, rapidly changing life style and other social factors not only disturb but disrupt these well established, conserved biological processes [3].

Herpesviruses easily adapted themselves to different animals, and through co-evolution with the given host an equilibrium has established for the compromise of both partners. The interaction is very intimate and varies by both herpesvirus species and the host macroorganism. That is one of the reasons why studies on herpesvirus pathogenesis has been hindered by the lack of appropriate animal models, and this is especially true for β-herpesvirinae and γ-herpesvirinae.

From these examples taken arbitrarily, it is conceivable that herpesviruses must not be regarded as conventional parasites, their existence in the body is neither mutualism nor commensalism, rather it is challenging to regard them as unconventional pathogens.

Author details

Joseph Ongrádi

Address all correspondence to: ongradi.jozsef@med.semmelweis-univ.hu

Institute of Medical Microbiology, Semmelweis University, Budapest, Hungary

References

[1] Morisette G, Flamand L: Herpesviruses and chromosomal integration. J. Virol. 2010; 84:12100–12109. DOI: 10.1128/JVI.01169-10

[2] Montoya JG, Neely MN, Gupta S, Lunn MR, Loomis KS, Prichett JC, Polsky B, Medveczky PG: Antiviral therapy of two patients with chromosomally-integrated human herpesvirus-6A presenting with cognitive dysfunction. J. Clin. Virol. 2012; 55:40–45. DOI: 10.1016/j.jcv.2012.05.016

[3] Ongrádi J, Stercz B, Kövesdi V, Nagy K, Prichett J, Ablashi D, Jacobson S: Human herpesvirus 6A, 6B, and 7 encephalitis. In: Singh SK, Ruzek D, editors. Neuroviral infections. Boca Raton, FL: Taylor & Francis Group/CRC Press; 2013. pp. 313–345. ISBN: 978-1-46-656719-1

[4] Anderson MR, Kashanchi F, Jacobson S: Exosomes in viral disease. Neurotherapeutics. 20 June, 2016. DOI: 10.1007/s13311-016-0450-6. Epub ahead of print.

[5] Brown N, Bhella D: Are viruses alive? Microbiol. Today. 2016; 43:58–61. www.microbiologysociety.org

[6] Reese TA: Coinfections: another variable in the herpesvirus latency—reactivation dynamic. J. Virol. 2016; 90:5534–5537. DOI: 10.1128/JVI.01865-15

[7] Ongrádi J, Kövesdi V, Nagy K, Matteoli B, Ceccherini-Nelli L, Ablashi DV: *In vitro* and *in vivo* transactivation of HIV by HHV-6. In: Chang TL, editor. HIV-host interactions. Vienna, Austria: InTech; 2011. pp. 257–298. ISBN: 978-953-307-442-9

Section 2

Novel Aspects of Human Herpesvirus Infections in Clinical Syndromes

Chapter 2

Herpes Simplex Virus Type 1 at the Central Nervous System

Carola Otth, Francisca Acuña-Hinrichsen,
Luis Leyton, Carolina Martin and
Margarita I. Concha

Additional information is available at the end of the chapter

http://dx.doi.org/10.5772/64130

Abstract

Herpes simplex virus type 1 (HSV-1) is a ubiquitous and neurotropic pathogen and is the most common cause of acute sporadic encephalitis in humans. This virus is characterized by establishing a persistent latent infection in neurons of its hosts for life. The pathogenic mechanisms of HSV-1 at the central nervous system (CNS) are not completely elucidated. Besides, evidences suggest that HSV-1 establish latency in the CNS in humans and that this condition would not be harmless, especially in people whose immune system is declined. This trait has been strongly suggested as a risk factor for the development of neurodegenerative pathologies such as Alzheimer's disease. Currently, it is unclear whether a neuron, which undergoes viral reactivation and produces infectious particles, survives and resumes latency, loses functionality, or is killed. These data highlight the need for more studies at cellular and molecular levels to understand the strategies used by the virus and the host cells during both productive and latent infection. The present chapter discusses the current investigations about HSV-1 infection at the CNS and the potential risk of neuronal dysfunction and chronic neurological diseases.

Keywords: HSV-1, AD, CNS infections, Neurovirulence, neuronal dysfunction, neuroepithelium

1. Introduction to herpes simplex virus

Human herpes viruses belong to the family *Herpesviridae* and are characterized by having a linear double-stranded DNA genome, an icosahedral capsid surrounded by a tegument—an amorphous layer of proteins that surround the capsid—and an envelope formed by polyamines, lipids, and glycoproteins. Herpes simplex virus (HSV) is distributed worldwide and has the ability to infect epithelial and neuronal cells establishing a latent persistent infection at the nervous system [1, 2].

HSV infection typically occurs during childhood, by direct inoculation of infected droplets from orolabial or nasal secretions onto susceptible mucosal surfaces or abraded skin, and infections mostly are asymptomatic and only 1–6% of primary infections are clinically recognized [3]. Initial infection typically occurs in the lip, but can also happen in the mucous membranes of the eyes or nose [1, 4].

In the productive infection, HSV expresses its genome, which is organized as immediate early, early and late genes producing viral particles progeny. For herpes simplex virus 1 (HSV-1), the initial step in the sequential viral gene expression is directed by VP16, a viral tegumental protein that enters into the nucleus associated to the capsids during infection (**Figure 1**). VP16 recruits the following transcription factors to the promoters of viral immediately early genes and several host proteins: host cell factor 1 (HCF1), octamer-binding protein 1 (Oct1), and lysine-specific demethylase 1 (LSD1). The immediate early genes are then transcribed, and among them the infected cell protein 0 (ICP0) is a key regulatory protein that commands different functions and regulates the expression of early and late viral genes [1, 5, 6].

Subsequently, during initial productive infection with HSV-1 on epithelial cells (see **Figure 1**), the viral progeny reaches the cell bodies of the sensory and sympathetic neurons in the trigeminal ganglia through retrograde transport, establishing latent infection, a characteristic of all herpes viruses.

In latent state, episomal HSV-1 DNA remains inside the nucleus of the peripheral neurons of the infected host, without production of infectious progeny lifelong. During latency, the latency-associated transcript (LAT) is abundantly transcribed in infected neurons in mice, rabbits, and humans and is predominantly detected in the nucleus, but can also be detected in the cytoplasm [7]. Splicing of the primary 8.3-kb LAT yields an abundant poly(A) and uncapped stable 2-kb LAT intron, which is necessary for the establishment and maintenance of latency [8]. In [9], the authors concluded that LAT is an miRNA precursor that encodes six miRNAs, one of these, miR-H6, downregulates immediate early ICP4 and ICP0 protein levels, which are involved in the initiation of productive HSV-1 infection or reactivation episodes.

Currently, it has been hypothesized that the establishment of latent state in neurons happens because HCF1 accumulates in the cytoplasm and is transported into the nuclei only in response to stress [5, 6, 10]. In addition, viral capsids, but not VP16, reach the nuclear pore through retrograde transport. Finally, in the absence of nuclear HCF1 and VP16, the immediately early HSV-1 genes are not expressed and the viral genome is fully silenced, except for LATs and miRNAs [1, 5, 6, 9–12].

Diverse nonspecific events (fever, stroke, hormonal cycle, physical or emotional stress, etc.), including immune system imbalance, can trigger HSV-1 reactivation. It has been suggested that in these situations, nuclear translocation of HCF1 is the triggering event involved in HSV-1 reactivation. Reactivated virus is transported back to the body surface to cause recurrent

http://dx.doi.org/10.5772/64130

lesions manifested as cold sores (herpes labialis) [1, 13]. In some cases, HSV-1 invades the central nervous system (CNS), where it replicates in neuronal cells [1, 10–15] causing devastating herpes simplex encephalitis (HSE) [1, 2], or providing a reservoir for virus production and shedding lifelong.

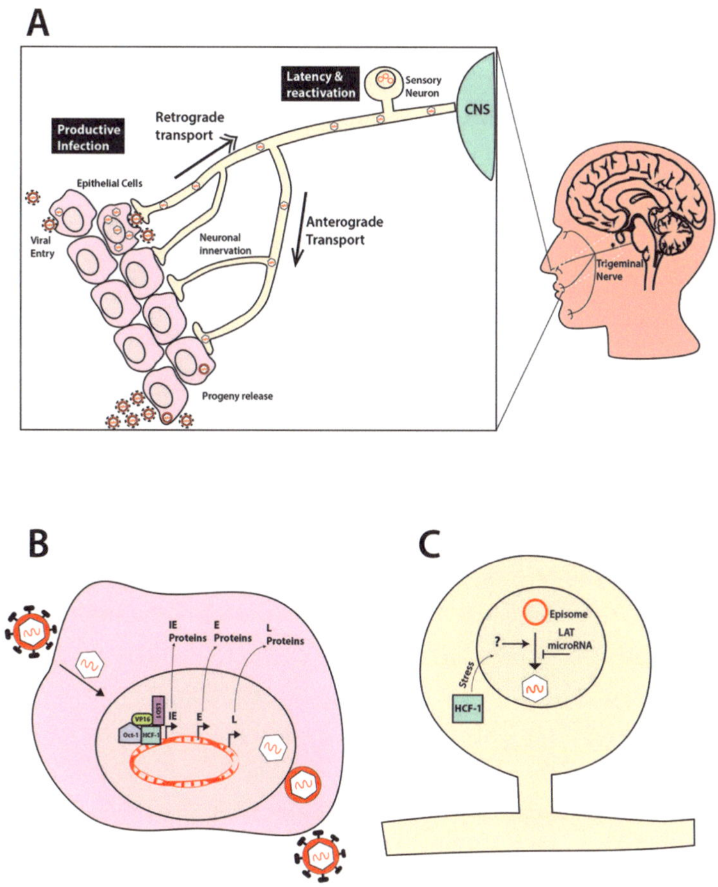

Figure 1. Productive infection and latency/reactivation of HSV-1 cycle. (**A**) The scheme shows that the viral progeny of HSV-1 productive infection at epithelial cells enters the axons that innerve this site of infection. Then, capsids travel by retrograde transport reaching the nucleus, located in the soma of the neuron at the trigeminal ganglia. At this place, HSV-1 genome enters the nucleus and remains as an episome in a latent state. Under stress conditions, HSV-1 reactivates expressing its genome, and initiating a controlled productive infection in neurons. Then, capsids travel back by anterograde transport reaching the initial site of infection at epithelial cells. The progeny released initiates a new productive infection at this place. (**B**) During productive infection, the initial step in the sequential viral gene expression program is directed by VP16, a viral tegumental protein that enters into the nucleus associated to the capsids during infection. VP16 recruits the following transcription factors to the promoters of viral immediately early genes and several host proteins: host cell factor 1 (HCF1), octamer-binding protein 1 (Oct1), and lysine-specific demethylase 1 (LSD1). The immediate early genes are then transcribed, and among them the infected cell protein 0 (ICP0) is a key regulatory protein that commands different functions and regulates the expression of early and late viral genes. (**C**) In neurons, HSV-1 latency transcripts (LATs and miRNA) silence the viral genome establishing a latent persistent infection. In this state, there is no production of viral particles. Nevertheless, under stressful conditions, the HSV-1 genome is reactivated by a mechanism that is suggested to involve the nuclear translocation of HCF1.

In animal models, there is evidence indicating that HSV-1 infection suppresses the hypothalamic-pituitary-adrenal axis during primary infection, suggesting that this stress-induced suppression has a role in virus reactivation [16].

HSV-1 is an endemic worldwide infection, with a population prevalence of 31% in children aged 6–14, 49% in people aged 14–49, and 80–90% in the population over 65 years old [4]. However, only 20–40% of infected people develop symptoms [17]. In spite of this, in [18], the authors showed that close to 35% of asymptomatic subjects were positive for HSV in eye and mouth swabs, showing higher HSV-1 genome copy numbers in saliva than in tears. Healthy humans are reservoirs of herpes viruses, and asymptomatic shedding is a major factor in the spread of the HSV-1.

2. Herpes simplex virus type 1 tropism

HSV attachment and entry are regulated by surface glycoproteins gC, gB, gD, and gH-gL. Attachment is a two-step process involving the primary interaction of gC and/or gB with heparan sulfate proteoglycans (HSPGs) present at cellular surfaces, followed by the secondary gD-mediated binding to its receptors, such as HVEM (herpes virus entry mediator), nectin-1, or 3-O-sulfated heparan sulfate. This interaction triggers the activation of gH-gL and gB, which leads to the fusion of viral envelope and plasma membrane of the host cell either at the surface or in endosomes [19]. The viral glycoprotein gD determines HSV tropism, and the conformational changes in gD upon binding to its receptors are critical in triggering an activation cascade [19]. HSV capsids are then delivered directly to the cytosol at the periphery of these cells, completing the entry process.

Several cell receptors for viral entry have been described, but numerous observations suggest that more receptors for HSV-1 might exist. In [20], a novel role for the proteolipid protein (PLP) in HSV-1 entry into the human oligodendrocytic cell line human oligodendroglioma (HOG) has been proposed. Oligodendrocytes (OLs) are the glial cells that produce myelin, the electrically insulating layer that surrounds axons in the CNS [21]. Proteolipid proteins, together with DM20, a smaller isoform generated by alternative splicing, are the most abundant proteins in the CNS myelin, comprising around 50% of total myelin proteins [22]. In addition, when PLP is transfected in cells infected with mutant virus unable to replicate, there is an increase in viral signal compared to cells without PLP. Additionally, a mouse monoclonal antibody against PLP drastically inhibited HSV-1 entry into HOG cells. Moreover, PLP and virions were shown to colocalize by confocal and electron microscopy analyses, suggesting that PLP might be involved in HSV-1 entry in human oligodendrocytes [20].

Viruses depend on cells for their replication and can differentially affect various signaling pathways during the course of infection [23]. Several gene products of HSV have been demonstrated to highjack signaling pathways such as protein kinase A (PKA), nuclear factor kappa B (NF-κB), PI3K/Akt, and mitogen-activated protein kinase (MAPK) [24–26]. Among them, the tegumental US3 protein kinase was shown to protect cells from apoptosis induced by a number of exogenous agents and stress [24, 27]. Although the precise mechanisms are still unclear [28–31], it has been proposed that US3 has a similar substrate range and specificity than protein kinase A [26]. More importantly, HSV-1 US3 plays a crucial role in the ability of the virus to invade the brain from the eyes and therefore constitutes a significant neuroinvasiveness factor in vivo [32]. In addition, US3 of the swine pseudorabies virus induces rearrangements in the actin cytoskeleton via activation of the PAK family of kinases, which leads to disassembly of actin stress fibers and induction of cellular protrusions [29].

Besides, some HSV-1 proteins control nuclear transcription to favor viral replication and immune evasion, where the immediately early viral protein ICP0 is the major HSV-1 protein dedicated to defeating host responses to infection [6]. Previous studies have demonstrated that ICP0 plays a key role in regulating the balance between lytic and latent infection. ICP0 has a zinc-stabilized RING finger domain that confers E3 ubiquitin ligase activity. This domain is essential for the core functions of ICP0 and its activity mediates the ubiquitination and proteasome-dependent degradation of several cellular proteins that are modified by the small ubiquitin-like SUMO family of proteins. Some of these proteins are involved in cellular defenses that restrict viral infection [33–37]. During the first 5 h after infection, ICP0 localizes and performs multiple functions in the nucleus. Nevertheless, after 7 h post infection, ICP0 accumulates in the cytoplasm where it modulates cell signaling [1]. Several functions of ICP0 linked to physical interactions with cytoplasmic proteins have been described. Thus, ICP0 interacts with EF-1δ and enhances translation efficiency and with CIN85 to recruit Cbl, which are involved in endocytosis and negative regulation of numerous receptor tyrosine kinases, depleting these receptors from the cell surface [38].

3. Herpes simplex virus type 1 at the central nervous system

Numerous and consistent reports note that there is a high percentage of the worldwide population with HSV-1 genetic material at the central nervous system [39–44]. However, the invasion mechanism used by this pathogen and its preference for infecting certain neuronal areas is not completely elucidated [8, 42, 45, 46]. Accordingly, the route of entry chosen by the virus to the brain could define the localization, distribution, and establishment of viral latency in certain areas of CNS. Faced with the above, the evidence points to the use of three different routes of viral entry: (1) through the trigeminal ganglia, (2) through vomeronasal system, and (3) the hematogenous route. In this way, HSV-1 travels centripetally from the trigeminal nerve to the meninges, finally reaching the temporal lobe. It also could use the neuronal flow provided by the vomeronasal system (olfactory nerve) and then be distributed in the hippocampus [47]; alternatively, it could travel through the hematogenous route in the presence of protein factors that can facilitate its entry into the brain [43, 44, 48].

The evidence on the latency at the CNS showed that 15.5% of olfactory bulbs [46, 49], and 72.5% of trigeminal nerves from human corpses at forensic post-mortem, and 35% of 40 autopsied human brains contained HSV-1 DNA [48]. At brain level, latent HSV-1 DNA was found in the olfactory bulbs, amygdala, hippocampus, brain stem, and trigeminal ganglia, even though, it is not known by which route HSV-1 entered the olfactory bulbs and brain. Nevertheless, olfactory bulb HSV-1 infection in mice [48] leads to virus migration into the brain amygdala and hippocampus via the olfactory nerve and locus coeruleus. Other herpes viruses, such as the human herpes virus 6 (HHV-6), also present high frequency of viral DNA in the olfactory bulb/tract region compared to the other brain regions examined in human autopsies, making it a possible route for CNS entrance [50]. The presence of HHV-6 in the nasal cavity and saliva was also a frequent observation, suggesting that both could represent in vivo reservoirs for the virus.

Most evidences are in favor of the olfactory route for neuroinvasion in humans. In this regard, HSV-1 antigens were detected in patients who died of HSE. The antigens were found in the olfactory tract and olfactory cortex, as well as in the limbic system, lower and middle temporal lobe, hippocampus, amygdala, insula, and cingulate gyrus, but not in regions related to the potential trigeminal invasion pathway [51–54]. Additionally, the presence of HSV-related histopathological alterations have been demonstrated in the olfactory neuroepithelium, olfactory nerve, and olfactory bulb [52, 53, 55], but not in the trigeminal ganglion [56]. The evidence supports that HSV-1 is able to establish a latent infection in the olfactory bulb and a particular set of limbic structures. This indicates that HSV reactivation may originate in the olfactory bulb as well as in limbic structures [47].

Furthermore, the information suggests that both primary infection and reactivation of latent virus in the brain may lead to damage of neurons involved in memory, learning, and behavior, as observed in infected mice models [55].

Independent of the route used by the virus, the infection at the CNS level can be localized or diffused and can cause acute neurological disorders as HSE or mild encephalitis, the latter being often imperceptible due to minimal symptoms [17]. Nevertheless, in most cases, the infectious process is asymptomatic, probably indicating that the virus establishes a latent infection in the CNS. This condition would not be harmless, especially in people whose immune system is compromised [55, 57].

Previously, HSV-1 DNA was detected in 1–30% of neurons of latently infected mouse ganglia [16, 58]. In addition, the latent HSV-1 DNA copy number in humans ranges from less than 300 copies/10^5 cells to over 10,000 copies/10^5 cells (in trigeminal ganglia) [16, 59]. Furthermore, another study found that the median HSV genome copy number per 10^5 cells for each ganglion was as follows: vestibular 83222 (4453–890217), geniculate 4307 (311–79518), cochlear 306 (86–32864), and trigeminal 111 (30– 20257) [16, 60].

Periodic but limited reactivation cycles in peripheral sensory neurons might facilitate invasion at CNS level. In this sense, in [47], the results showed that HSV-1 might suppress the apoptotic induction after a reactivation at the peripheral nervous system (PNS) (olfactory neuroepithelium and trigeminal ganglia) enhancing viral neuroinvasion. Besides, HSV-1 US3 has been shown to play a crucial role in the ability of the virus to block apoptosis, facilitating the brain invasion from the eyes and therefore constitutes a significant neuroinvasiveness factor in vivo [32].

Olfactory receptor neurons constitute a bipolar olfactory system, which has dendrites in the olfactory epithelium at the roof of the nasal-pharyngeal cavity. In addition, the olfactory nerve innervates the olfactory epithelium and the olfactory bulb ends in CNS. This system connects the environment with the nervous system, being a gateway to various pathogens to the CNS. Nevertheless, thanks to the presence of mucus- and pathogen-recognition receptors, the olfactory epithelium is protected from the most common infections [61, 62]. However, in laboratory models, olfactory portal can be used by several viruses (HSV-1, vesicular stomatitis virus, Borna disease virus, rabies virus, influenza A virus, parainfluenza viruses), and prions, to enter the CNS [47, 63]. Advances in the knowledge of the mechanisms involved in pathogen-host relationships, such as the route of entry and spread in the CNS, will provide tools for the development of more effective therapies and prevention programs. In addition, these studies will be very relevant in the case of new outbreaks of emerging zoonotic infections, involving pathogens that could use similar mechanisms to invade the CNS [62].

4. HSV-1 and risk of neurological diseases

HSV infection of the CNS can take place in newborns causing encephalitis, spread infection, or keratoconjunctivitis mostly associated to the genital herpes virus HSV-2 [2, 16, 64]. In adults and children older than 6 months, HSV-1 infection is the most common cause of sporadic and nonepidemic acute encephalitis by herpes simplex (HSE), followed by HHV-6 [65–67]. It is considered a devastating disease of the CNS causing fatal sporadic acute encephalitis, usually localized and with an incidence in the United States of two to four cases/million inhabitants per year [65–67]. This estimation is similar for the rest of the countries, and it affects equally both genders and its onset is likely to occur at any age but with two incidence peaks (under 20 and over 50 years old). Even under antiviral treatment, the mortality associated with HSE is 50–60%, and survivors show significant neuropsychological and neurobehavioral sequelae, which afflict patients for life even if they have been treated very early and have made a good recovery [2, 39, 67, 68]. A previous study demonstrated that HSV load in CSF was not associated with poor outcome in patients with HSE [69].

Neuroimaging findings in HSE patients showed abnormality on T2-weighted spin echo and T2-weighted FLAIR images, involving cortex and underlying white matter with predilection for the temporal and inferior frontal lobes, as well as the insular and cingulate cortexes. In early stages of HSE, these abnormalities are generally unilateral; however, they may progress to bilateral involvement, which can be asymmetric. Patchy areas of diffusion restriction indicating cytotoxic injury, particularly of cortex and deep-gray matter structures, are usually present and are key features of viral encephalitis [70]. The HSE-damaged regions of the CNS are related to the limbic system, which are associated with memory, cognitive and affective processes, and personality. The presence of HSV-1 viral antigens has been found in brains of patients dying of HSE, concentrated mainly in the inferior and middle temporal lobes, hippocampus, amygdala, olfactory cortex, insula, and cingulate gyrus [14, 65, 67].

Additionally, several studies suggest that the cellular damage and dysfunction due to repeated cycles of reactivation of HSV-1 may contribute to the development of chronic and degenerative neurological conditions, such as chronic psychiatric illness, epilepsy [71], dementia [17],

Alzheimer's disease (AD) [71–75], schizophrenia (SZ), bipolar disorder, multiple sclerosis [41], and Parkinson's disease [76]. This idea is mainly based on the evidence demonstrating the presence of HSV-1 genome in brain regions associated with such pathologies [77–82]. Concerning other herpes viruses, HHV-6 is frequently associated with neurologic diseases, including multiple sclerosis, mesial temporal lobe epilepsy (MTLE), encephalitis, and febrile illness [50].

Recently, it has been proposed that during reactivation, HSV-1 might affect neighboring neurons of PNS or CNS, through neuroinflammation or direct neuronal damage [4, 28, 82].

Additional findings established that cognitive functioning in individuals with schizophrenia is associated both with serological evidence of HSV-1 infection and with activated immune system, evidenced by elevated C-reactive protein (CRP) levels [83]. CRP is a pentameric protein generated in the liver, which plays a central role in the inflammatory process in humans. A previous study of 413 individuals with schizophrenia [84] found that those who had levels of CRP above 5.0 μg/ml had significantly lower cognitive scores than patients who did not have elevated CRP levels [84].

Genome-wide association studies (GWASs) have implicated single nucleotide polymorphisms (SNPs) on the human leukocyte antigen (HLA) region of chromosome 6p21.3-22.1, as common risk factors for schizophrenia [85]. Although studies indicate that exposure to HSV-1 is associated with impairment in specific cognitive domains among SZ patients and community-based control individuals [86], an association between HSV-1 exposure and SZ risk per se has not been convincingly demonstrated [85].

Given that the demonstration of the viruses in the host target tissues is difficult, the exposure to the infectious agent is measured indirectly using antibody titers in the serum, and serological assays indicate the infectious exposure, but do not reveal when it occurred. The timing of the exposure may be a critical determinant of viral effects on neurodevelopment thought to be relevant for SZ pathogenesis [86]. In [86], the authors suggested ominous effects of persistent infection that are particularly notable in SZ patients exposed to HSV-1: (1) structural damage in the cortical gray matter, (2) cognitive impairment, and (3) cognitive deterioration over time [86].

In addition, findings have established that limbic structures affected by HSE are the same as that affected in AD, hypothesizing that HSV-1 might be involved in the pathogenesis of this disease [75]. Two main pathological features in the brain characterize AD: senile plaques and neurofibrillary tangles (NFTs). Senile plaques are extracellular deposits of amyloid-β (Aβ) peptide, which are generated by amyloid-β protein precursor (APP) cleavage. Neurofibrillary tangles are intracellular clusters of abnormally phosphorylated tau protein, which is normally associated with microtubules in neurons, and contributes to AD pathology in its hyperphosphorylated state [87].

The loss of synapses and dying-back of axons are among the earliest detectable features in neurodegenerative diseases, which are accompanied by a decay of intracellular transport that correlates with the incipient loss of memory and brain functions [88]. In this regard, several triggering events such as oxidative stress, inflammatory cytokines, lack of growth factors, and Aβ peptide have been implicated in axonal and/or neuronal decay.

Additional support to the idea that HSV-1 could be a risk factor to AD comes from several studies, which have detected the viral genome inside neurons or in senile plaques and intranuclear inclusion bodies in astrocytes obtained from the brains of deceased persons from AD [68, 74, 75, 79, 88, 89]. Also, anti-HSV-1 antibodies have been found in cerebrospinal fluid (CSF) in 70% of people over age 50, but not in CSF of children under 7 years [72], suggesting that HSV-1 can cause neurological damage in these individuals [90]. A prospective population study showed that there is a significant risk of AD in older patients presenting IgM antibodies against HSV-1. Furthermore, an additional evidence for HSV-1 in AD involves the type-4 allele of the apolipoprotein E gene, known as APOE-ε4 or APOE4 [90, 91]. Currently, the APOE gene (located on chromosome 19) is the only gene identified related to the late onset of AD (LOAD). APOE at the molecular level is the gene that encodes for apolipoprotein E, which is a cholesterol carrier in the brain, helping to reduce amyloid aggregation and the clearing of deposits from the parenchyma of the brain. Thus, in the absence of function of this gene, excessive beta-amyloid deposits occur in the brain, which is one of the findings in patients with LOAD [91–93].

Interestingly, a significantly increased risk for sporadic AD is associated with the presence of both HSV-1 in brain and carriage of the APOE-ε4 allele [94]. In studies of AD post-mortem brains, neither HSV-1 nor the APOE-4 allele alone was found to be risky for AD; nevertheless, the virus with the allele APOE-4 together increased the risk for AD [95].

The APOE-ε4 allele with resultant ApoE4 phenotype influences the pathophysiology of AD by increasing the pathogen load in the brain specifically for HSV-1 and *Chlamydophila pneumoniae*. ApoE4 also interacts with pathogens to enhance the human innate pro-inflammatory response and contributes to the breakdown of the blood-brain barrier (BBB). HSV-1 may be a primary CNS infiltrative pathogen, and a possible treatment of HSV-1 and other pathogens present in AD brains and peripherally may be the most efficacious way to reduce CNS inflammation in the pathophysiology of AD [96].

In addition, an inverse correlation was found between the presence of IgM against HSV-1 and low plasma levels of peptide Aβ (usually generated by an increase in deposits of the peptide in the brain), which can be considered a marker of early risk of dementia [97]. More recent studies showed that an increase in anti HSV-1 IgG during reactivation correlates with cognitive impairment and prodromal phase of AD [96, 98]. Concerning the CSF biomarker profile, the total and phosphorylated (especially at Ser 181) tau proteins were significantly increased in AD and HSV-1 encephalitis compared to bacterial meningitis, human immunodeficiency virus (HIV)-associated dementia, and controls [99]. This evidence of high levels of total and phosphorylated tau proteins reflects cortical axonal degeneration and neurofibrillary pathology, respectively [99, 100].

Similarly, it has been observed that during HSV-1 infection, cellular distribution and processing of amyloid precursor protein (APP) in infected cells is altered, favoring an amyloidogenic cleavage [4, 96, 97, 101].

HSV-1 also enhances Alzheimer-type pro-inflammatory signaling pathways by inducing miRNA146a [102]. An exaggerated cytokine response, including increased tumor necrosis factor (TNF)-α, interleukin (IL)-6, and interferon (IFN)-γ levels, has been detected in CSF from individuals with HSE or AD compared with healthy controls [103]. In addition, astrocytosis represents a fundamental reaction of the CNS to diverse neurological disorders and brain injuries, where glial acidic fibrillary protein (GAFP) is high in CSF [103].

Additionally, it has been demonstrated that in vitro infection of neuronal cultures with HSV-1 generates a deterioration of neuritic processes, altered microtubule dynamics, hyperphosphorylation of tau protein and tau cleavage by active caspase-3, all characteristics associated with early events of neurodegeneration [13, 98, 104].

When brain swells, because of infection or normal damaging processes related to aging, there is a local activation of innate immune system. Contrary to other tissues, the CNS has practically no major histocompatibility complex (MHC) expression and is protected from antibodies, by the BBB [13]. That is why there must be a fast local response by microglial cells, in the detection of pathogen-associated molecular patterns (PAMPs) and toxic debris too (such as Aβ fibrils and other aggregated proteins) through several pattern-recognition receptors (PRRs) such as Toll-like receptors (TLRs) [105]. Growing evidence indicates that TLRs are pivotal mediating inflammatory responses in CNS pathologies. TLR-mediated intracellular signaling pathways converge to activate NF-κB, and c-Jun N-terminal kinases, which induce the transcription of many genes involved in the onset and/or regulation of this kind of responses, mostly cytokines and chemokines [13].

In this regard, HSV-1 has the ability to induce activation of signaling pathways dependent on Toll-like receptors (TLR2 and 4) in astrocytes [106]. Correspondingly, using an in vivo murine model of infection with HSV-1, we found hyperphosphorylation and cleavage of tau protein by activated caspase 3 during productive and latent infection, alterations that are mainly concentrated in the olfactory bulb and trigeminal nerve, and less extensive in regions of the cerebral cortex. Similarly, during latent infection with HSV-1 it was possible to observe a marked gliosis and increased expression of TLR-4 [55], suggesting repeated neuroinflammatory events that could result in neurodegenerative processes. Moreover, we have recently observed that during infection, the virus modulates differentially the stress sensors AMPK/Sirtuin 1 associated with apoptosis and mitochondrial biogenesis [23].

Even though the evidence reviewed here supports the hypothesis that recurrent infection by HSV-1 at the level of CNS would play a critical role in the development of diseases such as AD, it remains unanswered whether this virus is indeed a causative agent. Nonetheless, age is the main risk factor in the development of chronic and neurodegenerative diseases, coinciding with the decline of the immune system and therefore less restriction on the brain invasion of HSV-1.

In this regard, reports of the World Health Organization (WHO) and the International Federation of the AD (ADI) estimate that in 20 years, the number of people with AD will increase to approximately 66–67 million people and in subsequent years this number will double. Concomitantly, the world population has a greater life expectancy, so it is of great importance to establish possible genetic, environmental, and pathogenic factors that may have an impact on the development of diseases of the central nervous system, especially related to aging diseases [107].

Acknowledgements

This study was supported by grants FONDECYT REGULAR 1150574, CISNe-UACh, and DID-UACh.

Author details

Carola Otth[1,2*], Francisca Acuña-Hinrichsen[1,2], Luis Leyton[1], Carolina Martin[1] and Margarita I. Concha[3]

*Address all correspondence to: cotth@uach.cl

1 Institute of Clinical Microbiology, Faculty of Medicine, Austral University of Chile, Valdivia, Chile

2 Centro Interdisciplinario de Estudios del Sistema Nervioso (CISNe), Universidad Austral de Chile, Valdivia, Chile

3 Instituto de Bioquímica y Microbiología, Facultad de Ciencias, Universidad Austral de Chile, Valdivia, Chile

References

[1] Roizman B, Whitley RJ. An inquiry into the molecular basis of HSV latency and reactivation. Annu Rev Microbiol 2013;67:355–74. doi:10.1146/annurev-micro-092412-155654.

[2] Whitley RJ, Roizman B. Herpes simplex virus infections. Lancet 2001;357:1513–8. doi: 10.1016/S0140-6736(00)04638-9.

[3] Liesegang TJ. Herpes simplex virus epidemiology and ocular importance. Cornea 2001;20:1–13. doi:10.1017/CBO9781107415324.004.

[4] Bearer EL. HSV, axonal transport and Alzheimer's disease: in vitro and in vivo evidence for causal relationships. Future Virol 2012;7:885–99. doi:10.2217/fvl.12.81.

[5] Roizman B, Zhou G, Du T. Checkpoints in productive and latent infections with herpes simplex virus 1: conceptualization of the issues. J Neurovirol 2011;17:512–7. doi: 10.1007/s13365-011-0058-x.

[6] Zhou G, Du T, Roizman B. The role of the CoREST/REST repressor complex in herpes simplex virus 1 productive infection and in latency. Viruses 2013;5:1208–18. doi: 10.3390/v5051208.

[7] Li S, Carpenter D, Hsiang C, Wechsler SL, Jones C. Herpes simplex virus type 1 latency-associated transcript inhibits apoptosis and promotes neurite sprouting in neuroblastoma cells following serum starvation by maintaining protein kinase B (AKT) levels. J Gen Virol 2010;91:858–66. doi:10.1099/vir.0.015719-0.

[8] Perng G-C, Jones C. Towards an understanding of the herpes simplex virus type 1 latency- reactivation cycle. Interdiscip Perspect Infect Dis 2010;1–18. doi: 10.1155/2010/262415.

[9] Umbach JL, Kramer MF, Jurak I, Karnowski HW, M D, Cullen BR. MicroRNAs expressed by herpes simplex virus 1 during latent infection regulate viral mRNAs. Biol Chem 2008;454:780–3. doi:10.1038/nature07103.MicroRNAs.

[10] Du T, Zhou G, Khan S, Gu H, Roizman B. Disruption of HDAC/CoREST/REST repressor by dnREST reduces genome silencing and increases virulence of herpes simplex virus. Proc Natl Acad Sci USA 2010;107:15904–9. doi:10.1073/pnas.1010741107.

[11] Ball MJ, Mathews R, Steiner I, Hill JM, Wisner TW, Murdoch GH, et al. Latent HSV 1 virus in trigeminal ganglia: the optimal site for linking prevention of Alzheimer's disease to vaccination. Neurobiol Aging 2001;22:705–9. doi:10.1016/S0197-4580(01)00253-6.

[12] Bloom DC, Giordani N V, Kwiatkowski DL. Epigenetic regulation of latent HSV-1 gene expression. Biochim Biophys Acta 2010;1799:246–56. doi:10.1016/j.bbagrm.2009.12.001.

[13] Otth C, Zambrano A, Concha M. The possible link between herpes simplex virus type 1 infection and neurodegeneration. In R.B. Maccioni and G. Perry, editors. Current hypotheses and research milestones in Alzheimer's disease. SPRINGER -VERLAG, New York-Heidelberg; 2009. p181–191. DOI:10.1007/978-0-387-87995-6.

[14] Damasio AR, Van Hoesen GW. The limbic system and the localisation of herpes simplex encephalitis. J Neurol Neurosurg Psychiatry 1985;48:297–301. doi:10.1136/jnnp. 48.4.297.

[15] Saldanha J, Sutton RN, Gannicliffe A, Farragher B, Itzhaki RF. Detection of HSV1 DNA by in situ hybridisation in human brain after immunosuppression. J Neurol Neurosurg Psychiatry 1986;49:613–619. doi:10.1136/jnnp.49.6.613.

[16] Gilden DH, Mahalingam R, Cohrs RJ, Tyler KL. Herpesvirus infections of the nervous system. Nat Clin Pract Neurol 2007;3:82–94. doi:10.1038/ncpneuro0401.

[17] Dobson CB, Wozniak MA., Itzhaki RF. Do infectious agents play a role in dementia? Trends Microbiol 2003;11:312–7. doi:10.1016/S0966-842X(03)00146-X.

[18] Kaufman HE, Azcuy AM, Varnell ED, Sloop GD, Thompson HW, Hill JM. HSV-1 DNA in tears and saliva of normal adults. Investig Ophthalmol Vis Sci 2005;46:241–7. doi: 10.1167/iovs.04-0614.

[19] Zanjani NT, Miranda-Saksena M, Valtchev P, Diefenbach RJ, Hueston L, Diefenbach E, et al. Abalone hemocyanin blocks the entry of herpes simplex virus 1 into cells: a potential new antiviral strategy. Antimicrob Agents Chemother 2015;60:1003–12. doi: 10.1128/AAC.01738-15.

[20] Bello-Morales R, Crespillo AJ, Praena B, Tabarés E, Revilla Y, García E, et al. Role of proteolipid protein in HSV-1 entry in oligodendrocytic cells. PLoS One 2016;11:e0147885. doi:10.1371/journal.pone.0147885.

[21] Soldán MP, Pirko I. Biogenesis and significance of central nervous system myelin. Semin Neurol 2012;32:9–14. doi: 10.1055/s-0032-1306381.

[22] Greer JM, Lees MB. Myelin proteolipid protein—the first 50 years. Int J Biochem Cell Biol 2002;34:211–5. doi:10.1016/S1357-2725(01)00136-4.

[23] Martin C, Leyton L, Arancibia Y, Cuevas A, Zambrano A, Concha MI, et al. Modulation of the AMPK/Sirt1 axis during neuronal infection by herpes simplex virus type 1. J Alzheimer's Dis 2014;42:301–12. doi:10.3233/JAD-140237.

[24] Wagner MJ, Smiley JR. Herpes simplex virus requires VP11/12 to activate Src family kinase- phosphoinositide 3-kinase-Akt signaling. J Virol 2011;85:2803–12. doi:10.1128/JVI.01877-10.

[25] Benetti L, Roizman B. Protein kinase B/Akt is present in activated form throughout the entire replicative cycle of deltaU(S)3 mutant virus but only at early times after infection with wild-type herpes simplex virus 1. J Virol 2006;80:3341–8. doi: 10.1128/JVI.80.7.3341–3348.

[26] Benetti L, Roizman B. Herpes simplex virus protein kinase US3 activates and functionally overlaps protein kinase A to block apoptosis. Proc Natl Acad Sci USA 2004;101:9411–6. doi:10.1073/pnas.0403160101.

[27] Nishiyama Y. Herpes simplex virus gene products: the accessories reflect her lifestyle well. Rev Med Virol 2004;14:33–46. PMID: 14716690.

[28] Esaki S, Goshima F, Katsumi S, Watanabe D, Ozaki N, Murakami S, et al. Apoptosis induction after herpes simplex virus infection differs according to cell type in vivo. Arch Virol 2010;155:1235–45. doi:10.1007/s00705-010-0712-2.

[29] Favoreel HW, Van Minnebruggen G, Adriaensen D, Nauwynck HJ. Cytoskeletal rearrangements and cell extensions induced by the US3 kinase of an alphaherpesvirus

are associated with enhanced spread. Proc Natl Acad Sci USA 2005;102:8990–5. doi: 10.1073/pnas.0409099102.

[30] Galvan V. and Roizman B. Herpes simplex virus 1 induces and blocks apoptosis at multiple steps during infection and protects cells from exogenous inducers in a cell-type-dependent manner. Proc Natl Acad Sci USA 1998;95:3931–6. doi: 0027-8424/98/953931-6.

[31] Mori I. Herpes simplex virus type 1 persists in the aged brain through hypothetical expression of accessory genes. J Neurovirol 2010;16:203–7. doi: 10.3109/13550281003739040.

[32] Koyanagi N, Imai T, Arii J, Kato A, Kawaguchi Y. Role of herpes simplex virus 1 Us3 in viral neuroinvasiveness. Microbiol Immunol 2014;58:31–7. doi:10.1111/1348-0421.12108.

[33] Kalamvoki M, Roizman B. HSV-1 degrades, stabilizes, requires, or is stung by STING depending on ICP0, the US3 protein kinase, and cell derivation. Proc Natl Acad Sci USA 2014;111:E611–7. doi:10.1073/pnas.1323414111.

[34] Everett RD, Chiocca S, Orr A. The chicken adenovirus Gam1 protein, an inhibitor of the sumoylation pathway, partially complements ICP0-null mutant herpes simplex virus 1. J Virol 2014;88:5873–6. doi:10.1128/JVI.00080-14.

[35] Gu H, Poon AP, Roizman B. During its nuclear phase the multifunctional regulatory protein ICP0 undergoes proteolytic cleavage characteristic of polyproteins. Proc Natl Acad Sci USA 2009;106:19132–7. doi:10.1073/pnas.0910920106.

[36] Gu H, Roizman B. The two functions of herpes simplex virus 1 ICP0, inhibition of silencing by the CoREST/REST/HDAC complex and degradation of PML, are executed in tandem. J Virol 2009;83:181–7. doi:10.1128/JVI.01940-08.

[37] Gu H, Zheng Y, Roizman B. Interaction of herpes simplex virus ICP0 with ND10 bodies: a sequential process of adhesion, fusion, and retention. J Virol 2013;87:10244–54. doi: 10.1128/JVI.01487-13.

[38] Liang Y, Kurakin A, Roizman B. Herpes simplex virus 1 infected cell protein 0 forms a complex with CIN85 and Cbl and mediates the degradation of EGF receptor from cell surfaces. Proc Natl Acad Sci USA 2005;102:5838–43. doi:10.1073/pnas.0501253102.

[39] Kennedy PGE, Chaudhuri A. Herpes simplex encephalitis. J Neurol Neurosurg Psychiatry 2002;73:237–8. doi: 10.1136/jnnp.73.3.237.

[40] Itzhaki RF, Wozniak MA. Herpes simplex virus type 1 in Alzheimer's disease: the enemy within. J Alzheimers Dis 2008;13:393–405. PMID: 18487848.

[41] Sanders V, Felisan S. Detection of herpesviridae in postmortem multiple sclerosis brain tissue and controls by polymerase chain reaction. J Neurovirol 1996;2:249–58. PMID: 8799216.

[42] Mori I, Kimura Y, Naiki H, Matsubara R, Takeuchi T, Yokochi T, et al. Reactivation of HSV-1 in the brain of patients with familial Alzheimer's disease. J Med Virol 2004;73:605–11. doi:10.1002/jmv.20133.

[43] Burgos JS, Ramirez C, Sastre I, Alfaro JM, Valdivieso F. Herpes simplex virus type 1 infection via the bloodstream with apolipoprotein E dependence in the gonads is influenced by gender. J Virol 2005;79:1605–12. doi:10.1128/JVI.79.3.1605-1612.2005.

[44] Burgos JS, Alfaro JM, Sastre I, Valdivieso F. Hematogenous vertical transmission of herpes simplex virus type 1 in mice. Society 2006;80:2823–31. doi:10.1128/JVI.80.6.2823.

[45] Jamieson GA, Maitland NJ, Wilcock GK, Yates CM, Itzhaki RF. Herpes simplex virus type 1 DNA is present in specific regions of brain from aged people with and without senile dementia of the Alzheimer type. J Pathol 1992;167:365–8. doi:10.1002/path.1711670403.

[46] Liedtke W, Opalka B, Zimmermann CW, Lignitz E. Age distribution of latent herpes-simplex virus-1 and varicella-zoster virus genome in human nervous-tissue. J Neurol Sci 1993;116:6–11. PMID: 8389816.

[47] Mori I, Goshima F, Ito H, Koide N, Yoshida T, Yokochi T, et al. The vomeronasal chemosensory system as a route of neuroinvasion by herpes simplex virus. Virology 2005;334:51–8. doi:10.1016/j.virol.2005.01.023.

[48] Becker Y. HSV-1 brain infection by the olfactory nerve route and virus latency and reactivation may cause learning and behavioral deficiencies and violence in children and adults: a point of view. Virus Genes 1995;10:217–26. doi:10.1007/BF01701811.

[49] Baringer JR, Pisani P. Herpes simplex virus genomes in human nervous system tissue analyzed by polymerase chain reaction. Ann Neurol 1994;36:823–9. doi:10.1002/ana.410360605.

[50] Harberts E, Yao K, Wohler JE, Maric D, Ohayon J, Henkin R, Jacobson S. Human herpesvirus-6 entry into the central nervous system through the olfactory pathway. Proc Natl Acad Sci USA 2011;108:13734–9. doi:10.1073/pnas.1105143108.

[51] Esiri MM. Potential for HSV-1 vaccination to reduce risk of HSV-1 encephalitis and/or Alzheimer's disease? Neurobiol Aging 2001;22:711–3. doi:10.1016/S0197-4580(01)00248-2.

[52] Esiri MM. Viruses and Alzheimer's disease. J Neurol Neurosurg Psychiatry 1982;45:759–60. PMID: 6752349.

[53] Twomey JA, Barker CM, Robinson G. Howell DA. Olfactory mucosa in herpes simplex encephalitis.I. J Neurol Neurosurg Psychiatry 1979;42:983–7. doi:10.1029/2009GC.

[54] Dinn JJ. Transolfactory spread of virus in herpes simplex encephalitis. Br Med J 1980;22:281(6252):1392. PMID: 7437807.

[55] Martin C, Aguila B, Araya P, Vio K, Valdivia S, Zambrano A, et al. Inflammatory and neurodegeneration markers during asymptomatic HSV-1 reactivation. J Alzheimer's Dis 2014;39:849–59. doi:10.3233/JAD-131706.

[56] Ojeda VJ, Archer M, Robertson TA, Bucens MR. Necropsy study of the olfactory portal of entry in herpes simplex encephalitis. Med J Aust 1983;1:79–81. PMID: 6100934.

[57] Armien AG, Hu S, Little MR, Robinson N, Lokensgard JR, Low WC, Cheeran MC. Chronic cortical and subcortical pathology with associated neurological deficits ensuing experimental herpes encephalitis. Brain Pathol 2010;20(4):738–50. doi: 10.1111/j.1750-3639.2009.00354.

[58] Sawtell NM. Comprehensive quantification of herpes simplex virus latency at the single-cell level. J Virol 1997;71:5423–31. PMID: 9188614.

[59] Cohrs RJ, Randall J, Smith J, Gilden DH, Dabrowski C, van Der Keyl H, et al. Analysis of individual human trigeminal ganglia for latent herpes simplex virus type 1 and varicella-zoster virus nucleic acids using real-time PCR. J Virol 2000;74:11464–71. doi: 10.1128/JVI.74.24.11464-11471.2000.

[60] Vrabec JT, Alford RL. Quantitative analysis of herpes simplex virus in cranial nerve ganglia. J Neurovirol 2004;10:216–22. doi:10.1080/13550280490463569.

[61] Kalinke U, Bechmann I, Detje CN. Host strategies against virus entry via the olfactory system. Virulence 2011;2:367–70. doi:10.4161/viru.2.4.16138.

[62] Ludlow M, Kortekaas J, Herden C, Hoffmann B, Tappe D, Trebst C, et al. Neurotropic virus infections as the cause of immediate and delayed neuropathology. Acta Neuropathol 2015;131:1–26. doi:10.1007/s00401-015-1511-3.

[63] Detje CN, Meyer T, Schmidt H, Kreuz D, Rose JK, Bechmann I, et al. Local type I IFN receptor signaling protects against virus spread within the central nervous system. J Immunol 2009;182:2297–304. doi:10.4049/jimmunol.0800596.

[64] Tyler WJ, Petzold GC, Pal SK, Murthy VN. Experience-dependent modification of primary sensory synapses in the mammalian olfactory bulb. J Neurosci 2007;27:9427–38. doi:10.1523/JNEUROSCI.0664-07.

[65] Tyler KL. Emerging viral infections of the central nervous system. Arch Neurol 2009;66:1065–74. doi: 10.1001/archneurol.2009.189.

[66] Whitley R. Neonatal herpes simplex virus infection. Curr Opin Infect Dis 2002;17:243–6. PMID: 15166828.

[67] Tyler KL. Update on herpes simplex encephalitis. Rev Neurol Dis 2004;1:169–78. PMID: 16400278.

[68] Klapper PE, Cleator GM, Longson M. Mild forms of herpes encephalitis. J Neurol Neurosurg Psychiatry 1984;47:1247–50. doi:10.1136/jnnp.47.11.1247.

[69] Poissy J, Champenois K, Dewilde A, Melliez H, Georges H, Senneville E, et al. Impact of herpes simplex virus load and red blood cells in cerebrospinal fluid upon herpes simplex meningo-encephalitis outcome. BMC Infect Dis 2012;12:356. doi:10.1186/1471-2334-12-356.

[70] Soares BP, Provenzale JM. Imaging of herpesvirus infections of the CNS. Am J Roentgenol 2016;206:39–48. doi:10.2214/AJR.15.15314.

[71] Sanders VJ., Felisan SL, Waddell AE, Conrad AJ, Schmid P, Swartz BE, Kaufman M, Walsh GO, De Salles AA, Tourtellotte WW. Presence of herpes simplex DNA in surgical tissue from human epileptic seizure foci detected by polymerase chain reaction. Arch Neurol 1997;54:954–60. doi: 10.1001/archneur.1997.00550200020005.

[72] Wozniak MA, Shipley SJ, Combrinck M, Wilcock GK, Itzhaki RF. Productive herpes simplex virus in brain of elderly normal subjects and Alzheimer's disease patients. J Med Virol 2005;75:300–6. doi:10.1002/jmv.20271.

[73] Burgos JS, Ramirez C, Sastre I, Valdivieso F. Effect of apolipoprotein E on the cerebral load of latent herpes simplex virus type 1 DNA. J Virol 2006;80:5383–7. doi:10.1128/JVI.00006-06.

[74] Wozniak MA, Mee AP, Itzhaki RF. Herpes simplex virus type 1 DNA is located within Alzheimer's disease amyloid plaques. J Pathol 2009;217:131–8. doi:10.1002/path.

[75] Itzhaki RF, Lathe R, Balin BJ, Ball MJ, Bearer EL, Braak H, et al. Microbes and Alzheimer's Disease. J Alzheimer's Dis 2016:91–5. doi:10.3233/JAD-160152.

[76] Hemling N, Röyttä M, Rinne J, Pöllänen P, Broberg E, Tapio V, et al. Herpesviruses in brains in Alzheimer's and Parkinson's diseases. Ann Neurol 2003;54:267–71. doi: 10.1002/ana.10662.

[77] Schretlen DJ, Vannorsdall TD, Winicki JM, Mushtaq Y, Hikida T, Sawa A, Yolken R.H, Dickerson F.B, Cascella N.G. Neuroanatomic and cognitive abnormalities related to herpes simplex virus type 1 in schizophrenia. Schizophr Res 2010;118:224–31. doi: 10.1016/j.schres.2010.01.008.

[78] Itzhaki RF, Wozniak MA. Herpes simplex virus type 1, apolipoprotein E, and cholesterol: a dangerous liaison in Alzheimer's disease and other disorders. Prog Lipid Res 2006;45:73–90. doi:10.1016/j.plipres.2005.11.003.

[79] Piacentini R, Chiara G De, Domenica DLP, Ripoli C, Marcocci ME, Garaci E, et al. HSV-1 and Alzheimer's disease: more than a hypothesis. Front Pharmacol 2014;5:1–9. doi: 10.3389/fphar.2014.00097.

[80] Ball MJ, Lukiw WJ, Kammerman EM, Hill JM. Intracerebral propagation of Alzheimer's disease: strengthening evidence of a herpes simplex virus etiology. Alzheimers Dement 2013;9:169–75. doi:10.1016/j.jalz.2012.07.005.

[81] Chen SF, Huang CC, Wu HM, Chen SH, Liang YC, Hsu K Sen. Seizure, neuron loss, and mossy fiber sprouting in herpes simplex virus type 1-infected organotypic hippocampal cultures. Epilepsia 2004;45:322–32. doi:10.1111/j.0013-9580.2004.37403.x.

[82] Athmanathan S, Vydehi B V, Sundaram C, Vemuganti GK, Murthy JM. Neuronal apoptosis in herpes simplex virus - 1 encephalitis (HSE). Indian J Med Microbiol 2001;19:127–31. PMID: 17664814.

[83] Dickerson F, Stallings C, Origoni A, Vaughan C, Khushalani S, Yolken R. Additive effects of elevated C-reactive protein and exposure to herpes simplex virus type 1 on cognitive impairment in individuals with schizophrenia. Schizophr Res 2012;134:83–8. doi:10.1016/j.schres.2011.10.003.

[84] Dickerson F, Stallings C, Origoni A, Boronow J, Yolken R. C-reactive protein is associated with the severity of cognitive impairment but not of psychiatric symptoms in individuals with schizophrenia. Schizophr Res 2007;93:261–5. doi:10.1016/j.schres.2007.03.022.

[85] Bamne M, Wood J, Chowdari K, Watson AM, Celik C, Mansour H, et al. Evaluation of HLA polymorphisms in relation to schizophrenia risk and infectious exposure. Schizophr Bull 2012;38:1149–54. doi:10.1093/schbul/sbs087.

[86] Prasad KM, Watson AMM, Dickerson FB, Yolken RH, Nimgaonkar VL. Exposure to herpes simplex virus type 1 and cognitive impairments in individuals with schizophrenia. Schizophr Bull 2012;38:1137–48. doi:10.1093/schbul/sbs046.

[87] De-Paula VJ, Radanovic M, Diniz BS, Forlenza OV. Alzheimer's disease. Subcell Biochem 2012; 65:329–52. doi: 10.1007/978-94-007-5416-4_14.

[88] Mandelkow EM, Stamer K, Vogel R, Thies E, Mandelkow E. Clogging of axons by tau, inhibition of axonal traffic and starvation of synapses. Neurobiol Aging 2003;24:1079–85. doi:10.1016/j.neurobiolaging.2003.04.007.

[89] Itzhaki RF, Wozniak MA, Appelt DM, Balin BJ. Infiltration of the brain by pathogens causes Alzheimer's disease. Neurobiol Aging 2004;25:619–27. doi:10.1016/j.neurobiolaging.2003.12.021.

[90] Plentz A, Jilg W, Kochanowski B, Ibach B, Knöll A. Detection of herpesvirus DNA in cerebrospinal fluid and correlation with clinical symptoms. Infection. 2008;36(2):158–62. doi: 10.1007/s15010-007-6354-y.

[91] Letenneur L, Pérès K, Fleury H, Garrigue I, Barberger-Gateau P, Helmer C, et al. Seropositivity to herpes simplex virus antibodies and risk of Alzheimer's disease: a population-based cohort study. PLoS One 2008;3:1–5. doi:10.1371/journal.pone.0003637.

[92] Liu ST, Pham H, Pandol SJ, Ptasznik A. Src as the link between inflammation and cancer. Front Physiol 2014;4 Jan:2009–14. doi:10.3389/fphys.2013.00416.

[93] Cribbs DH, Azizeh BY, Cotman CW, LaFerla FM. Fibril formation and neurotoxicity by a herpes simplex virus glycoprotein b fragment with homology to the Alzheimer's Aβ peptide. Biochemistry 2000;39:5988–94. doi:10.1021/bi000029f.

[94] Itzhaki RF, Lin W, Shang D, Wilcock GK, Faragher B, Jamieson GA. Early reports Herpes simplex virus type 1 in brain and risk of Alzheimer' s disease. Lancet 1997;349:241–4. PMID: 9014911.

[95] Lin CY, Lucas M, Mazzone T. Endogenous apoE expression modulates HDL3 binding to macrophages. J Lipid Res 1998;39:293–301. PMID: 9507990.

[96] Harris SA, Harris EA. Herpes simplex virus type 1 and other pathogens are key causative factors in sporadic Alzheimer's disease. J Alzheimer's Dis 2015;48:319–53. doi: 10.3233/JAD-142853.

[97] Dartigues J, Féart C. Risk factors for Alzheimer disease. Neurology 2011;77:206–7. doi: 10.1212/WNL.0b013e31822550af

[98] Kobayashi N, Nagata T, Shinagawa S, Oka N, Shimada K, Shimizu A, Tatebayashi Y, Yamada H, Nakayama K, Kondo K. Increase in the IgG avidity index due to herpes simplex virus type 1 reactivation and its relationship with cognitive function in amnestic mild cognitive impairment and Alzheimer's disease. Biochem Biophys Res Commun 2013;430:907–11. doi:10.1016/j.bbrc.2012.12.054.

[99] Krut JJ, Zetterberg H, Blennow K, Cinque P, Hagberg L, Price RW, Studahl M, Gisslén M. Cerebrospinal fluid Alzheimer's biomarker profiles in CNS infections. J Neurol 2013;260:620–6. doi:10.1007/s00415-012-6688-y.

[100] Hampel H, Blennow K, Shaw LM, Hoessler YC, Trojanowski JQ. Total and phosphorylated tau protein as biological markers of Alzheimer's disease. Exp Gerontol 2011;45:1–21. doi:10.1016/j.exger.2009.10.010.

[101] Cheng S-B, Ferland P, Webster P, Bearer EL. Herpes simplex virus dances with amyloid precursor protein while exiting the cell. PLoS One 2011;6:e17966. doi:10.1371/journal.pone.0017966.

[102] Hill JM, Zhao Y, Clement C, Neumann DM, Lukiw WJ. HSV-1 infection of human brain cells induces miRNA-146a and Alzheimer-type inflammatory signalling. Neuroreport 2010;20:1500–5. doi:10.1097/WNR.0b013e3283329c05.HSV-1.

[103] Fagan AM, Perrin RJ. Upcoming candidate cerebrospinal fluid biomarkers of alzheimer's disease. Biomark Med 2013;6:455–76. doi:10.2217/bmm.12.42.

[104] Mancuso R, Baglio F, Agostini S, Cabinio M, Lagana MM, Hernis A, et al. Relationship between herpes simplex virus-1-specific antibody titers and cortical brain damage in Alzheimer's disease and amnestic mild cognitive impairment. Front Aging Neurosci 2014;6:285. doi:10.3389/fnagi.2014.00285.

[105] Griffiths M, Neal JW, Gasque P. Innate immunity and protective neuroinflammation: new emphasis on the role of neuroimmune regulatory proteins. Int Rev Neurobiol 2007;82:29–55. doi:10.1016/S0074-7742(07)82002-2.

[106] Villalba M, Hott M, Martin C, Aguila B, Valdivia S, Quezada C, et al. Herpes simplex virus type 1 induces simultaneous activation of Toll-like receptors 2 and 4 and expression of the endogenous ligand serum amyloid A in astrocytes. Med Microbiol Immunol 2012;201:371–9. doi:10.1007/s00430-012-0247- 0.

[107] Martin C, Concha MI, Otth C. Herpes simplex virus tipo 1 como factor de riesgo asociado con la enfermedad de Alzheimer. Rev Med Chil 2011;139:779–86. doi:/S0034-98872011000600013.

Chapter 3

Herpesviruses in Periapical Pathoses: An Updated Systematic Review

Aleksandar Jakovljević, Miroslav Andrić,
Aleksandra Knežević, Katarina Beljić-Ivanović,
Maja Miletić, Tanja Jovanović, Ljiljana Kesić and
Jelena Milašin

Additional information is available at the end of the chapter

http://dx.doi.org/ 10.5772/64004

Abstract

Apical periodontitis represents a chronic inflammation and destruction of periradicular tissue caused by polymicrobial infection of endodontic origin. The aim of this systematic review was to make an update on findings related to Epstein-Barr virus (EBV) and human cytomegalovirus (HCMV) presence in periapical pathoses and to correlate these findings with clinical, histopathological and radiographic features of periapical lesions. Methods were based on the preferred reporting items for systematic reviews and meta-analyses (PRISMA) statement. A search was performed using PubMed, Web of Science and SCOPUS. Search key words included the following medical subjects heading terms: (periapical disease OR apical periodontitis OR periapical lesions OR periapical abscess) AND (viruses OR herpesvir*). A manual search involved references from articles retrieved for possible inclusion. The search, evaluation, and critical appraisal of articles were performed by two independent judges. Collected data were analyzed using the measures of descriptive statistics. The final review has included twenty nine articles related to herpesviral presence periapical pathoses. Qualitative analysis indicated that EBV HCMV, and HHV-8 were the most prevalent species in periapical pathoses. Our findings suggest that there is wide variety of herpesviruses detection rates in periapical pathoses in relation to their clinical, histopathological and radiographic features.

Keywords: periapical disease, apical periodontitis, periapical abscess, human cytomegalovirus, Epstein–Barr virus

1. Introduction

Apical periodontitis represents an inflammatory process within the periapical tissues. It is characterized by chronic inflammation and destruction of tooth-supporting tissues around the apex of a tooth root [1]. It represents a remarkably prevalent condition [2]. In Europe, the prevalence of apical periodontitis is estimated at 34–61% of individuals and 2.8–4.2% of the teeth [3] and increases with age [4]. Although various chemical and physical factors are able to induce periapical inflammation, overwhelming evidences indicate that polymicrobial infection of endodontic origin is essential for its development [5, 6].

The relationship between periapical inflammation and root canal bacterial infection is well established [7–9]. In the classic study by Kakehashi et al. [7], rats subjected to surgical exposure and maintained in a conventional microbial environment uniformly developed pulpal necrosis and periapical inflammation. In contrast, germ-free animals exhibited no periapical destruction and formed reparative dentin at damaged sites. Subsequent study by Sundquist [8] confirmed the causative relationship between pulpal infection and periapical lesion development. He showed that traumatized but non-infected necrotic pulps did not result in periapical pathoses, whereas pulpal necrosis associated with pathogenic bacteria led to periapical breakdown [8]. These studies confirmed that pulpal infection appears to be an absolute essential for the development and progression of periapical inflammation.

Endodontic infection develops only in root canals of teeth devoid of vital pulp and their defence mechanisms. This may be consequence of pulpal necrosis because of dental caries, trauma to the tooth, attrition, abrasion, and iatrogenic operative procedures, but also due to removal of the pulp tissue for the previous root canal treatment [6]. Microorganisms can reach the pulp through various routes. The major pathways of pulpal contamination are direct pulp exposure, exposed dentinal tubules, lateral and apical accessory canals, and blood-transmitted bacteria. Once the infection is established in the root canal, bacteria may contact the periradicular tissues via apical and later foramina or root perforations and induce an acute or chronic inflammatory response [10].

Endodontic infections develop in a previously sterile place which does not contain any microorganisms. Therefore, any species found in the root canal has the potential to be an endodontic pathogen or at least to play a role in the ecology of the microbial community. However, the virulence and pathogenicity of individual species vary considerably and can be affected in the presence of other microbes [11]. Culture-dependent and culture-independent microbiological studies have identified more than 1000 different bacterial species/phylotypes in the oral cavity [12]. Subsequent studies by Siqueira [13, 14] revealed that over 460 different microbial species/phylotypes make the current list of endodontic pathogens. At high phylogenetic levels, endodontic bacteria fall into 15 phyla, with the most common species/phylotypes belonging to the phyla *Firmicutes*, *Bacteroides*, *Actinobacteria*, *Fusobacteria*, *Proteobacteria*, *Spirochetes*, and *Synergistetes* [15–17]. These microbiota are organized in a structure resembling biofilm [18, 19]. The biofilm community represents a complex biological system that is structurally and dynamically organized. Population of cells is strategically positioned for optimal metabolic interaction, and the resultant architecture favours the physiology and ecological role of the community [11].

Traditionally, endodontic infections have been classified as either primary or secondary. Primary root canal infection is caused by microorganisms that initially invade and colonize the necrotic pulp tissue, while secondary infection is caused by microorganisms that were not present in the primary infection, but were introduced in the root canal at some time after professional intervention. Additionally, persistent infection is caused by microorganisms that were members of primary or secondary infection which resisted intracanal antimicrobial procedures [6]. Secondary or persistent infections are the major causes of persistent apical periodontitis, which is basically a direct consequence of failure of endodontic treatment [13].

Periapical inflammation is a direct result of interactions between the bacteria inside the infected root canal system and the host's immune system. Apical inflammatory process serves two purposes: one is to try to remove the bacteria, while the other is to prevent microbial invasion into the periapical tissues [1, 10]. The initial response to bacterial presence will be an acute inflammatory reaction, known as acute apical periodontitis. It is of short duration and occurs within a previously healthy periapical region. If bacterial irritation in pulp and periapical tissues remains constant, it may then follow several possible courses such are further intensification, abscess formation, spreading of the infection through bone and/or soft tissues (i.e. cellulitis), or it may become chronic (i.e. chronic apical periodontitis). Continued presence of irritants in the apical part of the root canal system shifts acute inflammation gradually to a chronic inflammatory reaction, known histologically as a periapical granuloma [5, 20].

Histopathologically, the periapical granuloma consists of granulomatous tissue with inflammatory cells infiltrate, fibroblasts, and well-developed fibrous capsule [1, 10, 21]. Nair et al. [22, 23] performed serial sectioning of histological samples and had shown that more than 45% of all chronic apical granulomas were epithelialized.

The extra-epithelial tissues predominantly consist of inflammatory cells infiltrate [24–32]. Cellular composition of periapical lesions varies significantly, depending on the stage of lesion development and its progression, histological characteristics, presence or absence of clinical symptoms, and methods used for detection and quantification of inflammatory cells [33]. The main finding is that lymphocytes and macrophages are the predominant population of infiltrating cells. Among the lymphocytes, T cells are likely to be more numerous at certain stages than B cells [24–26], and CD4+ helper cells may outnumber CD8+ cytotoxic cells [29–31]. Additionally, T-helper type 1 (Th 1) lymphocytes characterize early forms of apical periodontitis. This suggests a role for Th 1 cells in the initiation and expansion of periapical lesions [34, 35]. The abundance of B lymphocytes, plasma cells, CD8+ cytotoxic/suppressor T cells, and Th 2 cells in late periapical granulation tissues suggests that these cells participate in lesion stabilization and possible healing [34, 35].

Periapical cysts (radicular cysts) are believed to be a direct sequel of chronic apical granulomas although not every granuloma develops into a cyst [1, 5, 36]. The reported incidence of cysts among apical periodontitis lesions varies from 6 to 55%. Although more than 50% of all lesions are epithelialized, investigation based on serial sectioning showed that the incidence of cysts among those lesions may be well below 20% [23, 37, 38]. There are two distinct categories of periapical cysts. A periapical pocket cyst is a sac-like epithelium-lined cavity that is open to and continuous with the root canal. On the other hand, a periapical true cyst has the cavity completely enclosed in an epithelial lining and there is no communication with the root canal [23, 38]. The four major histological components of true apical cysts are the cyst cavity, a complete epithelial lining of the cystic wall, extra-epithelial tissue and the collagenous capsule. The tissue between the epithelial lining and the fibrous capsule usually consists of numerous blood vessels and inflammatory cells [5, 26]. More than half of cystic lesions are true apical cysts, and the remainder are apical pocket cysts [23, 38].

Apart from its chronic forms, apical periodontitis can manifest itself in different clinical ways, including the development of an acute abscess [39]. An abscess is defined as a localized collection of pus inside the cavity formed by tissue liquefaction. The acute apical abscess is the most common form of dental abscess and is usually a sequel of an endodontic infection [40]. Along with Gram-negative dark-pigmented anaerobic bacteria of the genera *Prevotella, Porphyromonas,* and *Fusobacterium,* Gram-positive cocci, specifically peptostreptococci and streptococci, comprise the most frequently detected bacteria in apical abscess samples [41–44]. Apical abscesses may be either acute or chronic, and an acute apical abscess may be either a primary or secondary lesion. The purulent exudate formed in response to root canal infection spreads through the medullary bone to perforate the cortical bone and discharge into submucous or subcutaneous soft tissue. The spread of endodontic infections into fascial spaces is determined by the location of the root tip of the involved tooth in relation to its overlying buccal or lingual cortical plane, the thickness of the overlying bone, and the relationship of the apex to the attachments of surrounding muscles [45, 46]. Delayed or inappropriate treatment of acute apical abscess may result in spreading of infection and cause severe and/or life-threatening complications such are deep neck infections [47], mediastinitis [48], necrotizing fasciitis [49], orbital and brain abscess [50, 51], and cervical spondylodiscitis with spinal epidural abscess [52].

Although there is a clear implication of microbiological factors in the development of apical periodontitis, host-related factors, otherwise known as disease modifiers, are able to influence the outcomes of apical periodontitis. In this regard, the influence of various systemic conditions and genetic background of patients in the development of apical periodontitis have been extensively investigated [53, 54]. The results of studies conducted so far are not conclusive, but suggest an association between apical periodontitis and systemic disease such as diabetes mellitus. There is evidence associating diabetes mellitus with higher prevalence of apical periodontitis, greater size of periapical lesions, greater likelihood of asymptomatic infections, and delayed periapical repair [55–57]. On the other hand, some data suggest that chronic periapical disease may contribute to diabetic metabolic dyscontrol [58]. Although diabetic patients are apparently more prone to develop severe forms of apical periodontitis, no study so far reported the prevalence of endodontic abscesses in diabetic patients.

Genetic polymorphisms are another factor which can make individuals more prone to develop acute infections. Previously reported studies have hypothesized that polymorphisms in cytokine genes may contribute to an individual's increased susceptibility to periapical tissue destruction [59, 60]. Single nucleotide polymorphisms in variety of cytokine-encoding genes, including those for tumour necrosis factor (TNF)-α, interleukin (IL)-1β, IL-6, IL-8, IL-10, were correlated with clinical and radiographic features of apical periodontitis lesions and development of acute apical abscesses [61–63].

Apart from bacteria, various species of other microorganisms, including herpesviruses, have been associated with periapical pathosis. In 1958, Rauch [64] assumed that, apart from bacteria, another causative factor contributing to development of periapical granuloma may be a viral one. In this in vitro study, samples were taken from infected root canals and periapical tissue by means of paper point method. He used monkey kidney cells to inoculate them with the medium in which the paper points were stored. However, using this method, isolates from 10 patients were negative. Subsequent study by Shindell [65] analysed the presence of viruses in HeLa and human amnion cell cultures inoculated by periapical tissues of four patients. He also reported negative results from this experiment and concluded that based on his and previously reported results by Rauch, periapical granulomas are not associated with viral infection.

Over the past 25 years, data on possible involvement of herpesviruses in the development of periodontal tissue diseases have gradually accumulated in scientific literature. By the mid-1990s, Parra and Slots [66] and Contreras and Slots [67] detected several viral transcripts in periodontal pockets using polymerase chain reaction (PCR). They concluded that periodontal tissue breakdown occurs more frequently and progresses more rapidly in herpesvirus-infected that in herpesvirus-free periodontal sites. The same group of authors proposed herpesviruses as a putative pathogen in destructive periodontal disease. After these findings, Sabeti et al. [68, 69] hypothesized that concomitant herpes viral infection may contribute to the pathogenesis of apical periodontitis in the same way as it has been proposed for marginal periodontitis. Epidemiological studies carried out since the mid-2000s have identified Epstein–Barr virus (EBV) and human cytomegalovirus (HCMV) as the frequently detected species of the *Herpesviridae* family in apical periodontitis [70].

Of the approximately 120 identified herpesviruses, eight major types with distinct biological and clinical characteristics are known to infect humans, namely herpes simplex virus (HSV), varicella-zoster virus (VZV), EBV, HCMV, human herpesvirus (HHV)-6, HHV-7, and HHV-8 (Kaposi's sarcoma virus). The name of this virus family is derived from the Greek word *herpain*, meaning "to creep", which reflects the features of those viruses, namely latent and recurring infections. Till now, more than 5000 different strains of herpesviruses have been identified. Membership in the family Herpesviridae is based on a four-layer structure of the virion. The prototypical structure of herpesviruses consists of a double-strained DNA genome encased within an icosahedral capsid, a proteinaceous tegument, and a lipid-containing envelope embedded viral glycoproteins [71–73]. Of particular importance is that these viruses share the property to persist during the host lifetime and hold the ability to be reactivated at some point in time, under the influence of several stimuli. Humans are the only source of infection for these eight herpesviruses.

Despite the fact that numerous studies have analysed the relationship between herpesviral infection and apical periodontitis, its exact role in the etiopathogenesis of periapical lesions has not yet been completely elucidated. Up to now, two distinct theories have emerged. The findings of Slots et al. [74–76] within the past 15 years have established a hypothesis that herpesviruses may be implicated in the pathogenesis of apical periodontitis as a direct result of viral infections or as a result of a virally induced impairment of local host defence that favours bacterial overgrowth. These hypotheses are based on direct cytopathogenic effects of herpesviral infection on fibroblasts, keratinocytes, endothelial cells, inflammatory cells, and possibly bone cells. Study by Ongradi et al. [77] showed impaired functions of neutrophils in subjects who carried herpesviruses in oral lymphocytes and epithelial cells in comparison with virus-free persons. Moreover, it has been shown that fibroblast infected with herpesviruses may hamper tissue turnover and repair in regenerative periodontal therapy [78]. Herpesvirus infection induces host's antiviral innate and adaptive immune responses. These immune responses are incapable of eradicating viral infection, but they are effective in controlling viral replication and preventing clinical manifestations of a disease. Indirectly, herpesvirus-induced impairment of local host's defence causes upgrowth of resident bacteria in apical periodontium. Contreras and Slots [71] have reported that herpesviral proteins expressed on eukaryotic cells may act as new bacterial binding sites. Additionally, these interactions between herpesviruses and endodontic bacteria are probably bidirectional, since bacterial enzymes or other inflammatory-inducing factors have the potential to turn over herpesviral infection into active stage [76].

In contrast to herpesviral–bacterial hypothesis, Ferreira et al. [79, 80] hypothesized that the occurrence of herpesviruses might be just an epiphenomenon to bacterial infection that caused inflammation of periapical tissues and consequent influx of virus-infected inflammatory cells to the periapical area. Since herpesviruses can persistently occur in the human body by infecting defence cells, the mare presence of viral DNA in clinical samples does not necessarily imply a role in disease pathogenesis.

In our previous systematic review [70], herpesviral infection has been correlated with clinical features of apical periodontitis. Pooled results of six studies included in meta-analysis showed that the occurrence of HCMV or EBV did not significantly differ between symptomatic and asymptomatic apical periodontitis. The necessity for updated systematic review comes from several reasons. In the last 2 years, several studies reported new data on herpesviral occurrence in apical periodontitis lesions. Moreover, in previous systematic review, data of herpesviruses infection were not correlated with radiographic and histopathological features of apical periodontitis. Additionally, previous report did not analyse the occurrence of herpesviruses in samples of acute apical abscess.

All these issues pointed to the necessity to make an updated systematic review on herpesviral occurrence in periapical pathoses and to correlate these findings with clinical, histopathological, and radiographic features of apical periodontitis and acute apical abscess. In addition, the occurrence of herpesviral infection in relation to levels of proinflammatory mediators, the presence of different strains of herpesviruses and herpesviral–bacterial co-infection in periapical pathoses will be analysed.

2. Materials and methods

To address the research questions, we designed and implemented a systematic review based on the PRISMA (preferred reporting items for systematic reviews and meta-analyses) statement. The search, evaluation of relevant articles, and their critical appraisal were performed by two independent judges (A.J. and M.A.) blinded to each other.

In the first round, a comprehensive literature search was performed using electronic databases: PubMed, Web of Science, and Scopus. All mentioned databases provide the article title, abstract, and key words. Search key words included the following medical subjects heading (MeSH) terms: (periapical disease OR apical periodontitis OR periapical lesions OR periapical abscess) AND (viruses OR herpesvir*). A manual search involved reference lists from identified articles for possible inclusion of additional relevant studies. The language of the publication was restricted to English. Electronic and manual searches were last conducted on December 20, 2015.

In the second round, the title and abstract of retrieved articles were screened. For studies appearing to be relevant and for those with insufficient data in the title and abstract to make a clear decision, the full texts were obtained. After the full-text assessment, articles were submitted to final eligibility evaluation by the same two judges. Inclusion and exclusion criteria are presented in **Tables 1** and **2**. Only articles that met all eligibility criteria were marked as accepted and included in the third round.

- Article types: original scientifically papers, case series, and short communications
- Studies in which human subjects were in good general health (American Society of Anesthesiology status classification system I and II) and without immunosuppressive and antiviral therapy 6 months prior to examination
- Documented data of herpesviral infection in apical periodontitis and periapical abscess tissue samples
- Clear statement of the method (reverse transcriptase PCR, real-time PCR, nested PCR, multiplex PCR, immunohistochemistry, in situ hybridization, and flow cytometry) used for viral detection
- Studies with at least 5 patients without periodontally involved teeth (no probing depth >4 mm)

Table 1. Eligibility—inclusion criteria.

- Article types: in vitro study, animal study, case report, and review article
- The publication was based on a population that was part of another study
- Prevalence rates and data that allowed their calculation were absent

Table 2. Eligibility—exclusion criteria 1.

In the third round, each article was critically appraised by authors who were evaluating the methodological quality of all selected articles. Articles excluded from this phase and the reasons for exclusion are presented in **Table 3**. From remaining 29 articles, data on clinical, histopathological, and radiographic characteristics of study subjects, occurrence of herpesviruses among examined sample, viral diagnostic methods, etc. were extracted and tabulated. Collected data were qualitatively analysed using measures of descriptive statistics. Any different findings in each round were settled by discussion, and discrepancies between reviewers were resolved by consensus with a third party.

Reasons for exclusion	Author, year [reference numbers]
In vitro study design	Rauch 1958 [64]; Shindelle 1962 [65]
Case report study design	Gregory et al. 1975 [106];
No documented data of herpesviral DNA, cDNA, and/or mRNA	Goon et al. 1988 [107];
in tissue sample.	Wadden 1991 [108];
	Ramchandani et al. 2007 [109];
	Gupta et al. 2015 [110];

cDNA, complementary DNA; mRNA, messenger RNA.

Table 3. Articles excluded after critical appraisal.

3. Results

The electronic database and manual searches last updated on December 20, 2015, yielded 57 hits from PubMed, 63 hits from Web of Science and 87 hits from Scopus. The total number of articles after duplicates were removed was 150. A manual reference list search did not provide any relevant titles that were not found already by the electronic database research. Thirty-seven articles were considered relevant to the topic after abstract screening. Full texts of these 37 articles were evaluated using the eligibility criteria listed in **Tables 1** and **2**. Eight articles did not meet one or more of the eligibility criteria. These articles were excluded, and the reasons for exclusion are listed in **Table 3**. Twenty-nine articles were accepted for the final review (**Table 4**). Twenty-four articles were related to herpesviral finding in chronic periapical lesions, and five articles analysed the occurrence of herpesviruses in acute apical abscess lesions. A literature search flow diagram is presented in **Figure 1**. All studies in the final review were cross-sectional.

Author, year [reference numbers]	Specimens number and type	Specimens collected in conjunct with	Method of analysis
Rider et al. 1995 [81]	n = 20, radicular cysts	Cyst enucleation	Immunohistochemical analysis
Heling et al. 2001 [82]	n = 46, pulp tissue—irreversible pulpitis (11); pulp tissue—necrotic	Apicoectomy, Tooth extraction	PCR (DNA)

Author, year [reference numbers]	Specimens number and type	Specimens collected in conjunct with	Method of analysis
	pulp (17); periapical lesions (10); control pulpal tissue (8)		
Sabeti et al. 2003a [68]	n = 16, periapical lesions (14); control specimens (2)	Apicoectomy	RT-PCR (RNA, cDNA)
Sabeti et al. 2003b [69]	n = 14, periapical lesions;	Apicoectomy	RT-PCR (RNA, cDNA)
Sabeti et al. 2003c [83]	n = 5, periapical lesions;	Apicoectomy	RT-PCR (RNA, cDNA)
Sabeti et al. 2004 [84]	n = 34, periapical lesions;	Apicoectomy	RT-PCR (RNA, cDNA)
Slots et al. 2004 [85]	n = 44, periapical pathosis;	Apicoectomy	RT-PCR (RNA, cDNA)
Kabak et al. 2005 [86]	n = 57, periapical lesions;	Apicoectomy Tooth extraction	Immunohistochemical analysis
Yildirim et al. 2006 [87]	n = 24, granulomatous tissue (12); control pulpal tissue (12)	Tooth extraction	PCR (DNA)
Saboa-Dantas et al. 2007 [88]	n = 35, granulomas (n = 29); cysts (6)	Tooth extraction	Immunohistochemical analysis
Andric et al. 2007 [89]	n = 43, periapical cysts (n = 33); odontogenic keratocysts—control specimens (n = 10);	Apicoectomy	PCR (DNA)
Yazdi et al. 2008 [90]	n = 50, apical periodontitis;	Apicoectomy	RT-PCR (RNA, cDNA)
Sunde et al. 2008 [91]	n = 40, apical periodontitis;	Apicoectomy	Real-time PCR (DNA), In situ hybridization, Immunohistochemical analysis
Sabeti et al. 2009 [92]	n = 15, periapical lesions;	Tooth extraction	Flow cytometry
Li et al. 2009 [93]	n = 72, apical periodontitis (30); previously treated teeth with apical periodontitis (23); healthy pulp control (19)	Apicoectomy, Tooth extraction	RT-PCR (RNA, cDNA), Nested PCR, PCR (DNA)
Chen et al, 2009 [94]	n = 50, acute apical abscess (31); healthy pulp control (19)	Needle aspiration	PCR, Nested PCR (DNA)

Author, year [reference numbers]	Specimens number and type	Specimens collected in conjunct with	Method of analysis
Hernandi et al. 2010 [95]	n = 80, apical periodontitis (40); healthy pulp control (40)	Apicoectomy	RT-PCR (RNA, cDNA), Nested PCR, PCR (DNA)
Ferreira et al. 2011a [79]	n = 50, acute apical abscess (23); healthy pulp control (5)	Needle aspiration	PCR, Multiplex nested PCR (DNA)
Ferreira et al. 2011b [80]	n = 33, acute apical abscess (33)	Needle aspiration	PCR, Multiplex nested PCR (DNA)
Hernandi et al. 2011 [96]	n = 80, apical periodontitis (40); healthy pulp control (40)	Apicoectomy	RT-PCR (RNA, cDNA), Nested PCR, PCR (DNA)
Sabeti et al. 2012 [97]	n = 15, periapical lesions	Apicoectomy	Real-time RT-PCR (RNA, cDNA)
Hernandi et al. 2013 [98]	n = 78, apical periodontitis (58); gingival tissue (20);	Apicoectomy	Nested PCR, Real-time PCR (DNA)
Ozbek et al. 2013 [99]	n = 28, periapical lesions;	Apicoectomy	Real-time PCR (DNA)
Verdugo et al. 2015 [100]	n = 48, apical periodontitis (33); saliva (15);	Apicoectomy	PCR, Real-time PCR (DNA)
Ozbek et al. 2015a [101]	n = 33, acute apical abscess (27); healthy pulp control (6)	Needle aspiration	Real-time PCR (DNA))
Makino et al. 2015 [102]	n = 42, periapical lesions (32); gingival tissue (10);	Apicoectomy	Real-time PCR (DNA), In situ hybridization, Immunohistochemical analysis
Ozbek et al. 2015b [103]	n = 31, acute apical abscess (21); healthy pulp control (10);	Needle aspiration	Real-time PCR (DNA))
Popovic et al. 2015 [104]	n = 60, periapical lesions;	Tooth extraction	PCR (DNA)
Jakovljevic et al. 2015 [105]	n = 125, apical periodontitis (100); healthy pulp control (25)	Apicoectomy	PCR (DNA), RFLP

PCR, polymerase chain reaction; RT-PCR, reverse transcriptase polymerase chain reaction; HCMV, human cytomegalovirus; EBV, Epstein–Barr virus; DNA, deoxyribonucleic acid; cDNA, complementary deoxyribonucleic acid; mRNA, messenger ribonucleic acid.

Table 4. Articles included in the final review.

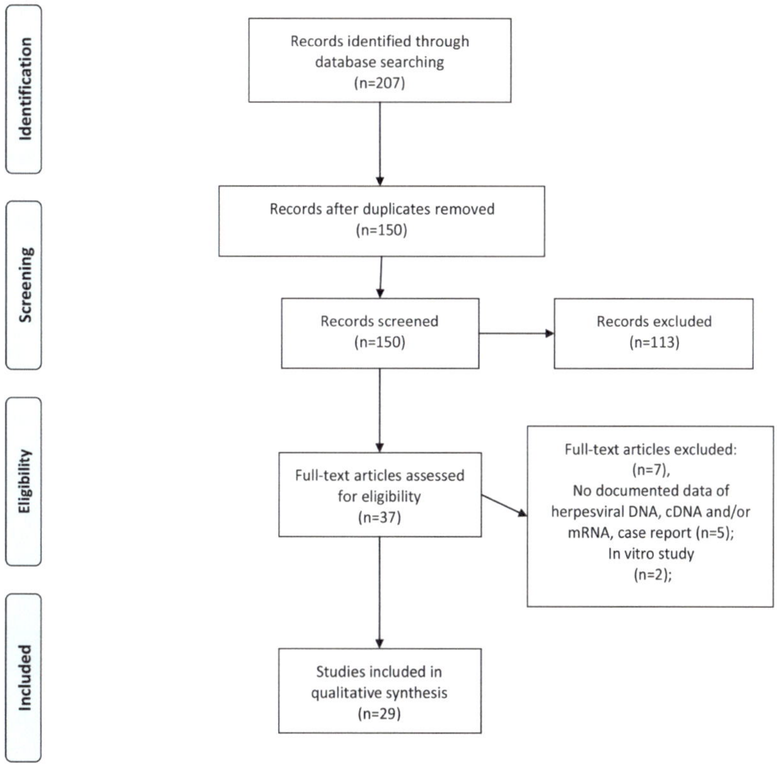

Figure 1. Flow diagram of systematic review process.

3.1. The occurrence of herpesviruses in samples of periapical pathoses compared to healthy control tissues

Twelve included studies investigated the occurrence of herpesviruses in samples of apical periodontitis lesions and healthy control tissues [68, 82, 87–89, 93, 95, 96, 98, 100, 103, 105]. Healthy pulp tissue samples, obtained from surgically extracted third molars or teeth extracted due to orthodontic reasons, were used as control specimen in the majority of studies [82, 87, 93, 95, 96, 105]. Few studies used gingival tissues as control specimens [98, 102]. Sabeti et al. [68] and Verdugo et al. [100] also reported usage of tissues from healthy periapical sites and saliva as controls.

Four studies [93, 95, 96, 105] reported significantly increased occurrence of herpesviruses in periapical lesions compared to control pulp tissues. Hernadi et al. [98] and Makino et al. [103] shown similar occurrence of herpesviruses between periapical lesions and gingival tissue.

Four studies compared the occurrence of herpesviruses between acute apical abscess samples and healthy pulp tissue [79, 94, 101, 103]. Although herpesviruses were more frequently detected in abscess samples compared to the pulp tissue samples, these differences were not significant (**Table 6**).

3.2. The occurrence of herpesviruses in symptomatic and asymptomatic apical periodontitis and acute apical abscesses

The majority of studies included in final review investigated the relationship between the presence of herpesviruses and clinical features of periapical lesions. The common approach was to compare the occurrence of herpesviruses in groups of symptomatic and asymptomatic lesions based on the presence of pain, sensitivity to percussion and palpation, and discomfort on biting at the time of sample collection. The summarized results of these studies are given in **Table 5**.

Author, year [reference number]	**Study group**	**Symptomatic lesions**	**Asymptomatic lesions**	**Control group**	**Lesion size**	**Dual infection**
Rider et al. 1995 [81]	n = 20, radicular cysts	HSV-1+ (0%) HSV-2+ (0%)		n = 2 HSV-positive controls—infected lung tissues		
Heling et al. 2001 [82]	n = 36, pulp tissue—irreversible pulpitis (11); necrotic pulp (17); periapical lesions (10);	HSV-1+ (0%) HSV-2+ (0%)		n = 8; control pulpal tissue; HSV-1+ (0%) HSV-2+ (0%)		
Sabeti et al. 2003a [68]	n = 14, periapical lesions;	n = 13 HCMV+ (92, 3%) EBV+ (61, 5%) HSV-1+ (0%)	n = 1 HCMV+ (100%) EBV+ (0%) HSV-1+ (0%)	n = 2; periapical tissue from healthy place; HCMV+ (0%) EBV+ (0%)	<5 × 7 mm HCMV+ (85, 7%) EBV+ (28, 6%) ≥5 × 7 mm HCMV+ (100%) EBV+ (85, 7%)	HCMV\EBV+ (57, 1%)
Sabeti et al. 2003b [69]	n = 14, periapical lesions;	n = 7 HCMV+ (100%) EBV+ (85, 7%)	n = 7 HCMV+ (14, 3%) EBV+ (14, 3%) HSV-1+ (14, 3%)		<5 × 7 mm HCMV+ (50%) EBV+ (0%) ≥5 × 7 mm	Symptomatic HCMV\EBV+ (100%)

Author, year [reference number]	Study group	Symptomatic lesions	Asymptomatic lesions	Control group	Lesion size	Dual infection
					HCMV+ (50%) EBV+ (66, 7%)	Asymptomatic HCMV\EBV+ (14, 3%)
Sabeti et al. 2003c [83]	n = 5, periapical lesions;	n = 5, HCMV+ (100%) EBV+ (100%) HSV-1+ (0%)			≥5 × 7 mm HCMV+ (100%) EBV+ (100%)	Symptomatic HCMV\EBV+ (100%)
Sabeti et al. 2004 [84]	n = 34, periapical pathosis;	n = 23, HCMV\EBV+ (69, 6%) HCMV\EBV- (0%)	n = 11, HCMV\EBV+ (36, 4%) HCMV\EBV - (54, 5%) HSV+ (18, 2%)		≥5 × 7 mm HCMV/ EBV + (79, 2%)	HCMV\EBV+ (58, 8%)
Slots et al. 2004 [85]	n = 44, periapical pathosis;	n = 25, HCMV+ (100%) EBV+ (76%)	n = 19, HCMV+ (37%) EBV+ (26%)		Range from 2 × 2 to 15 × 16 mm	Symptomatic HCMV\EBV+ (76%) Asymptomatic HCMV\EBV+ (26%)
Kabak et al. 2005 [86]	n = 57, periapical lesions;	n = 57, HSV-1+ (8, 8%)				
Yildirim et al. 2006 [87]	n = 12, granulomatous tissue;	n = 12, HCMV+ (58%) EBV+ (67%)		n = 12, control pulpal tissue; HCMV+ (8%) EBV+ (8%)		Symptomatic HCMV\EBV+ (33%)
Saboa–Dantas et al. 2007 [88]	n = 26, HIV-seronegative		n = 26, granulomas HCMV+	n = 9, HIV-seropositive;		HIV-seronegative HCMV\EBV+

Author, year [reference number]	Study group	Symptomatic lesions	Asymptomatic lesions	Control group	Lesion size	Dual infection
	granulomas (n = 22); cysts (n = 4);		(18, 75%) EBV+ (43, 75%); cysts HCMV+ (0%) EBV+ (0%);	granulomas HCMV+ (66, 7%) EBV+ (50%); cysts HCMV+ (50%) EBV+ (50%);		(7, 7%) HIV-seropositive HCMV\EBV+ (33, 3%)
Andric et al. 2007 [89]	n = 33, periapical cysts	n = 16, HCMV+ (38, 9%)	n = 17, HCMV+ (61, 1%)	n = 10, odontogenic keratocysts; HCMV+ (60%)	Range from 11 to 80 mm	
Yazdi et al. 2008 [90]	n = 50, apical periodontitis;	n = 28, HCMV+ (53, 6%) EBV+ (3, 6%)	n = 22, HCMV+ (22, 7%) EBV+ (4, 5%)		Average lesion size 4.55 × 4.8 mm	Symptomatic HCMV\EBV+ (0%) Asymptomatic HCMV\EBV+ (4, 5%)
Sunde et al. 2008 [91]	n = 40, apical periodontitis;	n = 18, HCMV+ (0%) EBV+ (72%)	n = 22, HCMV+ (0%) EBV+ (28%)			
Sabeti et al. 2009 [92]	n = 15, periapical lesions;	n = 15, HCMV+ (67%)			Range from 3.0 to 8.5 mm	
Li et al. 2009 [93]	n = 53, apical periodontitis (30); previously treated teeth	n = 32 HCMV DNA/ mRNA+ (15, 7%)/ (27, 5%) EBV DNA/ mRNA+	n = 21 HCMV DNA/ mRNA+ (16, 1%)/ (32, 3%) EBV DNA/ mRNA+	n = 19, healthy pulp control; HCMV DNA/ mRNA+ (42, 1%)/ (10, 5%)	≥5 mm HCMV DNA/ mRNA (13, 9%)/ (33, 3%) EBV DNA/ mRNA+ (50%)/ (36, 1%)	

Author, year [reference number]	Study group	Symptomatic lesions	Asymptomatic lesions	Control group	Lesion size	Dual infection
	with apical periodontitis (23);	(43, 1%)/ (21, 6%)	(45, 2%)/ (32, 3%)	EBV DNA/ mRNA+ (0%)/ (0%)	<5 mm HCMV DNA/ mRNA (0%)/ (29,4%) EBV DNA/ mRNA+ (47, 1%)/ (35,3%)	
Hernandi et al. 2010 [95]	n = 40, apical periodontitis;	n = 17, HCMV DNA/ mRNA+ (6%)/ (0%) EBV DNA/ mRNA+ (82%)/ (71%)	n = 13, HCMV DNA/ mRNA + (13%)/ (0%) EBV DNA/ mRNA+ (65%)/ (35%)	n = 40, healthy pulp control; HCMV DNA/ mRNA + (0%)/ (0%) EBV DNA/ mRNA+ (2, 5%)/ (2, 5%)	≥5 mm HCMV DNA/ mRNA (14%)/ (0%) EBV DNA/ /mRNA+ (91%)/ (76%) ≤5 mm HCMV DNA/ mRNA (0%)/(0%) EBV DNA/ mRNA+ (53%)/(21%)	Symptomatic HCMV\EBV DNA+ (6%) Asymptomatic HCMV\EBV DNA+ (9%) Control group HCMV \EBVDNA+ (0%)
Hernandi et al. 2011 [96]	n = 40, apical periodontitis;	n = 17, HHV 6+ (29, 4%) HCMV+ (2, 5%) EBV+ (35%)	n = 23, HHV 6+ (13%) HCMV+ (7, 5%) EBV+ (37, 5%)	n = 40, healthy pulp control; HHV 6+ (2, 5%) HCMV+ (0%) EBV+ (2, 5%)	≥5 mm n = 21 HHV 6+ (23, 8%) HCMV+ (14, 8%) EBV+ (90, 5%) ≤5 mm n = 19 HHV 6+ (15, 8%) HCMV+ (5, 3%) EBV+ (52, 6%)	HHV 6\EBV+ (17, 5%) HCMV\EBV+ (7, 5%)

Author, year [reference number]	Study group	Symptomatic lesions	Asymptomatic lesions	Control group	Lesion size	Dual infection
Sabeti M et al. 2012 [97]	n = 15, periapical lesions;	n = 9, HCMV+ (55%) EBV+ (88, 9%)	n = 6, HCMV+ (0%) EBV+ (0%)			Symptomatic HCMV\EBV+ (44, 4%)
Hernandi et al. 2013 [98]	n = 58, apical periodontitis;	n = 28, HCMV+ (14, 3%) EBV+ (89, 3%)	n = 30, HCMV+ (10%) EBV+ (63, 3%)	n = 20, gingival tissue; HCMV+ (0%) EBV+ (10%)	≥5 mm n = 31 HCMV+ (16, 1%) EBV+ (93, 5%) ≤5 mm n = 27 HCMV+ (7, 4%) EBV+ (55, 6%)	
Ozbek et al. 2013 [99]	n = 28, apical periodontitis;	n = 16, HCMV + (37, 5%) EBV+ (18, 7%)	n = 12, HCMV + (25%) EBV+ (8, 3%)		≤5 mm Symptomatic HCMV+ (37, 5%) EBV+ (18, 7%) Asymptomatic HCMV+ (25%) EBV+ (8, 3%)	Symptomatic HCMV\EBV+ (25%) Asymptomatic HCMV\EBV+ (16, 7%)
Verdugo et al. 2015 [100]	n = 33, apical periodontitis;	n = 20, HCMV+ (15%) EBV+ (70%)	n = 13, HCMV+ (0%) EBV+ (38, 5%)	n = 15, saliva; HCMV+ (6, 7%) EBV+ (40%)		Symptomatic HCMV\EBV+ (15%)
Makino et al. 2015 [102]	n = 32, apical periodontitis;	n = 32, granulomas; EBV+ (78, 1%)		n = 20, gingival tissue; EBV+ (0%)		
Popovic et al. 2015 [104]	n = 60, apical periodontitis;	n = 31, HCMV + (70, 9%)	n = 29, HCMV + (24, 1%) EBV+ (0%)		≤5 mm Symptomatic HCMV+ (12, 5%)	Symptomatic HCMV\EBV+ (35, 5%)

http://dx.doi.org/ 10.5772/64004

Author, year [reference number]	Study group	Symptomatic lesions	Asymptomatic lesions	Control group	Lesion size	Dual infection
		EBV+ (41, 9%)			EBV+ (12, 5%) Asymptomatic HCMV+ (0%) EBV+ (0%) >5 mm Symptomatic HCMV+ (91, 3%) EBV+ (52, 2%) Asymptomatic HCMV+ (38, 9%) EBV+ (0%)	
Jakovljevic et al. 2015 [105]	n = 100, apical periodontitis;	n = 34,HCMV+ (52, 9%) EBV+ (79, 4%)	n = 66, HCMV + (54, 5%)EBV+ (74, 2%)	n = 25, healthy pulp control; HCMV+ (28%)EBV+ (24%)	>5 mm n = 69 HCMV+ (57, 9%) EBV+ (78, 3%) ≤5 mm n = 31 HCMV+ (54, 8%) EBV+ (71%)	HCMV\EBV+ (41%)

[68]*($p = 0.03$; Chi-squared test)—dual HCMV/EBV infection in lesions of 5 mm × 7 mm or grater in radiographic size.*
[69]*($p = 0.007$; $p = 0.04$; Chi-squared test, Yates')—dual HCMV/ EBV infection in symptomatic periapical lesions.*
[84]*($p < 0.001$; Chi-squared test)—presence of herpesviruses more in large versus small size periapical lesions.*
[84]*($p < 0.001$; Chi-squared test)—dual HCMV/ EBV infection in large periapical lesions.*
[85]*($p < 0.0001$; Chi-squared test)—dual HCMV/ EBV infection in symptomatic versus asymptomatic periapical lesion.*
[87]*($p < 0.040$; $p < 0.040$ Mann–Whitney U-test)—dual HCMV/ EBV infection in periapical lesions versus healthy pulpal control.*
[88]*($p = 0.001$; Chi-squared test, Yates')—HCMV infection in periapical lesions of HIV-positive versus HIV-negative patients.*
[90]*($p = 0.03$; Chi-squared test)—HCMV infection in symptomatic versus asymptomatic periapical lesions.*
[91]*($p = 0.025$; Chi-squared test)—EBV infection in symptomatic versus asymptomatic periapical lesions.*
[93]*($p < 0.05$; Chi-squared test)—EBV DNA and RNA in endodontic pathoses versus healthy pulp control.*
[95]*($p < 0.0001$; $p < 0.0001$; Chi-squared test, Yates')—EBV DNA and RNA in apical periodontitis lesions versus healthy pulp control.*
[95]*($p < 0.0001$; $p < 0.0001$; Chi-squared test, Yates')—EBV DNA and RNA in symptomatic versus asymptomatic periapical lesions.*
[95]*($p = 0.02$; $p = 0.002$; Chi-squared test, Yates')—both EBV DNA and RNA in large versus small size periapical lesions.*
[96]*($p = 0.03$; Fisher exact test)—HHV-6 DNA in apical periodontitis versus control group.*
[96]*($p = 0.018$; Logistic regression analysis)—Correlation between HHV-6 DNA occurrence and lesion size.*
[96]*($p = 0.008$; Logistic regression analysis)—HHV-6 DNA in symptomatic versus asymptomatic periapical lesions.*
[96]*($p < 0.01$; Fisher exact test)—HHV-6B DNA versus HHV-6A DNA in symptomatic large-sized lesions.*

[97]*($p = 0.048$; $p = 0.002$; Mann–Whitney U test)—dual HCMV/ EBV infection in symptomatic versus asymptomatic periapical lesion.*
[98]*($p < 0.000001$; Chi-squared test, Yates)—EBV infection in apical periodontitis lesions versus control group.*
[98]*($p < 0.05$; Chi-squared test, Yates)—EBV infection in symptomatic versus asymptomatic periapical lesions.*
[98]*($p = 0.002$; Chi-squared test)—EBV infection more in large versus small size periapical lesions.*
[100]*($p < 0.01$; Chi-squared test)—EBV copies more in symptomatic versus asymptomatic periapical lesions.*
[100]*($p = 0.07$; Chi-squared test)—EBV infection more in symptomatic versus asymptomatic periapical lesions.*
[103]*($p < 0.0001$; Mann–Whitney U test)—EBV DNA copies in apical periodontitis versus healthy gingival tissues.*
[104]*($p < 0.001$; Chi-squared test)—HCMV infection in symptomatic versus asymptomatic periapical lesions.*
[104]*($p < 0.001$; Chi-squared test)—EBV infection in symptomatic versus asymptomatic periapical lesions.*
[104]*($p < 0.001$; Chi-squared test)—HCMV/EBV dual infection in symptomatic versus asymptomatic periapical lesions.*
[104]*($p < 0.001$; Chi-squared test)—HCMV infection in large symptomatic versus small symptomatic periapical lesions.*
[104]*($p < 0.001$; Chi-squared test)—HCMV infection in large asymptomatic versus small asymptomatic periapical lesions.*
[105]*($p = 0.020$; Chi-squared test)—EBV infection in periapical lesions versus healthy pulpal control.*
[105]*($p = 0.001$; Chi-squared test)—EBV-1 versus EBV-2 infection in periapical lesions versus healthy pulpal control.*
[105]*($p = 0.020$; Chi-squared test)—HCMV infection in periapical lesions versus healthy pulpal control.*
[105]*($p = 0.036$; Chi-squared test)—HCMV gB 1 versus gB 2 infection in periapical lesions versus healthy pulpal control.*
[105]*($p = 0.038$; Chi-squared test)—HCMV/EBV dual infection in large-sized versus small-sized periapical lesions.*

Table 5. The occurrence of herpesviruses among apical periodontitis lesions and control specimens.

Author, year [reference numbers]	Study group	Control group	Co-infection	Lesion size
Chen et al. 2009 [94]	n = 31 HCMV+ (29%) EBV+ (6.5%) HSV+ (3.2%) VZV+ (0%)	n = 19 healthy pulp HCMV+ (42.1%) EBV+ (0%) HSV+ (5.3%) VZV+ (0%)		≥5 mm HCMV+ (26.1%) EBV+ (4.3%) HSV+ (4.3%) <5 mm HCMV+ (37.5%) EBV+ (12.5%)
Ferreira et al. 2011a [79]	n = 23 HCMV+ (0%) EBV+ (0%) HSV+ (4%) VZV+ (9%) HHV 6+ (9%) HHV 7+ (4%) HHV 8+ (48%) HPV+ (13%)	n = 5 healthy pulp HCMV+ (0%) EBV+ (0%) HSV+ (0%) VZV+ (0%) HHV 6+ (0%) HHV 7+ (20%) HHV 8+ (40%) HPV+ (0%)	VZV+ (8.7%) HSV+ (8.7%) HHV 6+ (4.3%) HHV 7+ (4.3%) HHV 8 (21.7%)	
Ferreira et al. 2011b [80]	n = 33 HCMV+ (0%) EBV+ (6%) VZV+ (6%) HHV 6+ (6%) HHV 7+ (3%) HHV 8+ (54.5%) HSV+ (3%) HPV+ (9%)		HHV 8 (15.2%) VZV+ (6.1%) HPV+ (6.1%) HSV+ (3%) EBV+ (3%) HHV 6 + (3%) HHV 7 + (3%) HHV 8, HPV -bacterial co-infection	
Ozbek et al. 2015a [101]	n = 27 HCMV+	n = 6 healthy pulp	Dual HCMV/EBV (4%)	

Author, year [reference numbers]	Study group	Control group	Co-infection	Lesion size
	(22.2%)EBV+ (11.1%) HPV+ (7.4%)	HCMV+ (0%) EBV+ (0%) HPV+ (0%)		
Ozbek et al. 2015b [103]	n = 21 HCMV+ (19%) EBV+ (14%) HHV 6+ (5%) HPV+ (5%)	n = 10 healthy pulp HCMV+ (0%) EBV+ (0%) HHV 6+ (0%) HPV+ (0%)	Dual HCMV/EBV (4.8%) Dual HCMV/HHV 6 (4.8%)	≥5 mm HCMV+ (27%) EBV+ (18%) HHV 6+ (9%) HPV+ (9%) <5 mm HCMV+ (10%) EBV+ (10%) HHV 6+ (0%) HPV+ (0%)

HCMV, human cytomegalovirus; EBV, Epstein–Bar virus; HHV, human herpesvirus; HPV, human papillomavirus; VZV, Varicella-zoster virus; HSV, Herpes simplex virus.

Table 6. The occurrence of herpesviruses among acute apical abscess lesions and control specimens.

Fourteen studies compared the occurrence of herpesviruses between the symptomatic and asymptomatic periapical lesions [68, 69, 84, 85, 90, 91, 93, 95–100, 104, 105]. The most investigated herpesviruses were EBV and HCMV. An overall analysis of EBV and HCMV presence showed variability in their occurrence.

The results of analysed studies revealed that EBV was the most prevalent herpesvirus in samples of apical periodontitis lesions [91, 93, 95–98, 100, 105]. Six studies shown that EBV infection was found in an increased percentage among symptomatic periapical lesions. Among these studies, five of them reported that EBV occurrence was significantly more common in symptomatic compared to asymptomatic periapical lesions [91, 95, 98, 100, 104].

Additionally, HCMV infection was also found in large percentage among symptomatic periapical lesions [68, 69, 85, 90, 104]. Yazdi et al. [90] and Popovic et al. [104] reported significant difference in HCMV occurrence between symptomatic and asymptomatic periapical lesions ($P = 0.03$, $P < 0.001$, respectively).

All studies of apical abscesses analysed the occurrence of herpesviruses in patients with acute and developed form of disease [79, 80, 94, 101, 103] (**Table 6**). They were characterized by rapid onset, spontaneous pain, tenderness of the tooth to pressure, pus formation, and associated swelling. The results of analysed studies have shown that HHV-8 and HCMV were the most frequently detected herpesviruses in cases of acute apical abscess. Two studies of Ferreira et al. [79, 80] have reported remarkably high occurrence of HHV-8 compared to other analysed herpesviruses. Oppositely, Chen et al. [94] and Ozbek et al. [101, 103] have found that HCMV was the most prevalent herpesvirus in abscess samples. Although herpesviruses were more prevalent in abscess lesions, their occurrence was not significantly different compared to control pulp tissues [79, 80, 94, 101, 103].

3.3. Findings of herpesviral infections among large- and small-sized apical periodontitis lesions

Clinical investigations use different radiographic methods to confirm the presence of periapical pathoses and to determine their size. The size of the periapical lesions is important prognostic parameter because it indicates the level of periapical bone resorption. Numerous studies investigated the occurrence of herpesviruses in periapical lesions regarding their size, estimated by conventional radiography. The common approach was to compare the occurrence of herpesviruses in groups of large- (≥5 × 7 mm) and small-sized (<5 × 7 mm) lesions based on its mesiodistal and craniocaudal diameter. The summarized results of relevant studies are given in **Table 5**.

Eight studies investigated the occurrence of herpesviruses among small- and large-sized periapical lesions [68, 69, 93, 95, 96, 98, 104, 105]. The most frequently analysed herpesviruses were EBV and HCMV. Similarly, an overall analysis of EBV and HCMV presence in apical periodontitis lesions with different size showed variability in their occurrence.

All eight studies reported that EBV infection was found in an increased percentage among large-sized periapical lesions [68, 69, 93, 95, 96, 98, 104, 105]. Two studies of Hernadi et al. [95, 98] have shown that EBV infection was significantly more frequent in large-sized compared to small-sized periapical lesions (P = 0.02, P = 0.002, respectively).

Moreover, five studies showed that HCMV infection was found in large percentage among large-sized periapical lesions [68, 69, 96, 104, 105]. Popovic et al. [104] reported that HCMV was detected significantly more often in large-sized compared to small-sized periapical lesions (P < 0.001). In opposite to these findings, several studies reported that EBV [95, 96, 98, 105] and HCMV [68, 69, 105] could be found in large percentage among small-sized periapical lesions.

Beside EBV and HCMV infection, Hernadi et al. [96] also found that HHV-6 significantly correlates with increasing periapical lesion size (P = 0.018).

Only two studies [94, 103] analysed the occurrence of herpesviruses among acute apical abscesses with different size. HCMV was the most frequently detected herpesvirus in both groups of lesions without significant difference in relation to their size (**Table 6**).

3.4. Findings of herpesviral infections in periapical granulomas and radicular cysts

Four studies analysed the presence of herpesviruses in apical periodontitis lesions in relation to their histopathological features [86, 88, 93, 105]. The common approach was to compare the occurrence of herpesviruses between periapical granulomas and radicular cysts.

In study of Kabak et al. [86], the immunohistochemistry analysis showed the presence of HSV in five radicular cysts, while none of the periapical granulomas were positive. Saboia-Dantas et al. [88] compared the presence of HCMV and EBV between 29 periapical granulomas and 6 radicular cysts. Statistical analysis did not reveal significant difference between HCMV and EBV presence in examined groups. Additionally, subsequent studies by Li et al. [93] and Jakovljevic et al. [105] did not report significant differences in the occurrence of herpesviruses between periapical granulomas and radicular cysts (**Table 5**).

3.5. Findings of multiple herpesviral infections and co-infection with bacteria in periapical pathoses

Fifteen included studies reported the presence of dual herpesviral infection in apical periodontitis samples [68, 69, 83–85, 87, 88, 90, 95–97, 99, 100, 104, 105].

Dual infection including HCMV and EBV was the most commonly investigated. Only one study reported dual infection of EBV and HHV-6 in 17, 5% of investigated sample [95]. Majority of studies compared the presence of dual infection in relation to clinical and radiographic features of apical periodontitis. Three studies [68, 84, 105] showed that dual infection was detected significantly more often in large-sized compared to small-sized periapical lesions ($P = 0.03$, $P < 0.001$, $P = 0.038$, respectively). Moreover, the results of four other studies [83, 86, 97, 104] indicated that dual herpesviral infection was significantly more common in symptomatic in comparison with asymptomatic apical periodontitis ($P = 0.007$, $P < 0.001$, $P = 0.048$, $P < 0.0001$, respectively) (**Table 5**).

Two studies investigated the presence of herpesviral–bacterial co-infection in samples of apical periodontitis [84, 100]. Sabeti et al. [84] showed that *Fusobacterium* species, *Streptococcus* species, and *Parvimonas micra* were the most common bacterial species in co-infection with herpesviruses in these lesions. Additionally, Verdugo et al. [100] reported that *Tannerella forsythia, Porphyromonas gingivalis,* and *Prevotella nigrescens* were the most common bacterial species found in concomitant infection with EBV (**Table 5**).

Four studies investigated the presence of multiple herpesviral infections in samples of acute apical abscesses [79, 80, 101, 103]. Studies of Ferreira et al. [79, 80] reported multiple infections with several herpesviruses. The most prevalent herpesviruses in multiple infections of acute apical abscess were HHV-8, HSV, and VZV (**Table 6**). Additionally, Ozbek et al. [101, 103] showed the presence of dual infection between HCMV and EBV, and HCMV and HHV-6 in samples of large acute apical abscesses. Ferreira et al. [80] investigated the presence of herpesviral–bacterial co-infection in acute apical abscess. They have shown that the most prevalent bacterial species were *Tannerella forsythia* (70%), *Tannerella forsythia* (67%), *Porphyromonas endodontialis* (67%), *Dialister invisus* (61%), and *Dialister pneumosintes* (57, 5%). Their findings indicate that HHV-8 was positively associated with seven of the target bacterial species, but all these associations were weak (**Table 6**).

3.6. Findings of different herpesviral genotypes in periapical pathoses

Four studies investigated the presence of different genotypes of herpesviruses in periapical pathoses [93, 94, 96, 105].

Li et al. [93] analysed the presence of EBV BLR F2 gene product genotypes (type 1 and type 2) in apical periodontitis lesions. Although, 50.1% of samples were EBV positive, authors did not report the frequencies of investigated genotypes. They were not able to distinguish EBV strains because the sequences of the amplified region were too similar.

Hernadi et al. [96] reported the presence of different genotypes of HHV-6 in samples of apical periodontitis. They analysed the occurrence of two variants (type A and B) of the immediate early fragment sequence of HHV-6. They did not find significant difference between HHV-6 type A and B in samples of apical periodontitis and control group. On the other side, HHH-6B was significantly associated with symptomatic and large-sized lesions ($P < 0.01$).

Jakovljevic et al. [105] analysed the occurrence of EBV EBNA-2 (type 1 and 2) and HCVM gB (types I–IV) genotypes in apical periodontitis samples. They have reported that EBV type 1 was more frequently detected compared to EBV type 2 in both periapical lesions and healthy pulp tissues (74 versus 6% and 24 versus 4%, $P = 0.001$). In addition, authors have reported that only two out of four HCMV gB genotypes (type I and II) were detected. HCMV gB-II was more frequently detected among periapical lesions and healthy pulp tissue compared to gB-1 (42 versus 12%, 28 versus 0%, $P = 0.036$) Significant differences were not observed in the distribution of HCMV and EBV genotypes regarding clinical and radiographic features of periapical lesions.

Analysing the samples of acute apical abscess, Chen et al. [94] showed the presence of EBV type 1 in two examined samples. These findings were not correlated with clinical and radiographic features of acute apical abscess.

3.7. Quantitative herpesviral analysis in apical periodontitis lesions

The quantification of herpesviruses in apical periodontitis samples has been reported in four studies [91, 97, 100, 102]. All studies reported the number of HCMV and/or EBV copies/mL in samples of apical periodontitis using the real-time PCR method.

Sunde et al. [91] analysed the number of HCMV and EBV copies in samples of apical periodontitis. EBV was detected in 50% of sample, while HCVM was not detectable. They reported low average levels of EBV copies in symptomatic and asymptomatic apical periodontitis (300 versus 970 copies/mL) without any significant difference between the analysed groups.

Sabeti et al. [97] analysed the number of HCMV and EBV copies in symptomatic and asymptomatic apical periodontitis. Four out of nine symptomatic lesions were positive for HCMV, and the average number of HCMV copies was 874.000/mL. Eight out of nine symptomatic lesions exhibited the presence of EBV. The average number of EBV copies in samples was 2.162.500/mL. In contrast, HCMV and EBV were not detected in asymptomatic lesions. They have reported significant difference in the occurrence of HCMV and EBV between symptomatic and asymptomatic periapical lesions ($P = 0.048$, $P = 0.002$, respectively).

Similarly, Verdugo et al. [100] demonstrated the presence of increased number of EBV copies in symptomatic in comparison with asymptomatic periapical lesions. They reported that the average number of EBV copies in symptomatic lesions (391.903/mL) was significantly higher than the average copy numbers of EBV in asymptomatic lesions (623/mL) ($P<.01$). Additionally, HCVM was detected in only 3 out of 20 symptomatic lesions (at average number of 124.076 copies/mL).

Makino et al. [102] reported the difference in EBV DNA copies between samples of periapical granulomas and healthy gingival tissue. They have shown that EBV was positive in 78.1% of sample and the median EBV DNA copy number was 8.688/μg total DNA. In contrast, EBV was not detected in control group and that difference was statistically significant ($P = 0.0001$).

3.8. Levels of proinflammatory mediators in relation to herpesviral infection in apical periodontitis

The relationship between herpesviral infection and levels of proinflammatory mediators in apical periodontitis has been analysed in three studies [87, 97, 98].

Yildirim et al. [87] investigated a possible relationship between the presence of HCMV and EBV in apical periodontitis samples and increased levels of bone resorption-inducing cytokines. They analysed the presence of HCMV and EBV DNA and the expression of mRNA transcripts of receptor activator of nuclear factor (NF-kB) ligand (RANKL), osteoprotegerin, core binding factor α-1, colony-stimulating factor-1, transforming growth factor (TGF)-3, and monocyte chemoattractant protein-1. Only, the RANKL expression revealed statistically significant difference between periapical lesions and healthy pulpal tissue ($P < 0.04$). No correlation was found between herpesvirus presence and cytokine expression in apical periodontitis sample.

Sabeti et al. [97] correlated the occurrence of HCMV and EBV infection in periapical tissues with the expression of mRNA transcripts of TNF-α, γ-interferon (IFN), IL-1β, IL-6, IL-10, and IL-12. They found significant direct correlation between EBV, HCMV and TNF-α, γ-IFN, IL-1β, and IL-12 in symptomatic periapical lesions.

Hernadi et al. [98] evaluated the association between TNF-α and TGF-β and the clinical, radiologic, and virologic characteristics of the lesions. They compared the levels of these cytokines in relation to EBV, HCVM, HHV-6, and HHV-8 infection in apical periodontitis. They showed that the levels of TNF-α were significantly higher in periapical lesions with EBV infection in comparison with lesions without EBV infection (1.1×10^{-2} versus 6.8×10^{-3}, $P = 0.032$). All other comparisons between levels of cytokines and features of periapical lesions were insignificant.

4. Discussion

The emerging role of herpesviruses in the development and progression of apical periodontitis changes previous concepts of etiopathogenesis of destructive periapical disease. The hallmark of herpesviral infection is impairment of immune system. Most herpesviruses are ubiquitous agents. They are often acquired early in life and capable of infecting individuals from diverse geographical and economic backgrounds [71]. The initial herpesviral infection is followed by a latent phase in host cells, which ensures the survival of the viral genome throughout the lifetime of the infected individual. The α herpesviruses establish latency in long-living non-dividing neuronal cells of sensory ganglia. The β herpesviruses establish latency in bone marrow-derived myeloid progenitor cells, while the γ herpesviruses are latent in B lymphocytes [72]. Herpesvirus reactivation may occur spontaneously or as a result of psychosocial and physical stress, hormonal changes, infections, immunosuppressive medication, and other events impairing the host immune defence [73]. After activation, they can infect monocytes/ macrophages, T and B lymphocytes, epithelial cells, endothelial cells, fibroblasts, and other mammalian cells [73].

Cell-mediated immune responses are the key defence mechanisms against herpesviral infection [71–73]. Cytotoxic T lymphocytes and natural killer cells are the most important effector cells responsible for suppression of viral replication and maintenance of herpesviruses in latent state. The T-lymphocyte response to herpesviruses changes over time from a predominantly CD4+ response early in infection, to a CD8+ response during latent phase [71–73].

In response to antiviral host defences, herpesviruses have developed a number of immunosubversive mechanisms to ensure persistent infections in the host [71–73]. Herpesviruses can affect toll-like receptors function thus interfering with antigen presentation process [111]. In addition, they have the ability to inhibit the expression of the major histocompatibility complex (MHC) class I and II on the surface of macrophages [112]. These actions allow them to evade cytotoxic T-cell recognition [113] and natural killer cell lysis [114]. Moreover, herpesviruses can inhibit migration of dendritic cells [115] and decrease chemotaxis of polymorphonuclear leukocytes [116]. Herpesviruses infection induces production of proinflammatory cytokines [117] but also impairs antiviral cytokine responses [113, 118]. Although IFN-γ, TNF-α, and IL-6 exert high antiviral activity, some herpesviruses encode unique homologs of IL-10 capable to inhibit production of these cytokines in macrophages and monocytes [119–121]. Additionally, some herpesviral genes protect cells from undergoing apoptosis in order to prolong the life of infected cells [113].

As already mentioned, tissues of periapical granuloma and radicular cysts are characterized by inflammatory cells infiltration [24–33]. However, these inflammatory cells are also the host cells for herpesviruses [72]. In proposed herpesviral–bacterial hypothesis, bacterial infection of the pulp causes herpesviral-infected inflammatory cells to enter pulpal tissue through the periapical region. Bacterial infection causes subsequent herpesviral reactivation. Reactivated herpesviruses in pulp and periapical tissues may induce development of periapical pathoses as a direct result of viral infection or as a result of virally induced damage to the host defence. Although primary bacterial infection in periapical region may induce herpesviral reactivation, herpesviral infection also possesses mechanisms to induce upgrowth of bacterial pathogens in the periodontium [75, 76]. Previous results suggest that herpesviral infection in apical periodontitis was associated with *Fusobacterium* species, *Tannerella forsythia, Porphyromonas gingivalis, Parvimonas micra,* and *Streptococcus* species [84, 100]. Additionally, Ferreira et al. [80] reported positive association between HHV-8 and several bacteria in acute apical abscess. Using the animal model, Stern et al. [122] have shown that co-infection of murine CMV and *Porphyromonas gingivalis* is characterized with decreased level of antiviral IFN-γ. Moreover, interaction between EBV and *Porphyromonas gingivalis* may also be bidirectional [123]. Herpesviral proteins on infected cells may serve as a new attachment sites for bacteria [124], while some bacterial products may facilitate herpesviral entry into cells and activate intracellular signalling pathways [125].

In contrast to proposed model of herpesviral–bacterial interaction, Ferreira et al. [79, 80] hypothesized that occurrence of herpesviruses might be just an epiphenomenon to bacterial infection that caused inflammation of periapical tissue and consequent influx of virus-infected inflammatory cells. Those authors believed that the presence of viral DNA in clinical samples does not necessarily imply a role in disease pathogenesis [79, 80]. Both theories suggest that virus-infected inflammatory cells, in which herpesviruses maintained their latency, could be attracted to periapical area. Histological analyses confirmed that these inflammatory cells constitute regular infiltrate of periapical granuloma and radicular cysts. Obviously, the essential difference between proposed hypotheses is whether herpesviruses may or may not be reactivated in periapical region and subsequently induce tissue breakdown.

Viral activation may be assessed by molecular techniques identifying transcription of genes associated with viral reactivation, immunologic methods to detect viral proteins, and by electron microscopy demonstrating the presence of intact virions inside the cells [126]. Li et al. [93] pointed out that the detection of herpesviral DNA *per se* is not sufficient to distinguish latent episomal viral DNA from genomic viral DNA contained in virus particles that would be indicative of an active infection. Herpesvirus virion genes are replicated in a specific order: immediate–early, early, and late genes [72]. Slots [71–73] proposed that the transcription of late genes can be used as an indicator of viral replication and active infection. Therefore, several studies have used detection of complementary DNA of genes transcribed late during the infectious cycle of herpesviruses [68, 69, 83–85, 90, 93, 95, 96]. The majority of those studies [68, 69, 83–85, 90] reported high occurrence of herpesviral infection in their samples. Moreover, the authors concluded that their findings suggest the presence of an active herpesviral infection at apical periodontitis sites. Although studies of Li et al. [93] and Hernadi et al. [95, 96] have employed the same reverse-transcription (RT) PCR technique for complementary DNA herpesviral detection, they failed to report such high percentage of periapical lesions exhibiting active replication of EBV and HCMV. Those findings could be explained by different prevalence of herpesviruses due to geographic, socio-economic, and racial/ethnical factors [71–76].

Quantification of herpesviruses by real-time PCR can also be used as a marker of active infection [126, 127]. Previously reported studies showed that increased viral load of herpesviruses correlates positively with progression of marginal periodontitis [126–128]. Based on these findings, Sunde et al. [91] suggested that increased number of viral copies of HCMV and EBV could possibly correlate with clinical features of apical periodontitis. However, their results did not reveal any significant differences between HCMV and EBV copies in symptomatic and asymptomatic periapical lesions. On the other hand, Sabeti et al. [97] and Verdugo et al. [100] have found significant differences in HCMV and EBV copy number between symptomatic and asymptomatic lesions. Makino et al. [102] have shown that the number of EBV copies was significantly increased in periapical lesions compared to healthy pulp controls. These results are in accordance with previous reports of Kubar et al. [126, 127], and their statement that increased herpes viral load may represent an important characteristic of active herpesvirus infection.

Statistical analysis of pooled data in our previous review [70] suggested that there is no significant correlation between the occurrence of HCMV and EBV and clinical features of apical periodontitis. These results are based on analysis of studies which used RT-PCR technique for complementary DNA herpesviral detection [68, 69, 85, 90, 93, 95]. In addition, studies included in this review used immunohistochemical [81, 82, 86] or single-PCR [104, 105] method to identify herpesviruses in symptomatic and asymptomatic periapical lesions. One of the aims of this study was to analyse the occurrence of herpesviruses in relation to histopathological and radiographic features of periapical lesions. Only four studies [86, 88, 93, 105] have compared the presence of herpesviruses in periapical granulomas and radicular cysts and concluded that there were no significant differences between these two groups. Although radicular cysts are related to more intensive bone resorption in periapical area compared to periapical granulomas, the fact that both types of lesions are characterized by intensive inflammatory cells infiltrate might explain these results [129].

The analysis of correlation between herpesviral infection and size of apical periodontitis lesions gave inconclusive results. Only 8 out of 24 studies [68, 69, 93, 95, 96, 98, 104, 105] analysed the occurrence of herpesviruses in small- and large-sized periapical lesions. We did not conduct meta-analysis of these studies because they employed different techniques to identify herpesviral presence (**Table 4**). Only one study [104] reported significantly increased detection rates of HCMV in large-sized compared to small-sized periapical lesions. Also, Hernadi et al. [95, 98] showed that EBV infection was more frequent in large-sized compared with small-sized periapical lesions. Additionally, Hernadi et al. [96] reported positive correlation between the occurrence of HHV-6 and increased periapical lesion size.

During primary HCMV infection, the host responds by production of IL-1β, IL-6, IL-12, TNF-α, IFN-γ, and prostaglandin E_2 (PGE_2) [117]. EBV infection stimulates the production of IL-1β, IL-1 receptor agonist (IL-1Ra), IL-6, IL-8, IL-10, IL-12, TNF-α, IFN-γ, etc. [117]. In addition, increased production of proinflammatory cytokines induces bone resorption in periapical area [130–132]. Sabeti et al. [97] found significant correlation between EBV and HCMV infection and TNF-α, IFN-γ, IL-1β, and IL-12 in symptomatic periapical lesions. Similar results were reported by Hernadi et al. [98]. They detected increased levels of TNF-α in apical periodontitis lesions infected with EBV in comparison with a lesion without EBV infection [98]. Although disturbed balance between RANKL and OPG has been correlated with increased periapical bone resorption [133], Yildirim et al. [87] did not find correlation between herpesviral presence and increased RANKL expression in apical periodontitis samples.

Growing knowledge about herpesviruses indicates that there is a great diversity of viral strains which might influence the course and severity of infection. Until now, researchers have identified more than 5000 different strains of herpesviruses. Different herpesviral genotypes possess specific pathogenic abilities due to differences in cell tropism and specific interactions with the host's immune system [71–73, 134].

Although, HCMV and EBV were the most investigated herpesviruses in periapical pathoses, only one study [105] analysed the occurrence of different HCMV gB and EBV EBNA-2 genotypes in apical periodontitis. Subtype classification of HCMV is mostly based on the gB gene which encodes a glycoprotein with high immune reactivity incorporated in the viral envelope. This glycoprotein is required for HCMV infectivity because it regulates viral penetration into cells, transmission of infection, and modulation of cellular transcription [135,

136]. Based on the nucleotide sequence of gB genes, all HCMV genotypes belong to one of four variants (gB I-gB IV) [137] with evidently different geographical distribution [138]. Depending on the sequence of EBV EBNA-2 gene, two types of EBV can be distinguished, EBV-1 and EBV-2. EBNA-2 acts as a transcription factor inducing the expression of viral latent membrane protein genes. EBNA-2 is also required for continued proliferation of lymphoblastoid cell lines in which the latent viral genome is maintained [139].

Our previous research [105] indicated that gB-II was more frequently detected than gB-I in both periapical lesions (42 versus 12%) and healthy control group (28 versus 0%) (P = 0.036). Additionally, EBV-1 was also more frequently detected compared to EBV-2 in both periapical lesions (74 versus 6%) and healthy control group (24 versus 4%) (P = 0.001). Our results were in accordance with previously reported occurrence of HCMV gB and EBV EBNA-2 genotypes in generalized chronic periodontitis and peri-implantitis tissues [140, 141]. On the other hand, our findings did not reveal significant differences between HCMV and EBV genotypes and clinical or histopathological features of apical periodontitis lesions. Also, Hernadi et al. [96] investigated the occurrence of HHV-6 subtypes (type A and B) in apical periodontitis. They have reported that subtype A was found in small-sized, asymptomatic lesions and in a control pulp sample, whereas subtype B was significantly associated with large sized symptomatic lesions.

The rates of herpesviral detection in acute apical abscess vary among analysed studies (**Table 6**). In studies of Chen et al. [94] and Ozbek et al. [101, 103], HCMV and EBV were the most frequently detected herpesviruses in acute apical abscesses. However, no significant differences were noted compared to healthy pulp controls and between small- and large-sized lesions [94, 101, 103] (**Table 6**). In contrast to these findings, Ferreira et al. [79, 80], reported very low occurrence of HCMV and EBV infection in acute apical abscesses among Brazilian population. Analysing the occurrence of all members of *Herpesviridae* family in acute apical abscess samples, they reported the increased detection rate of HHV-8 [79, 80].

HHV-8 was first described in Kaposi's sarcoma tissues from an HIV-positive individual [142]. Since then, epidemiological and molecular studies suggested that HHV-8 is the etiological agents of all subtypes of Kaposi's sarcoma and two B-cell lymphomas, i.e. primary effusion lymphoma and multicentric Castelman's disease [143–145]. HHV-8 DNA sequence have also been found in association with other diseases, such as pemphigus, various skin diseases, salivary gland tumours, multiple myeloma, and non-neoplastic lymphadenopathies of immunocompetent individuals, but the role of this virus in these diseases remains uncertain [146]. Until now, only these two studies [79, 80] investigated the occurrence of HHV-8 in periapical pathoses. Data from periodontal literature are also scarce and inconclusive, but it has been suggested that HHV-8 in immunocompetent patients may reduce the host defences and thereby contribute to destructive periodontal disease by mechanism similar to other herpesviruses [147, 148].

Assessing the studies included in this review, it is obvious that there is a wide variety in the detection rates of herpesviruses. Such discrepancies are mainly due to different methodological approaches for virus detection. In previous reports, Slots [76] claimed that observed variations in detection rates of herpesviruses can be caused by different inclusion criteria and clinical status of study individuals, use of different diagnostic methods, or geographic differences in herpesvirus occurrence.

Replacing classical viral diagnostic techniques, the PCR method has become the standard methodology for the detection of herpesvirus nucleic acids [149]. Included studies used different variants of PCR method (**Table 4**). When discussing the results of the PCR analyses, several issues should be taken into consideration, including the selection of PCR method, the selection of primers, the high sensitivity of this technique, and the possible false-positive and false-negative results [70, 149].

Single stage or end-point PCR is a gel-based technique that identifies the target nucleic acid as either present or absent. Nested PCR, as one of the variants of classical PCR method, is used to increase the sensitivity and specificity of the PCR assay [149]. However, the results of this method should be taken with precaution because it may detect herpesviruses at copy counts too low to be of clinical significance. Additionally, it must be stressed that single stage and nested PCR cannot distinguish latent episomal viral DNA from genomic viral DNA. Oppositely to other variants of PCR methods, RT-PCR assay can detect and quantify RNA expression and may identify active herpesvirus infection [149]. That is the reason why RT-PCR method should be recommended as method of choice in herpesviruses detection. In addition, real-time PCR assay has been used to quantify herpesviruses at diseased periapical site. Increased viral load detected by real-time PCR can also be indicative of viral replication and active viral infection [127].

The sensitivity of PCR techniques is determined by the selection of primer pairs used in the PCR. Possible reason for different detection rates of herpesviruses among included studies may be due to the use of different primers [150]. The majority of studies [68, 69, 83–85, 90, 93, 95–97] tested the coding sequence of HCMV pp65 matrix protein which is transcribed late during the infectious cycle. On the other hand, two other studies [87, 89] reported different, immediate early gene primers for HCMV transcript detection. Similarly, identification of EBV products in analysed samples was not uniform. The PCRs in 10 studies [68, 69, 83–85, 87, 90, 97, 104, 105] were performed with amplification of genome encoding for the EBNA-2. Oppositely, studies by Li et al. [93] and Hernadi et al. [95, 96] reported different primers for the BLR F2 gene product and the Bam H1-W fragment of the EBV genome.

Such variations in use of different primers were not observed for HSV, HHV-6, and HHV-8 detection. Primers for glycoprotein D, as major component of the virion envelope and infected cell membranes, were used to analyse HSV infection in samples of periapical pathoses [68, 69, 83, 84]. HHV-6 was detected by amplification of the immediate early fragment that is conservative regulator region in its genome [96]. Additionally, Chen et al. [94] and Ferreira et al. [79, 80] reported the amplification of ORF26 gene of HHV-8 that represents a minor capsid protein.

In addition, it is important to be aware of possible false-negative and false-positive results using the PCR techniques. False-negative PCR results may be caused by inadequate sampling technique or by inhibitory effects of components of the amplification process. However, false-positive results may be caused by cross-contamination among samples or the contamination of samples by saliva.

http://dx.doi.org/ 10.5772/64004

Other related factors that influence the prevalence of herpesviruses are race/ethnicity and socio-economic status of individuals [151–153]. Epidemiological results show that as a country becomes more developed, the occurrence of herpesviruses may decrease. Herpesviruses seroprevalence tended to be the highest in South America, Africa, and Asia and the lowest in Western Europe and the United States [154–156]. Most of the studies analysed in this review were performed on North American [68, 69, 81, 83–85, 92–94, 97, 100] and European populations [86, 87, 89, 91, 95, 96, 99, 101, 103–105]. Results of these studies are in accordance with the herpesviruses seroprevalence in the United States [156] and Europe [157–162]. Moreover, data on herpesvirus seroprevalence among organ recipients in Iran [163], patients with HSV infection of the peripheral nervous system in Israel [164], patients with head and neck carcinomas in Japan [165], and patients with hematologic disorders in Brazil [166] are in line with results of herpesvirus detection rates in specimens of periapical pathoses.

All studies included in the final review were cross-sectional. A significant limitation of all the microbiological studies of endodontic infections is their cross-sectional nature. Given results of any cross-sectional study preclude any strong conclusions about involvement of certain identified microbiota in causation of disease. As a consequence, these results may only suggest possible association between certain microbial species and development of disease, and they cannot be used for determination of cause-and-effect relationship between them [40].

In conclusion, this study provides an updated review of the occurrence of herpesviruses in periapical pathoses with different clinical, histopathological, and radiographic features. HCMV and EBV were the most prevalent herpesviruses in apical periodontitis lesions, followed by HHV-8 in samples of acute apical abscesses. Several studies reported positive correlation between the occurrence of herpesviruses and clinical and histopathological features of apical periodontitis, but overall results are still controversial.

Presented results place periapical pathoses into a context of complex aetiology, with many aspects still remaining to be elucidated. It might be concluded that the etiopathogenesis of periapical pathoses involves specific bacteria and viruses, protective and destructive host immune responses, modifiable and non-modifiable environmental factors, and genetic and epigenetic factors.

It is well known that herpesviral infection can cause focal immunosuppression, but the specific molecular mechanisms by which herpesviruses may cause or exacerbate periapical pathoses still have to be identified. Further studies on experimental animal models or controlled longitudinal trials with potential antiviral therapy and quantification of viral copies as prognostic markers should provide more data on herpesviruses as a factor in the pathogenesis of the periapical inflammation.

Acknowledgements

Supported by Grants 175075 and 175073 from the Ministry of Education, Science and Technological Development of the Republic of Serbia.

Author details

Aleksandar Jakovljević[1,4*], Miroslav Andrić[1], Aleksandra Knežević[2], Katarina Beljić-Ivanović[3], Maja Miletić[4], Tanja Jovanović[2], Ljiljana Kesić[5] and Jelena Milašin[6]

*Address all correspondence to: dr.sasuli@hotmail.com

1 Clinic of Oral surgery and Implantology, School of Dental Medicine, University of Belgrade, Belgrade, Serbia

2 Department of Virology, Institute of Microbiology and Immunology, Faculty of Medicine, University of Belgrade, Belgrade, Serbia

3 Clinic of Restorative Dentistry and Endodontics, School of Dental Medicine, University of Belgrade, Belgrade, Serbia

4 Department of Pathophysiology, School of Dental Medicine, University of Belgrade, Belgrade, Serbia

5 Department of Oral Medicine and Periodontology, Clinic of Dentistry, Medical Faculty, University of Nis, Nis, Serbia

6 Department of Human Genetics, School of Dental Medicine, University of Belgrade, Belgrade, Serbia

References

[1] Nair PN. Pathogenesis of apical periodontitis and the causes of endodontic failure. Crit Rev Oral Biol Med. 2004;15:348–391. doi:10.1177/154411130401500604.

[2] Figdor D. Apical periodontitis: a very prevalent problem. Oral Surg Oral Med Oral Pathol Oral Radiol Endod. 2002;94:651–652. doi:10.1067/moe.2002.130322.

[3] Jiménez-Pinzón A, Segura-Egea JJ, Poyato-Ferrera M, Velasco-Ortega E, Ríos-Santos JV. Prevalence of apical periodontitis and frequency of root-filled teeth in an adult Spanish population. Int Endod J. 2004;37:167–173. doi:10.1111/j.0143-2885.2004.00759.x.

[4] Eriksen HM. Epidemiology of apical periodontitis. In: Ørstavik D, Pitt Ford TR, editors. Essential endodontology. Prevention and treatment of apical periodontitis. 1st ed. London: Blackwell Science;1998. pp. 179–191.

[5] Nair PN. Apical periodontitis: a dynamic encounter between root canal infection and host response. Periodontol 2000. 1997;13:121–148. doi:10.1111/j.1600-0757.1997.tb00098.x.

[6] Siqueira JF Jr. Endodontic infections: concepts, paradigms, and perspectives. Oral Surg Oral Med Oral Pathol Oral Radiol Endod. 2002;94:281–293. doi:10.1067/moe.2002.126163.

[7] Kakehashi S, Stanley HR, Fitzgerald RJ. The effects of surgical exposures of dental pulps in germ-free and conventional laboratory rats. Oral Surg Oral Med Oral Pathol. 1965;20:340–349. doi:10.1016/0030-4220(65)90166-0.

[8] Sandquist G. Bacteriological studies of necrotic dental pulps [thesis]. Umea (Sweden): University of Umea; 1976.

[9] Möller AJ, Fabricius L, Dahlén G, Ohman AE, Heyden G. Influence on periapical tissues of indigenous oral bacteria and necrotic pulp tissue in monkeys. Scand J Dent Res. 1981;89:475–484.

[10] Stashenko P, Teles R, D'Souza R. Periapical inflammatory responses and their modulation. Crit Rev Oral Biol Med. 1998;9:498–521. doi:10.1177/10454411980090040701.

[11] Siqueira JF Jr, Rocas IN, Ricucci D. Biofilms in endodontic infection. Endod Topics. 2012;22:33–49. doi:10.1111/j.1601-1546.2012.00279.x.

[12] Paster BJ, Dewhirst FE. Molecular microbial diagnosis. Periodontology 2000. 2009;51:38–144.

[13] Siqueira JF Jr, Rôças IN. Diversity of endodontic microbiota revisited. J Dent Res. 2009;88:969–81. doi:10.1177/0022034509346549.

[14] Siqueira JF Jr, Alves FR, Rôças IN. Pyrosequencing analysis of the apical root canal microbiota. J Endod. 2011;37:1499–503. doi:10.1016/j.joen.2011.08.012.

[15] Saito D, Leonardo Rde T, Rodrigues JL, Tsai SM, Höfling JF, Gonçalves RB. Identification of bacteria in endodontic infections by sequence analysis of 16S rDNA clone libraries. J Med Microbiol. 2006;55:101–7. doi:10.1099/jmm.0.46212-0.

[16] Munson MA, Pitt-Ford T, Chong B, Weightman A, Wade WG. Molecular and cultural analysis of the microflora associated with endodontic infections. J Dent Res. 2002;81:761–6. doi:10.1177/154405910208101108.

[17] Rôças IN, Siqueira JF Jr. Root canal microbiota of teeth with chronic apical periodontitis. J Clin Microbiol. 2008;46:3599–606. doi:10.1128/JCM.00431-08.

[18] Nair PNR. Light and electron microscopic studies of root canal flora and periapical lesions. J Endod. 1987;13:29–39.

[19] Ricucci D, Siqueira JF Jr. Biofilms and apical periodontitis: study of prevalence and association with clinical and histopathologic findings. J Endod. 2010;36:1277–88. doi:10.1016/j.joen.2010.04.007.

[20] Metzger Z, Abramovitz I. Periapical lesions of endodontic origin. In: Ingle JI, Bakland LK, Baumgartner JC, editors. Ingle's endodontics. 6th ed. Hamilton: BC Decker Inc. 2008. p. 494.

[21] Langeland K, Block RM, Grossman LI. A histopathologic and histobacteriologic study of 35 periapical endodontic surgical specimens. J Endod. 1977;3:8–23. doi:10.1016/S0099-2399(77)80217-3.

[22] Nair PNR, Schmid-Meier E. An apical granuloma with epithelial integument. Oral Surg Oral Med Oral Pathol. 1986;62:698–703. doi:10.1016/0030-4220(86)90266-5.

[23] Nair PNR, Pajarola G, Schroeder HE. Types and incidence of human periapical lesions obtained with extracted teeth. Oral Surg Oral Med Oral Pathol Oral Radiol Endod. 1996;81:93–102.

[24] Cymerman JJ, Cymerman DH, Walters J, Nevins AJ. Human T lymphocyte subpopulations in chronic periapical lesions. J Endod. 1984;10:9–11. doi:10.1016/S0099-2399(84)80246-0.

[25] Nilsen R, Johannessen AC, Skaug N, Matre R. In situ characterization of mononuclear cells in human dental periapical inflammatory lesions using monoclonal antibodies. Oral Surg Oral Med Oral Pathol. 1984;58:160–5. doi:10.1016/0030-4220(84)90131-2.

[26] Torabinejad M, Kettering JD. Identification and relative concentration of B and T lymphocytes in human chronic periapical lesions. J Endod. 1985;11:122–5. doi:10.1016/S0099-2399(85)80230-2.

[27] Yu SM, Stashenko P. Identification of inflammatory cells in developing rat periapical lesions. J Endod. 1987;13:535–40.

[28] Gao Z, Mackenzie IC, Rittman BR, Korszun AK, Williams DM, Cruchley AT. Immunocytochemical examination of immune cells in periapical granulomata and odontogenic cysts. J Oral Pathol. 1988;17:84–90. doi:10.1111/j.1600-0714.1988.tb01512.x.

[29] Barkhordar RA, Desouza YG. Human T-lymphocyte subpopulations in periapical lesions. Oral Surg Oral Med Oral Pathol. 1988;65:763–6.

[30] Lukic A, Arsenijević N, Vujanić G, Ramić Z. Quantitative analysis of the immunocompetent cells in periapical granuloma: correlation with the histological characteristics of the lesions. J Endod. 1990;16:119–22.

[31] Piattelli A, Artese L, Rosini S, Quaranta M, Musiani P. Immune cells in periapical granuloma: morphological and immunohistochemical characterization. J Endod. 1991;17:26–9. doi:10.1016/S0099-2399(07)80157-9.

[32] Márton IJ, Kiss C. Characterization of inflammatory cell infiltrate in dental periapical lesions. Int Endod J. 1993;26:131–6. doi:10.1111/j.1365-2591.1993.tb00555.x.

[33] Márton IJ, Kiss C. Overlapping protective and destructive regulatory pathways in apical periodontitis. J Endod. 2014;40:155–63.

[34] Rodini CO, Lara VS. Study of the expression of CD68+ macrophages and CD8+ T cells in human granulomas and periapical cysts. Oral Surg Oral Med Oral Pathol Oral Radiol Endod. 2001;92:221–7.

[35] Colić M, Gazivoda D, Vucević D, Vasilijić S, Rudolf R, Lukić A. Proinflammatory and immunoregulatory mechanisms in periapical lesions. Mol Immunol. 2009;47:101–13.

[36] Nair PNR. Non-microbial endodontic disease. In: Ingle JI, Bakland LK, Baumgartner JC, editors. Ingle's endodontics. 6th ed. Hamilton: BC Decker Inc. 2008. p. 309.

[37] Nair PN. New perspectives on radicular cysts: do they heal? Int Endod J. 1998;31:155–60. doi:10.1046/j.1365-2591.1998.00146.x.

[38] Simon JH. Incidence of periapical cysts in relation to the root canal. J Endod. 1980;6:845–8. doi:10.1016/S0099-2399(80)80039-2.

[39] Torabinejad M, Shabahang S. Pulp and periapical pathosis. In: Torabinejad M, Walton RE, editors. Endodontics. Principles and practice. 4th ed. St. Louise: Saunders/Elsevier; 2009. pp. 49–67.

[40] Siqueira JF Jr, Rôças IN. Microbiology and treatment of acute apical abscesses. Clin Microbiol Rev. 2013;26:255–73. doi:10.1128/CMR.00082-12.

[41] Williams BL, McCann GF, Schoenknecht FD. Bacteriology of dental abscesses of endodontic origin. J Clin Microbiol. 1983;18:770–4.

[42] Brook I, Frazier EH, Gher ME. Aerobic and anaerobic microbiology of periapical abscess. Oral Microbiol Immunol. 1991;6:123–5. doi:10.1111/j.1399-302X.1991.tb00464.x.

[43] Külekçi G, Inanç D, Koçak H, Kasapoglu C, Gümrü OZ. Bacteriology of dentoalveolar abscesses in patients who have received empirical antibiotic therapy. Clin Infect Dis. 1996;23 Suppl 1:S51–3. doi:10.1093/clinids/23.Supplement_1.S51.

[44] Rôças IN, Siqueira JF Jr. Detection of novel oral species and phylotypes in symptomatic endodontic infections including abscesses. FEMS Microbiol Lett. 2005;250:279–85.

[45] Larawin V, Naipao J, Dubey SP. Head and neck space infections. Otolaryngol Head Neck Surg. 2006;135:889–93. doi:10.1016/j.otohns.2006.07.007.

[46] Moghimi M, Baart JA, Karagozoglu KH, Forouzanfar T. Spread of odontogenic infections: a retrospective analysis and review of the literature. Quintessence Int. 2013;44:351–61.

[47] Daramola OO, Flanagan CE, Maisel RH, Odland RM. Diagnosis and treatment of deep neck space abscesses. Otolaryngol Head Neck Surg. 2009;141:123–30. doi:10.1016/j.otohns.2009.03.033.

[48] Pappa H, Jones DC. Mediastinitis from odontogenic infection. A case report. Br Dent J. 2005;198:547–8.

[49] Umeda M, Minamikawa T, Komatsubara H, Shibuya Y, Yokoo S, Komori T. Necrotizing fasciitis caused by dental infection: a retrospective analysis of 9 cases and a review of the literature. Oral Surg Oral Med Oral Pathol Oral Radiol Endod. 2003;95:283–90. doi: 10.1067/moe.2003.85.

[50] Kim IK, Kim JR, Jang KS, Moon YS, Park SW. Orbital abscess from an odontogenic infection. Oral Surg Oral Med Oral Pathol Oral Radiol Endod. 2007;103:e1–6. doi: 10.1016/j.tripleo.2006.07.002.

[51] Corson MA, Postlethwaite KP, Seymour RA. Are dental infections a cause of brain abscess? Case report and review of the literature. Oral Dis. 2001;7:61–5. doi:10.1034/j.1601-0825.2001.70112.x.

[52] Pasqualini L, Mencacci A, Scarponi AM, et al. Cervical spondylodiscitis with spinal epidural abscess caused by *Aggregatibacter aphrophilus*. J Med Microbiol. 2008;57:652–5. doi:10.1099/jmm.0.47614-0.

[53] Márton IJ. How does the periapical inflammatory process compromise general health? Endodonic Topics. 2004;8:3–14. doi:10.1111/j.1601-1546.2004.00095.x.

[54] Segura-Egea JJ, Martín-González J, Castellanos-Cosano L. Endodontic medicine: connections between apical periodontitis and systemic diseases. Int Endod J. 2015;48:933–51. doi:10.1111/iej.12507.

[55] Segura-Egea JJ, Jiménez-Pinzón A, Ríos-Santos JV, Velasco-Ortega E, Cisneros-Cabello R, Poyato-Ferrera M. High prevalence of apical periodontitis amongst type 2 diabetic patients. Int Endod J. 2005;38:564–9. doi:10.1111/j.1365-2591.2005.00996.x.

[56] López-López J, Jané-Salas E, Estrugo-Devesa A, Velasco-Ortega E, Martín-González J, Segura-Egea JJ. Periapical and endodontic status of type 2 diabetic patients in Catalonia, Spain: a cross-sectional study. J Endod. 2011;37:598–601. doi:10.1016/j.joen.2011.01.002.

[57] Marotta PS, Fontes TV, Armada L, Lima KC, Rôças IN, Siqueira JF Jr.Type 2 diabetes mellitus and the prevalence of apical periodontitis and endodontic treatment in an adult Brazilian population. J Endod. 2012;38:297–300. doi:10.1016/j.joen.2011.11.001.

[58] Segura-Egea JJ, Castellanos-Cosano L, Machuca G, et al. Diabetes mellitus, periapical inflammation and endodontic treatment outcome. Med Oral Patol Oral Cir Bucal. 2012;17:e356–61. doi:10.4317/medoral.17452.

[59] Morsani JM, Aminoshariae A, Han YW, Montagnese TA, Mickel A. Genetic predisposition to persistent apical periodontitis. J Endod. 2011;37:455–9. doi:10.1016/j.joen.2011.01.009.

[60] Aminoshariae A, Kulild JC. Association of functional gene polymorphism with apical aeriodontitis. J Endod. 2015;41:999–1007.

[61] de Sá AR, Moreira PR, Xavier GM, et al. Association of CD14, IL1B, IL6, IL10 and TNFA functional gene polymorphisms with symptomatic dental abscesses. Int Endod J. 2007;40:563–72.

[62] Menezes-Silva R, Khaliq S, Deeley K, Letra A, Vieira AR. Genetic susceptibility to periapical disease: conditional contribution of MMP2 and MMP3 genes to the development of periapical lesions and healing response. J Endod. 2012;38:604–7. doi:10.1016/j.joen.2012.02.009.

[63] Amaya MP, Criado L, Blanco B, et al. Polymorphisms of pro-inflammatory cytokine genes and the risk for acute suppurative or chronic nonsuppurative apical periodontitis in a Colombian population. Int Endod J. 2013;46:71–8. doi:10.1111/j.1365-2591.2012.02097.x.

[64] Rauch B. Attempts to isolate a virus from infected root canals and periapical tissue using monkey kidney cells cultures. J Can Dent A. 1958;24:404–10.

[65] Shindell E. Studies on the possible presence of a virus in subacute and chronic periapical granulomas. Oral Surg Oral Med Oral Pathol. 1962;15:1382–4. doi:10.1016/0030-4220(62)90359-6.

[66] Parra B, Slots J. Detection of human viruses in periodontal pockets using polymerase chain reaction. Oral Microbiol Immunol. 1996;11:289–93. DOI:10.1111/j.1399-302X.1996.tb00183.x.

[67] Contreras A, Slots J. Mammalian viruses in human periodontitis. Oral Microbiol Immunol 1996;11:381–6. doi:10.1111/j.1399-302X.1996.tb00199.x.

[68] Sabeti M, Valles Y, Nowzari H, et al. Cytomegalovirus and Epstein–Barr virus DNA transcription in endodontic symptomatic lesions. Oral Microbiol Immunol 2003a; 18:104–8. doi:10.1034/j.1399-302X.2003.00055.x.

[69] Sabeti M, Simon JH, Slots J. Cytomegalovirus and Epstein–Barr virus are associated with symptomatic periapical pathosis. Oral Microbiol Immunol 2003b;18:327–8. doi:10.1034/j.1399-302X.2003.00079.x.

[70] Jakovljevic A, Andric M. Human cytomegalovirus and Epstein–Barr virus in etiopathogenesis of apical periodontitis: a systematic review. J Endod 2014;40:6–15. doi:10.1016/j.joen.2013.10.001.

[71] Contreras A, Slots J. Herpesviruses in human periodontal disease. J Periodontal Res. 2000a;35:3–16. doi:10.1034/j.1600-0765.2000.035001003.x.

[72] Slots J. Herpesviruses in periodontal diseases. Periodontol 2000. 2005;38:33–62. doi:10.1111/j.1600-0757.2005.00109.x.

[73] Slots J. Human viruses in periodontitis. Periodontol 2000. 2010a;53:89–110. doi:10.1111/j.1600-0757.2009.00325.x.

[74] Slots J, Sabeti M, Simon JH. Herpesviruses in periapical pathosis: an etiopathogenic relationship? Oral Surg Oral Med Oral Pathol Oral Radiol Endod. 2003;96:327–31. doi: 10.1016/S1079-2104(03)00352-4.

[75] Slots J. Herpesviral-bacterial synergy in the pathogenesis of human periodontitis. Curr Opin Infect Dis. 2007;20:278–83. doi:10.1097/QCO.0b013e3280964da0.

[76] Slots J. Herpesviral-bacterial interactions in periodontal diseases. Periodontol 2000. 2010b;52:117–40.

[77] Ongrádi J, Sallay K, Kulcsár G. The decreased antibacterial activity of oral polymorphonuclear leukocytes coincides with the occurrence of virus-carrying oral lymphocytes and epithelial cells. Folia Microbiol (Praha). 1987;32:438–47.

[78] Smith MacDonald E, Nowzari H, Contreras A, Flynn J, Morrison J, Slots J. Clinical and microbiological evaluation of a bioabsorbable and a nonresorbable barrier membrane in the treatment of periodontal intraosseous lesions. J Periodontol. 1998;69:445–53.

[79] Ferreira DC, Rôças IN, Paiva SS, et al. Viral-bacterial associations in acute apical abscesses. Oral Surg Oral Med Oral Pathol Oral Radiol Endod 2011a;112:264–71. doi: 10.1016/j.tripleo.2011.01.029.

[80] Ferreira DC, Paiva SSM, Carmo FL, et al. Identification of herpesviruses types 1 to 8 and human papillomavirus in acute apical abscesses. J Endod 2011b;37:10–6. doi: 10.1016/j.joen.2010.09.009.

[81] Rider CA, Rupkalvis R, Miller AS, Chen SY. Search for evidence of three viral agents in radicular (periapical) cysts with immunohistochemistry. Oral Surg Oral Med Oral Pathol Oral Radiol Endod. 1995;80:87–91. doi:10.1016/S1079-2104(95)80022-0.

[82] Heling I, Morag-Hezroni M, Marva E, Hochman N, Zakay-Rones Z, Morag A. Is herpes simplex virus associated with pulp/periapical inflammation? Oral Surg Oral Med Oral Pathol Oral Radiol Endod. 2001;91:359–61. doi:10.1067/moe.2001.113162.

[83] Sabeti M, Simon JH, Nowzari H, et al. Cytomegalovirus and Epstein–Barr virus active infection in periapical lesions of teeth with intact crowns. J Endod 2003c;29:321–3. doi: 10.1097/00004770-200305000-00002.

[84] Sabeti M, Slots J. Herpesviral-bacterial coinfection in periapical pathosis. J Endod 2004;30:69–72. doi:10.1097/00004770-200402000-00001.

[85] Slots J, Nowzari H, Sabeti M. Cytomegalovirus infection in symptomatic periapical pathosis. Int Endod J 2004;37:519–24. doi:10.1111/j.1365-2591.2004.00816.x.

[86] Kabak SL, Kabak YS, Anischenko SL. Light microscopic study of periapical lesions associated with asymptomatic apical periodontitis. Ann Anat. 2005;187:185–94. doi: 10.1016/j.aanat.2004.05.001.

[87] Yildirim S, Yapar M, Kubar A, et al. Human cytomegalovirus, Epstein–Barr virus and bone resorption-inducing cytokines in periapical lesions of deciduous teeth. Oral Microbiol Immunol 2006;21:107–11. doi:10.1111/j.1399-302X.2006.00268.x.

[88] Saboia-Dantas CJ, Coutrin de Toledo LF, Sampaio-Filho HR, et al. Herpesviruses in asymptomatic apical periodontitis lesions: an immunohistochemical approach. Oral Microbiol Immunol 2007;22:320–5. doi:10.1111/j.1399-302X.2007.00362.x.

[89] Andric M, Milasin J, Jovanovic T, et al. Human cytomegalovirus is present in odontogenic cysts. Oral Microbiol Immunol 2007;22:347–51. doi:10.1111/j.1399-302X.2007.00369.x.

[90] Yazdi KA, Sabeti M, Jabalameli F, et al. Relationship between human cytomegalovirus transcription and symptomatic apical periodontitis in Iran. Oral Microbiol Immunol 2008;23:510–4. doi:10.1111/j.1399-302X.2008.00471.x.

[91] Sunde PT, Olsen I, Enersen M, et al. Human cytomegalovirus and Epstein–Barr virus in apical and marginal periodontitis: a role in pathology? J Med Virol 2008;80:1007–11. doi:10.1002/jmv.21180.

[92] Sabeti M, Daneshmand A, Simon JH, et al. Cytomegalovirus-infected inflammatory cells in dental periapical lesions. Oral Microbiol Immunol 2009;24:434–6. doi:10.1111/j.1399-302X.2009.00540.x.

[93] Li H, Chen V, Chen Y, et al. Herpesviruses in endodontic pathoses: association of Epstein–Barr virus with irreversible pulpitis and apical periodontitis. J Endod 2009;35:23–9. doi:10.1016/j.joen.2008.09.017.

[94] Chen V, Chen Y, Li H, Kent K, Baumgartner JC, Machida CA. Herpesviruses in abscesses and cellulitis of endodontic origin. J Endod. 2009;35:182-8. DOI: 10.1016/j.joen.2008.11.018.

[95] Hernádi K, Szalmás A, Mogyorósi R, et al. Prevalence and activity of Epstein–Barr virus and human cytomegalovirus in symptomatic and asymptomatic apical periodontitis lesions. J Endod 2010;36:1485–9. doi:10.1016/j.joen.2010.06.008.

[96] Hernádi K, Csoma E, Adám B, et al. Association of human herpesvirus 6 subtypes with symptomatic apical periodontitis. Oral Surg Oral Med Oral Pathol Oral Radiol Endod. 2011;112:401–6. doi:10.1016/j.tripleo.2011.02.007.

[97] Sabeti M, Kermani V, Sabeti S, et al. Significance of human cytomegalovirus and Epstain-Bar virus in inducing cytokine expression in periapical lesions. J Endod 2012;38:47–50.

[98] Hernádi K, Gyöngyösi E, Mészáros B, et al. Elevated tumor necrosis factor-alpha expression in periapical lesions infected by Epstein–Barr virus. J Endod 2013;39:456–60. doi:10.1016/j.joen.2012.12.028.

[99] Ozbek SM, Ozbek A , Yavuz MS. Detection of human cytomegalovirus and Epstein–Barr virus in symptomatic and asymptomatic apical periodontitis lesions by real-time PCR. Med Oral Patol Oral Cir 2013;18:811–6. doi:10.4317/medoral.18905.

[100] Verdugo F, Castillo A, Simonian K, et al. Periodontopathogen and Epstein–Barr virus-associated periapical periodontitis may be the source of retrograde infectious peri-implantitis. Clin Implant Dent Relat Res 2015;17:199–207. doi:10.1111/cid.12083.

[101] Ozbek A, Ozbek SM. Detection of herpesviruses and human papillomavirus in acute apical abscesses by real-time PCR. Clin Oral Investig. 2015a;19:343–7. doi:10.1007/s00784-014-1251-0.

[102] Makino K, Takeichi O, Hatori K, Imai K, Ochiai K, Ogiso B. Epstein–Barr virus infection in chronically inflamed periapical granulomas. PLoS One. 2015;10:e0121548. doi: 10.1371/journal.pone.0121548.

[103] Ozbek SM, Ozbek A, Demiray T. Prevalence of several herpesviruses and human papillomavirus in acute apical abscesses. Int Endod J. 2015b. doi:10.1111/iej.12482.

[104] Popovic J, Gasic J, Zivkovic S, et al. Prevalence of Human cytomegalovirus and Epstein–Barr virus in chronic periapical lesions. Intervirology. 2015;58:271–7. doi: 10.1159/000441208.

[105] Jakovljevic A, Andric M, Knezevic A, et al. Human cytomegalovirus and Epstein–Barr Virus genotypes in apical periodontitis lesions. J Endod. 2015;41:1847–51. doi:10.1016/j.joen.2015.08.027.

[106] Gregory WB Jr, Brooks LE, Penick EC. Herpes zoster associated with pulpless teeth. J Endod. 1975;1:32–5. doi:10.1016/S0099-2399(75)80248-2.

[107] Goon WW, Jacobsen PL. Prodromal odontalgia and multiple devitalized teeth caused by a herpes zoster infection of the trigeminal nerve: report of case. J Am Dent Assoc. 1988;116:500–4. doi:10.14219/jada.archive.1988.0301.

[108] Wadden JV. Extensive endodontic involvement following herpes zoster attack to facial area: report of a case. Northwest Dent. 1991;70:31.

[109] Ramchandani PL, Mellor TK. Herpes zoster associated with tooth resorption and periapical lesions. Br J Oral Maxillofac Surg. 2007;45:71–3. doi:10.1016/j.bjoms.2005.05.008.

[110] Gupta S, Sreenivasan V, Patil PB. Dental complications of herpes zoster: Two case reports and review of literature. Indian J Dent Res. 2015;26:214–9. doi: 10.4103/0970-9290.159175.

[111] Cai MS, Li ML, Zheng CF. Herpesviral infection and Toll-like receptor 2. Protein Cell. 2012;3:590–601.

[112] Wagner M, Gutermann A, Podlech J, Reddehase MJ, Koszinowski UH. Major histocompatibility complex class I allele-specific cooperative and competitive interactions

between immune evasion proteins of cytomegalovirus. J Exp Med. 2002;196:805–16. doi:10.1084/jem.20020811.

[113] Tortorella D, Gewurz BE, Furman MH, Schust DJ, Ploegh HL. Viral subversion of the immune system. Annu Rev Immunol. 2000;18:861–926. doi:10.1146/annurev.immunol. 18.1.861.

[114] Rossini G, Cerboni C, Santoni A, et al. Interplay between human cytomegalovirus and intrinsic/innate host responses: a complex bidirectional relationship. Mediators Inflamm. 2012;2012:607276. doi:10.1155/2012/607276.

[115] Varani S, Frascaroli G, Homman-Loudiyi M, Feld S, Landini MP, Söderberg-Nauclér C. Human cytomegalovirus inhibits the migration of immature dendritic cells by down-regulating cell-surface CCR1 and CCR5. J Leukoc Biol. 2005;77:219–28. doi:10.1189/jlb. 0504301.

[116] Bale JF Jr, Kern ER, Overall JC Jr, Baringer JR. Impaired migratory and chemotactic activity of neutrophils during murine cytomegalovirus infection. J Infect Dis. 1983;148:518–25.

[117] Mogensen TH, Paludan SR. Molecular pathways in virus-induced cytokine production. Microbiol Mol Biol Rev. 2001;65:131–50. doi:10.1128/MMBR.65.1.131-150.2001.

[118] Alcami A, Koszinowski UH. Viral mechanisms of immune evasion. Trends Microbiol. 2000; 8:410–8. doi:10.1016/S0966-842X(00)01830-8.

[119] Thomassen MJ, Divis LT, Fisher CJ. Regulation of human alveolar macrophage inflammatory cytokine production by interleukin-10. Clin Immunol Immunopathol. 1996;80:321–4. doi:10.1006/clin.1996.0130.

[120] Kotenko SV, Saccani S, Izotova LS, Mirochnitchenko OV, Pestka S. Human cytomegalovirus harbors its own unique IL-10 homolog (cmvIL-10). Proc Natl Acad Sci USA. 2000;97:1695–700. doi:10.1073/pnas.97.4.1695.

[121] Salek-Ardakani S, Arrand JR, Mackett M. Epstein–Barr virus encoded interleukin-10 inhibits HLA-class I, ICAM-1, and B7 expression on human monocytes: implications for immune evasion by EBV. Virology. 2002;304:342–51. doi:10.1006/viro.2002.1716.

[122] Stern J, Shai E, Zaks B, et al. Reduced expression of gamma interferon in serum and marked lymphoid depletion induced by Porphyromonas gingivalis increase murine morbidity and mortality due to cytomegalovirus infection. Infect Immun. 2004;72:5791–8. doi:10.1128/IAI.72.10.5791-5798.2004.

[123] Sugano N, Ikeda K, Oshikawa M, et al. Relationship between *Porphyromonas gingivalis*, Epstein–Barr virus infection and reactivation in periodontitis. J Oral Sci. 2004;46:203–6. doi:10.2334/josnusd.46.203.

[124] Teughels W, Sliepen I, Quirynen M, et al. Human cytomegalovirus enhances A. actinomycetemcomitans adherence to cells. J Dent Res. 2007;86:175–80. doi: 10.1177/154405910708600213.

[125] Dai L, DeFee MR, Cao Y, et al. Lipoteichoic acid (LTA) and lipopolysaccharides (LPS) from periodontal pathogenic bacteria facilitate oncogenic herpesvirus infection within primary oral cells. PLoS One. 2014;9:e101326. doi:10.1371/journal.pone.0101326.

[126] Kubar A, Saygun I, Yapar M, Ozdemir A, Slots J. Real-time PCR quantification of cytomegalovirus in aggressive periodontitis lesions using TaqMan technology. J Periodontal Res. 2004;39:81–6. doi:10.1111/j.1600-0765.2004.00707.x.

[127] Kubar A, Saygun I, Ozdemir A, Yapar M, Slots J. Real-time polymerase chain reaction quantification of human cytomegalovirus and Epstein–Barr virus in periodontal pockets and the adjacent gingiva of periodontitis lesions. J Periodontal Res. 2005;40:97–104. doi:10.1111/j.1600-0765.2005.00770.x.

[128] Konstantinidis A, Sakellari D, Papa A, Antoniadis A. Real-time polymerase chain reaction quantification of Epstein–Barr virus in chronic periodontitis patients. J Periodontal Res. 2005;40:294–8. doi:10.1111/j.1600-0765.2005.00796.x.

[129] Radics T. The role of inflammatory and immunological processes in the development of chronic apical periodontitis [thesis]. Debrecen (Hungary): University of Debrecen; 2004.

[130] Gazivoda D, Dzopalic T, Bozic B, Tatomirovic Z, Brkic Z, Colic M. Production of proinflammatory and immunoregulatory cytokines by inflammatory cells from periapical lesions in culture. J Oral Pathol Med 2009;38:605–11.

[131] Teixeira-Salum TB, Rodrigues DB, Gervasio AM, Souza CJ, Rodrigues V Jr, Loyola AM. Distinct Th1, Th2 and Treg cytokines balance in chronic periapical granulomas and radicular cysts. J Oral Pathol Med 2010;39:250–6. doi:10.1111/j.1600-0714.2009.00863.x.

[132] Jakovljevic A, Knezevic A, Karalic D, et al. Pro-inflammatory cytokine levels in human apical periodontitis: correlation with clinical and histological findings. Aust Endod J. 2015;41:72–7. doi:10.1111/aej.12072.

[133] Belibasakis GN, Rechenberg DK, Zehnder M. The receptor activator of NF-kB ligand-osteoprotegerin system in pulpal and periapical disease. Int Endod J. 2013;46:99–111. doi:10.1111/j.1365-2591.2012.02105.x.

[134] Puchhammer-Stöckl E, Görzer I. Cytomegalovirus and Epstein–Barr virus subtypes—the search for clinical significance. J Clin Virol. 2006;36:239–48. doi:10.1016/j.jcv.2006.03.004.

[135] Navarro D, Paz P, Tugizov S, et al. Glycoprotein B of human cytomegalovirus promotes virion penetration into cells, transmission of infection from cell to cell, and fusion of infected cells. Virology 1993;197:143–58. doi:10.1006/viro.1993.1575.

[136] Simmen KA, Singh J, Luukkonen BG, et al. Global modulation of cellular transcription by human cytomegalovirus is initiated by viral glycoprotein B. Proc Natl Acad Sci USA 2001;98:7140–5. doi:10.1073/pnas.121177598.

[137] Chou SW, Dennison KM. Analysis of interstrain variation in cytomegalovirus glycoprotein B sequences encoding neutralization-related epitopes. J Infect Dis 1991;163:1229–34. doi:10.1093/infdis/163.6.1229.

[138] Zipeto D, Hong C, Gerna G, et al. Geographic and demographic differences in the frequency of human cytomegalovirus gB genotypes 1-4 in immunocompromised patients. AIDS Res Hum Retroviruses 1998;14:533–6. doi:10.1089/aid.1998.14.533.

[139] Dambaugh T, Hennessy K, Chamnankit L, et al. U2 region of Epstein–Barr virus DNA may encode Epstein–Barr nuclear antigen 2. Proc Natl Acad Sci USA 1984;81:7632–6. doi: 10.1073/pnas.81.23.7632.

[140] Wu YM, Yan J, Ojcius DM, et al. Correlation between infections with different genotypes of human cytomegalovirus and Epstein–Barr virus in subgingival samples and periodontal status of patients. J Clin Microbiol 2007;45:3665–70.

[141] Jankovic S, Aleksic Z, Dimitrijevic B, et al. Correlation between different genotypes of human cytomegalovirus and Epstein–Barr virus and peri-implant tissue status. Aust Dent J 2011;56:382–8. doi:10.1111/j.1834-7819.2011.01360.x.

[142] Chang Y, Cesarman E, Pessin M.S, et al. Identification of herpesvirus-like DNA sequences in AIDS-associated Kaposi's sarcoma. Science. 1994;265:1865–1869.

[143] Cesarman E, Chang Y, Moore PS, Said JW, Knowles DM. Kaposi's sarcoma-associated herpesvirus-like DNA sequences in AIDS-related body-cavity-based lymphomas. N Engl J Med.1995;332:1186–1191.

[144] Cesarman E, Knowles DM. The role of Kaposi's sarcoma-associated herpesvirus (KSHV/HHV-8) in lymphoproliferative diseases. Semin Cancer Biol. 1999;9:165–74. doi: 10.1006/scbi.1998.0118.

[145] Soulier J, Grollet L, Oksenhendler E, et al. Kaposi's sarcoma-associated herpesvirus-like DNA sequences in multicentric Castleman's disease. Blood. 1995;86:1276–80.

[146] Ablashi DV, Chatlynne LG, Whitman JE Jr, Cesarman E. Spectrum of Kaposi's sarcoma-associated herpesvirus, or human herpesvirus 8, diseases. Clin Microbiol Rev. 2002;15:439–64. doi:10.1128/CMR.15.3.439-464.2002.

[147] Mardirossian A, Contreras A, Navazesh M, Nowzari H, Slots J. Herpesviruses 6, 7 and 8 in HIV- and non-HIV-associated periodontitis. J Periodontal Res. 2000;35:278–84. doi: 10.1034/j.1600-0765.2000.035005278.x.

[148] Contreras A, Nowzari H, Slots J. Herpesviruses in periodontal pocket and gingival tissue specimens. Oral Microbiol Immunol. 2000b;15:15–8. doi:10.1034/j.1399-302x.2000.150103.x.

[149] Slots J. Periodontal herpesviruses: prevalence, pathogenicity, systemic risk. Periodontol 2000. 2015;69:28–45. doi:10.1111/prd.12085.

[150] Haque T, Crawford DH. PCR amplification is more sensitive than tissue culture methods for Epstein–Barr virus detection in clinical material. J Gen Virol. 1997;78:3357–60. doi:10.1099/0022-1317-78-12-3357.

[151] Stadler LP, Bernstein DI, Callahan ST, et al. Seroprevalence of cytomegalovirus (CMV) and risk factors for infection in adolescent males. Clin Infect Dis. 2010;51:e76–81. doi: 10.1086/656918.

[152] Stadler LP, Bernstein DI, Callahan ST, et al. Seroprevalence and risk factors for cytomegalovirus infections in adolescent females. J Pediatric Infect Dis Soc. 2013;2:7–14. doi:10.1093/jpids/pis076.

[153] Stowe RP, Peek MK, Perez NA, Yetman DL, Cutchin MP, Goodwin JS. Herpesvirus reactivation and socioeconomic position: a community-based study. J Epidemiol Community Health. 2010;64:666–71. doi:10.1136/jech.2008.078808.

[154] Looker KJ, Garnett GP. A systematic review of the epidemiology and interaction of herpes simplex virus types 1 and 2. Sex Transm Infect. 2005;81:103–7. doi:10.1136/sti.2004.012039.

[155] Maeda A, Sato T, Wakiguchi H. Epidemiology of Epstein–Barr virus (EBV) infection and EBV-associated diseases. Nihon Rinsho. 2006;64:609–12.

[156] Cannon MJ, Schmid DS, Hyde TB. Review of cytomegalovirus seroprevalence and demographic characteristics associated with infection. Rev Med Virol. 2010;20:202–13. doi:10.1002/rmv.655.

[157] Varga M, Görög D, Kári D, et al. Cytomegalovirus seroprevalence among solid organ donors in Hungary: correlations with age, gender, and blood group. Transplant Proc. 2011;43:1233–5. doi:10.1016/j.transproceed.2011.03.067.

[158] Mutlu B, Günlemez A, Türker G, Gökalp AS, Willke A. Is serologic screening necessary in the donor bloods for cytomegalovirus seronegative blood transfusion to risky patients? Mikrobiyol Bul. 2008;42:337–41.

[159] Pejcic A, Kesic L, Milasin J. Association between periodontopathogens and CRP levels in patients with periodontitis in Serbia. J Dent Res Dent Clin Dent Prospects. 2011;5:10–6.

[160] Petrović SM, Zelić K, Milasin J, Popović B, Pucar A, Zelić O. Detection of herpes simplex virus type 1 in gingival crevicular fluid of gingival sulcus/periodontal pocket using polymerase chain reaction. Srp Arh Celok Lek. 2014;142:296–300.

[161] Djuric M, Jankovic L, Jovanovic T, et al. Prevalence of oral herpes simplex virus reactivation in cancer patients: a comparison of different techniques of viral detection. J Oral Pathol Med. 2009;38:167–73. doi:10.1111/j.1600-0714.2008.00684.x.

[162] Banko A, Lazarevic I, Cupic M, Stevanovic G, Boricic I, Jovanovic T. Carboxy-terminal sequence variation of LMP1 gene in Epstein–Barr-virus-associated mononucleosis and tumors from Serbian patients. J Med Virol. 2012;84:632–42. doi:10.1002/jmv.23217.

[163] Taherimahmoudi M, Ahmadi H, Baradaran N, et al. Cytomegalovirus infection and disease following renal transplantation: preliminary report of incidence and potential risk factors. Transplant Proc. 2009;41:2841–4. doi:10.1016/j.transproceed.2009.07.027.

[164] Steiner I. Herpes virus infection of the peripheral nervous system. Handb Clin Neurol. 2013;115:543–58. doi:10.1016/B978-0-444-52902-2.00031-X.

[165] Deng Z, Uehara T, Maeda H, et al. Epstein–Barr virus and human papillomavirus infections and genotype distribution in head and neck cancers. PLoS One. 2014;9:e113702. doi:10.1371/journal.pone.0113702.

[166] de Matos SB, Meyer R, Lima FW. Seroprevalence and serum profile of cytomegalovirus infection among patients with hematologic disorders in Bahia State, Brazil. J Med Virol. 2011;83:298–304. doi:10.1002/jmv.21965.

Chapter 4

Ectopic Expression of Human Herpesvirus 1 Thymidine Kinase Induces Male Infertility

Mo Chen, Li-yi Cai, Takako Kato and Yukio Kato

Additional information is available at the end of the chapter

http://dx.doi.org/10.5772/64390

Abstract

The herpesvirus family comprises several widespread infectious pathogens. They infect a variety of animal hosts, including humans and cause complex clinical outcomes. Recently, the possible correlation between genital infection by human herpesviruses (HHVs) and male infertility has attracted considerable attention. In this chaper, we investigated the mechanism of HHV-1-induced infertility in transgenic (Tg) rats and its possible correlation with infertility in human males. Ectopic expression of HHV-1 thymidine kinase (TK) in the testis of Tg rats increased male infertility. In addition, truncated TK proteins were found in postmeiotic spermatids of Tg rat testis, leading to progressive degeneration of germ cells and vacuolization of the seminiferous epithelium. These findings suggest the possibility that a similar process occurs within HHV-infected human germ cells.

Keywords: herpesvirus, thymidine kinase, genital infection, male infertility, spermatogenesis

1. Introduction

Herpesviruses belong to a family of double-stranded DNA (dsDNA) viruses commonly causing herpes in animals. They present a unique four-layered structure. The outermost layer corresponds to the envelope, a lipid bilayer membrane interspersed with glycoproteins. This encases the tegument, a protein coat that surrounds the icosahedral nucleocapsid containing the viral linear DNA genome (**Figure 1**) [1]. At present, over 130 herpesvirus species have been identified, eight of which are known as human herpesviruses (HHVs): HHV-1 and HHV-2 (commonly called herpes simplex virus-1 and -2; HSV-1 and HSV-2), HHV-3 (varicella-zoster virus; VZV), HHV-4 (Epstein-Barr virus; EBV), HHV-5 (cytomegalovirus; CMV), HHV-6 (human herpesvirus 6, including HHV-6A and HHV-6B), HHV-7 (human herpesvirus 7), and HHV-8 (Kaposi's sarcoma-associated herpesvirus; KSHV). HHVs are divided into three subfamilies (α-, β- and γ-herpesviruses) based on their unique properties (**Table 1**) [2]. HHVs are widespread among humans to the extent that more than 90% of adults are thought to be infected with at least one variety [2]. HHVs generally infect ectoderm-derived tissues, such as skin, mucoepithelial tissue and nervous tissue; however, they usually show preference for specific target cells/tissues and ensuing clinical outcomes (**Table 1**) [2]. In addition, many people carrying the virus may be asymptomatic due to the latency of associated transcripts, which help HHVs evade the host's immune response [3]. Moreover, HHVs hide in specific cells during latent infection periods (**Table 1**).

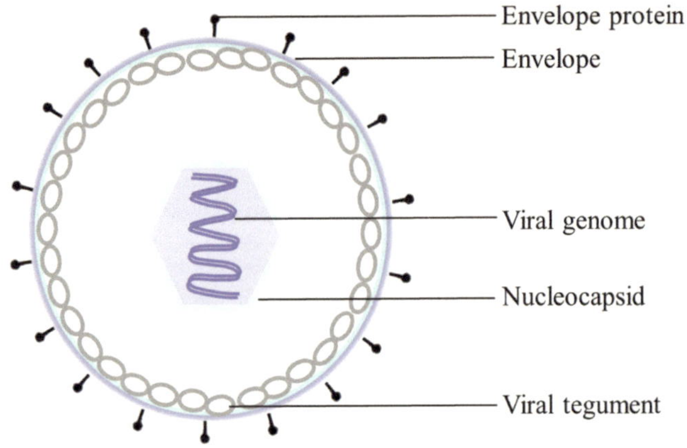

Figure 1. HHVs structure. HHVs have a unique four-layered structure: a core of double-stranded DNA is surrounded by the nucleocapsid, which is enclosed by the envelope. The envelope is attached to the capsid through the tegument. Glycoproteins cover the surface of the envelope.

During the last decade, numerous studies have demonstrated that genital infections are often associated with human infertility, especially in males [4]. Most recently, genital infections caused by herpesviruses have attracted considerable attention [5–7]. Although herpes genitalis can be mainly caused by HHV-1 and HHV-2 [8], other HHVs have also been frequently detected in the genital organs of infertile male patients [9–11]. Although not fully demonstrated, there is a possible correlation between human male infertility and HHVs.

Our laboratory recently developed a line of transgenic (Tg) rats expressing a chimeric gene with the promoter of porcine follicle-stimulating hormone β subunit (FSHβ) and the open reading frame of HHV-1 thymidine kinase (TK). Unexpectedly, we observed that Tg rats showed infertility upon ectopic expression of HHV-1-TK in the testis, independent of the FSHβ promoter [12]. Indeed, we found that the accumulation of HHV-1-TK protein in postmeiotic spermatids was the cause of male infertility [13]. In this study, we used the Tg rat model to elucidate the HHV-mediated mechanism responsible for male infertility.

http://dx.doi.org/10.5772/64390

Virus	Common name	Major target	Diseases	Clinical syndromes	Site of latency
HHV-1[α]	HSV-1 Herpes simplex virus-1	Mucoepithelial	Oral herpes, genital herpes	Oral and genital herpes, gingivostomatitis, keratoconjunctivitis, encephalitis, pneumonitis, esophagitis, hepatitis	Sensory and cranial nerve ganglia
HHV-2[α]	HSV-2 Herpes simplex virus-2	Same as above	same as above	Oral and genital herpes herpes, gingivostomatitis, keratoconjunctivitis, meningitis, encephalitis, pneumonitis, esophagitis, hepatitis	Same as above
HHV-3[α]	VZV Varicella zoster virus	Same as above	Chickenpox, shingles	Shingles (extradermatomal), pneumonitis, disseminated infection, hepatitis, retinitis, meningitis, hemolysis, leukopenia, thrombocytopenia	Same as above
HHV-4[γ]	EBV Epstein-Bar virus	B cells and epithelial cells	Infectious mononucleosis, Burkitt's lymphoma, CNS lymphoma, posttransplant lymphoproliferative syndrome (PTLD), nasopharyngeal carcinoma, HIV-associated hairy leukoplakia	Mononucleosis, posttransplant lymphoproliferative disorders, pneumonitis, hepatitis, encephalitis, hemolysis, leukopenia, thrombocytopenia	Memory B cells
HHV-5[β]	CMV Cytomegalovirus	Monocyte, lymphocyte and epithelial cells	Infectious mononucleosis-like syndrome, retinitis	Lymphadenopathy, hepatitis, pneumonitis, cns vasculitis/ encephalitis, retinitis, esophagitis, hemolysis, leukopenia, thrombocytopenia	Monocytes, macrophages, lymphocytes, others

Virus	Common name	Major target	Diseases	Clinical syndromes	Site of latency
HHV-6A/B[β]		T cells, NK cell, epithelial cells and others	HHV-6A: multiple sclerosis, encephalitis, glioma HHV-6B: sixth disease (roseola infantum or exanthem subitum), multiple sclerosis, encephalitism, hepatitis, pneumonitis, glioma	HHV-6A: meningoencephalitis, encephalitis, perceptual-motor dysfunction, hemiplegia, lymphoproliferative disorder HHV-6B: rash, fever, meningoencephalitis, encephalitis, perceptual-motor dysfunction, hemiplegia, lymphoproliferative disorder, pneumonitis, hepatitis, thrombocytopenia, leukopenia,	T, B, NK cells, monocytes, macrophages, liver, salivary endothelial, neuronal cells
HHV-7[γ]		T cells	Sixth disease (roseola infantum or exanthem subitum), pityriasis rosea	Rash, fever, encephalitis?, hepatitis?	CD4+ T cells, salivary epithelial, lung, skin cells
HHV-8[γ]	KSHV Kaposi's sarcoma-associated herpesvirus	Lymphocyte and others	Kaposi's sarcoma, primary effusion lymphoma, some types of multicentric Castleman's disease	Fever, mononucleosis, skin lesions, encephalitis?	B cells

1. α-herpesvirus: rapid reproduction and cell lysis in vitro, rapid cell lysis and spread in vivo, primary target mucoepithelial cells, latency in sensory ganglia.

2. β-herpesvirus: long replication cycle in vivo and in vitro, limited host range, large infected cells, latency in mononuclear cells, secretory cells, some epithelial cells, and others.

3. γ-herpesvirus: replication in lymphoblastoid cells, lytic cycle in some fibroblasts and epithelial cells.

Table 1. Main characteristics of HHVs.

2. HHVs infection and male human infertility

Human infertility is a widespread problem that has been increasing in recent decades. It affects 20–30% of couples in the world [14], and 40–50% is attributed to male infertility [15, 16]. Many risk factors can disrupt male reproductive capacity and cause infertility. Among these are infections with pathogens [17], such as viruses [7], mycoplasma [18], chlamydia [19], and bacteria [20].

Recently, a number of studies have detected HHVs in the semen and/or spermatozoa of ~90% of infertile male patients, although regional variations must be taken into account (**Table 2**) [6, 9–11, 21–31]. Many investigators have tried to confirm the relationship between male infertility and HHVs infection by combining viral infection rates with statistical analysis of semen and/or sperm samples derived from PCR-based viral DNA analysis, antigen-antibody reaction, and immunocytochemistry of spermatozoa. However, only in a few cases, a significant difference in sperm counts, motility, and/or abnormality has been found between HHVs carriers and non-carriers [6, 9, 11, 27].

Although many studies have revealed a high prevalence of HHVs in male infertility patients, it is still difficult to conclude that HHVs infection is the causative agent. To address this issue, the capacity of HHVs to infect the testis and interfere with spermatogenesis should be proven regardless of the presence or absence of HHVs in the semen and spermatozoa. This would require direct evidence of a molecular mechanism for HHV-induced infertility. In this respect, studies in Tg animal models offer the opportunity to better understand human male infertility.

Country or area (year)	**Carrier% (carrier/ subject)**	**HHV-1**	**HHV-2**	**HHV-3**	**HHV-4**	**HHV-5**	**HHV-6A/B**	**HHV-7**	**HHV-8**
		(HSV-1)	**(HSV-2)**	**(VZV)**	**(EBV)**	**(CMV)**			
Italian (1999) [22]	91 (30/33)	–	–	–	–	–	–	–	91
Germany (2001) [6]	17.1 (43/252)	3.2	0	7.1	3.6	4	0.4*	0	
Athens (2003) [9]	56.6 (64/113)	49.5	–	16.8	7.1	–	–	–	
UK (2006) [25]	3 (1/33)				3				
USA (2007) [10]	18.7 (45/241)	3.7	–	0.4	8.7	3.7	–	–	
Coast (2007) [31]	14.3 (9/63)					14.3			
Greece (2009) [11]	–	2.1	–	3.2	39.1	56.5	66.3	0	–
Germany (2009) [23]	6.5 (11/170)					6.5			

Country or area (year)	Carrier% (carrier/ subject)	HHV-1 (HSV-1)	HHV-2 (HSV-2)	HHV-3 (VZV)	HHV-4 (EBV)	HHV-5 (CMV)	HHV-6A/B	HHV-7	HHV-8
Russia (2011) [26]	11 (10/91)	–	–	–	–	11	–	–	–
Spain (2012) [24]	54 (59/109)	29	–	45	43	8.2	3.6	–	
Denmark (2012) [28]	27.8 (55/198)	0.4	0.1	0	6.3	2.7	13.5	4.2	0
China (2013) [21]	38.5 (59/153)	25.4	–	–	3.9	21.6	1.9	–	–
Iran (2013) [27]	22.9 (16/70)	22.9	14.3	–	–	–	–	–	–
France (2015) [29]	1.7 (3/184)	–	–	–	–	–	1.7	–	–
Russia (2014) [30]	17.7 (41/232)	–	–	–	3.4	5.2	6.5	–	–

HHV-6A/B does not discriminate between HHV-6A and HHV-6B in all of the references.

* Significant difference of sperm count or sperm motility in infertile and fertile group.

Table 2. Summary of HHVs infection profiles from selected studies.

3. HHV-1-TK as a reporter system

TK (EC 2.7.1.21) is a key enzyme in the pyrimidine salvage pathway that catalyzes the transfer of the ATP γ-phosphate to thymidine to produce dTMP. HHV-1-TK is a phosphotransferase specifically required for viral DNA synthesis. HHV-1-TK shows broad substrate specificity, including pyrimidines (thymidine, deoxycytidine) and their analogs (azidothymidine), as well as purines (guanosine) and their analogs (acyclovir, ganciclovir [GCV], buciclovir and penciclovir). The ability to transform synthetic precursors, such as GCV, into toxic nucleotide analogs has resulted in effective cancer therapy agents [32, 33]. GCV consists of a guanine linked to an acyclic sugar moiety at position 3′. HHV-1-TK converts GCV into GCV-monophosphate, which is further phosphorylated into GCV-triphosphate by the host's kinases. GCV-triphosphate has high affinity for DNA polymerase and functions as a competitive inhibitor of guanosine triphosphate (dGTP), becoming incorporated into the nascent DNA strand (**Figure 2**). GCV causes a distortion in the DNA sugar phosphate backbone, which

http://dx.doi.org/10.5772/64390

blocks DNA replication [34–36] and induces cell apoptosis, thus selectively eliminating HHV-1-TK-positive cells [37, 38]. Moreover, HHV-1-TK-expressing cells trigger apoptosis of neighboring cells due to the transfer of GCV-triphosphate via gap junctions in a phenomenon called "bystander killing" [39]. Therefore, HHV-1-TK can be used as a marker/reporter gene for removing specific target cells.

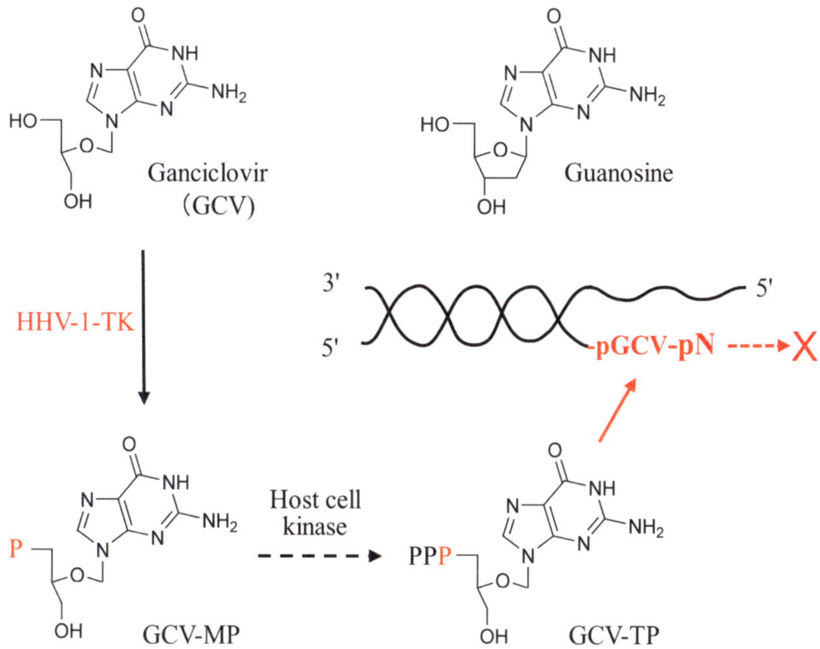

Figure 2. Incorporation of GCV disrupts extension of replicating DNA strands. In HHV-1-TK-positive cells, GCV is phosphorylated into GCV-monophosphate and then converted into GCV-triphosphate. GCV-triphosphate has high affinity for DNA polymerase and is utilized as a dGTP analog. However, the acyclic sugar moiety distorts the sugar phosphate backbone, resulting in irregular extension of the replicating DNA strand.

4. Infertility in HHV-1-TK in Tg animals

4.1. Ectopic expression of HHV-1-TK

The use of HHV-1-TK offers a valuable tool for the ablation of specific cell types as well as in gene therapy. In the early 1990s, Tg rats were engineered to express HHV-1-TK under the control of the FSHβ promoter (**Figure 3A**) in the anterior lobe of the pituitary gland [12]. However, the experiment was interrupted due to observed infertility of male rats. The same happened with Tg mice [40]. Moreover, Ellison and Bishop showed that ectopic expression of HHV-1-TK fused to the human immunodeficiency virus long terminal repeat (HIV-1-LTR) gene caused male infertility in Tg mice [41]. In the present work, we observed ectopic expression of HHV-1-TK gene in the testis of Tg rats (**Figure 3B**).

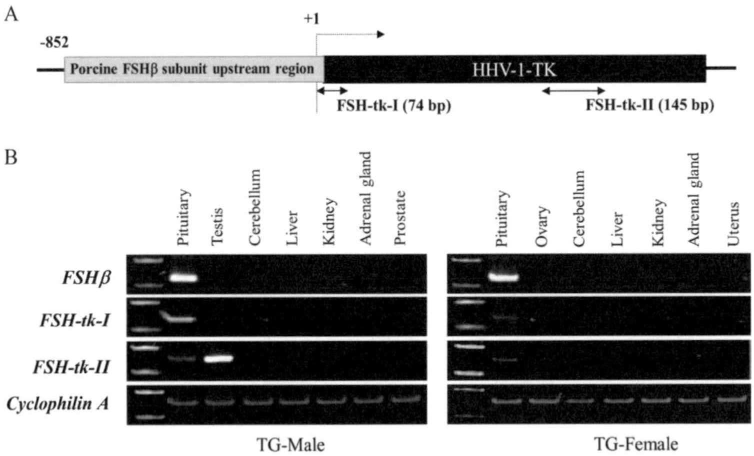

Figure 3. Ectopic expression of HHV-1-TK in transgenic (Tg) rats. (A) HHV-1-TK (blue box) was fused to the 5′-upstream region (-852/+10 bp) of porcine FSHβ (light blue). Arrows indicate the region amplified using specific primer sets (FSH-tk-I and FSH-tk-II); product sizes are shown in parentheses. (B) Total RNAs of pituitary, gonads (testis and ovary), cerebellum, liver, kidney, adrenal glands, prostate, and uterus of Tg rats (male and female) were analyzed by real-time polymerase chain reaction (RT-PCR) using specific primers for rat FSHβ subunit, HHV-1-TK (I), HHV-1-TK (II) and cyclophilin A (control). Reproduced and modified from [12] with permission from the Society for Reproduction and Development.

Whereas the testes of 3-month-old normal rats exhibited morphologically normal germ cells through all stages of maturation, histological analysis of Tg rats revealed developmentally

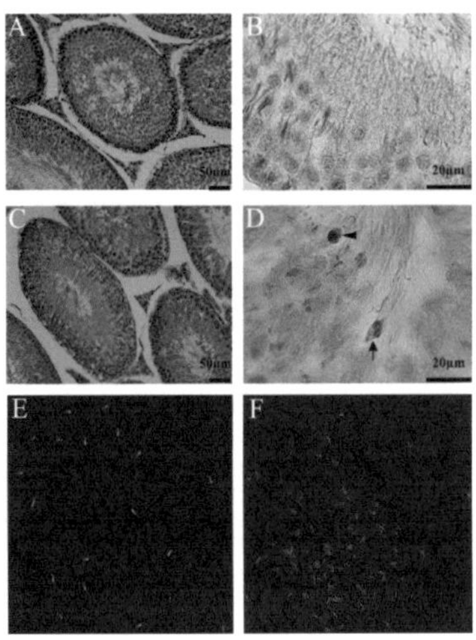

Figure 4. Histological analysis of rat testis and motility of epididymal spermatozoa. (A–D) Sections stained with hematoxylin and eosin showing testicular spermatogenesis in normal (A and B) and Tg (C and D) 3-month-old rats. Arrowhead, elongated arrested round spermatid; arrow, multinucleated cell. (E and F) Spermatozoa obtained from the epididymis of normal (E) and Tg (F) rats stained with SYBR-14 and propidium iodide from a LIVE/DEAD sperm viability kit. Green and red indicate live and dead spermatozoa, respectively. Reproduced and modified from [12] with permission from the Society for Reproduction and Development.

arrested spermatozoa and multinuclear cells, together with altered elongated spermatozoa (**Figure 4**) [12]. Loss of sperm motility and viability was also observed (**Figure 4F**). Compared with normal rats, testis and epididymis weights were also decreased by 35 and 57%, respectively. In contrast, prostate and seminal vesicles weights were similar [12].

4.2. Disruption of spermatogenesis

Histological analysis revealed that in Tg rats abnormal spermatogenesis could be observed as early as 3 months in development. Although spermatocytogenesis and meiosis seemed to progress normally (**Figure 5B**), the number of spermatozoa in the epididymis decreased dramatically (**Figure 5F**). Furthermore, large numbers of degenerated germ cells

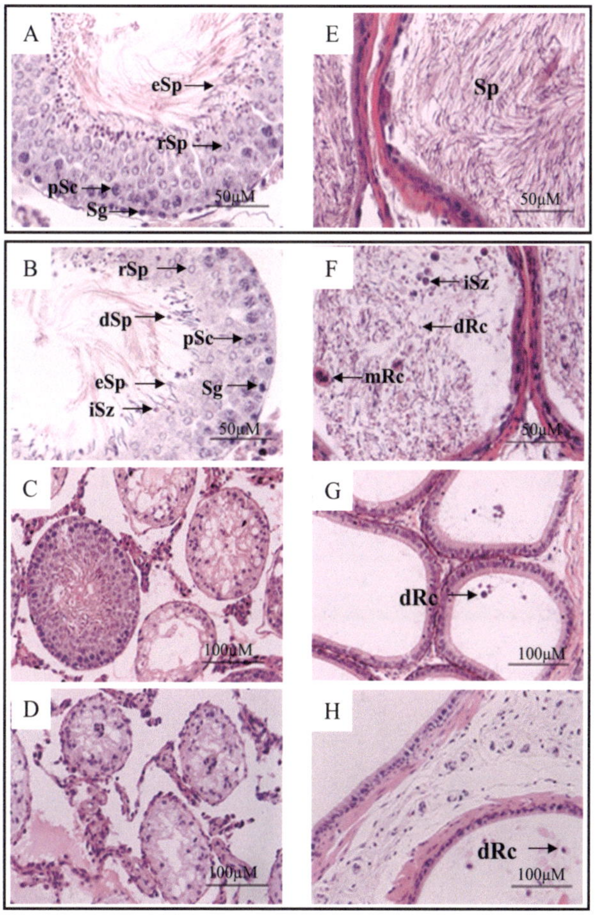

Figure 5. Histological analysis of testis and epididymis in normal and Tg rats. A–D. Sections of normal (A) and 3-, 6-, and 12-month-old (B–D, respectively) Tg rat testis stained with hematoxylin and eosin. (E–H) Sections of normal (E) and 3-, 6- and 12-month-old (F–H, respectively) Tg rat epididymis stained with hematoxylin and eosin. *Abbreviations*: spermatogonium (Sg), pachytene spermatocyte (pSc), immature spermatozoon (iSz), spermatid (Sp), round spermatid (rSp), elongated spermatid (eSp), degenerated spermatid (dSp), multinucleated round cell (mRc), and degenerated round cell (dRc). Reproduced and modified from [13] with permission from the European Teratology Society.

and immature/malformed spermatozoa were present (**Figure 5F**), indicating that maturation was likely to be disrupted. Degenerated germ cells with large vacuoles and cells lost throughout the tubules were observed in the testis of 6-month-old Tg rats (**Figure 5C**). In 12-month-old Tg rats there was a complete loss of germ cells and only Sertoli cells remained in the tubules (**Figure 5D**). In the epididymis of 6- and 12-month-old Tg rats, spermatozoa could hardly be observed (**Figure 5G–H**). Thus, Tg rats showed a spermatid-stage-specific defect in maturation and an age-dependent loss of germ cells.

4.3. HHV-1-TK accumulation increases the number of apoptotic germ cells

Whereas spermatocytogenesis and meiosis were confirmed in Tg rats, degeneration of germ cells by necrosis and apoptosis was frequently observed in the seminiferous tubules. In addition, terminal deoxynucleotidyl transferase dUTP nick end labeling (TUNEL) assay showed a stage-independent increase in TUNEL-positive tubules and cells (**Figure 6**).

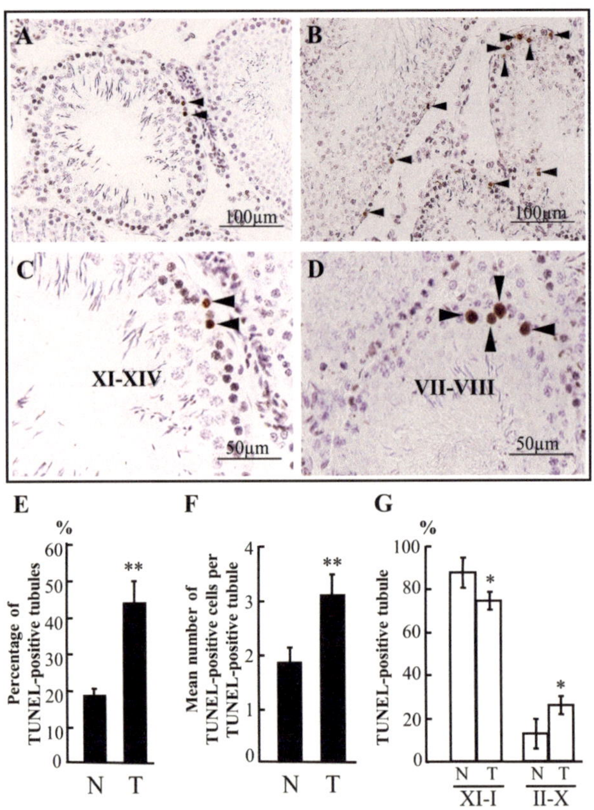

Figure 6. Terminal deoxynucleotidyl transferase dUTP nick end labeling (TUNEL) assay of spermatozoa. (A–D) TUNEL assay of normal (A and C) and Tg (B and D) 3-month-old rats. Representative TUNEL-positive cells are indicated by arrowheads. (E) Percentage of TUNEL-positive tubules. (F) Mean number of TUNEL-positive cells per TUNEL-positive tubule (**$p < 0.01$). (G) TUNEL-positive tubules of normal (N) and Tg (T) rats at stages XI-I and II-X (*$p < 0.05$). Reproduced and modified from [13] with permission from the European Teratology Society.

4.4. HHV-1-TK accumulation in postmeiotic spermatids

Tg rat testes (3- and 6-month-old) were simultaneously stained with anti-HHV-1-TK and nuclear DAPI stain (**Figure 7**). We observed that HHV-1-TK protein accumulated in the cytoplasm of postmeiotic spermatids while it was absent from spermatogonia, spermatocytes, Leydig cells and Sertoli cells. Furthermore, germ cells were obviously reduced in 6-month-old Tg rat testes (**Figure 7B-C**).

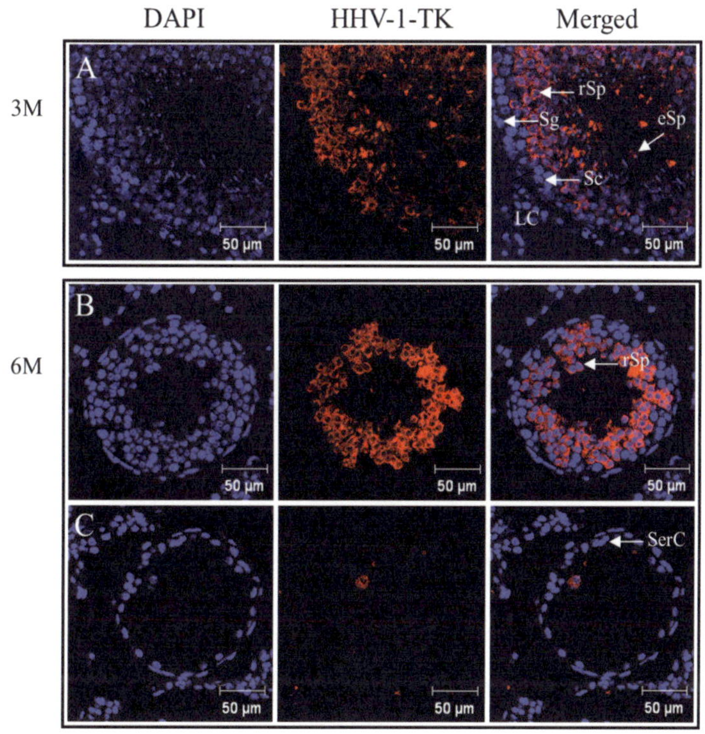

Figure 7. Immunohistochemistry of Tg rat testis. Immunostaining of 3-month-old Tg rat testis with anti-HHV-1-TK antibody and nuclear DAPI stain. HHV-1-TK localizes to the cytoplasm of round spermatids, but not to other testis cells. (B and C). Immunostaining of 6-month-old Tg rat testis. Germ cells decrease markedly. HHV-1-TK is observed in round spermatids (B) but not in Sertoli cells (C). *Abbreviations*: spermatogonium (Sg), spermatocyte (Sc), elongated spermatid (eSp), round spermatid (rSp), Leydig cell (LC), and Sertoli cell (SerC). Reproduced and modified from [13] with permission from the European Teratology Society.

5. Mechanism of ectopic expression of HHV-1-TK

Ectopic expression of HHV-1-TK protein was confirmed in postmeiotic spermatids by immunohistochemistry. This suggested the existence of alternative promoters directing specific and ectopic expression in postmeiotic spermatids. Western blot analysis of HHV-1-TK in Tg rat testis revealed for the first time two bands at 37 and 39 kDa, corresponding to truncated products of the full-size 43 kDa HHV-1-TK protein (**Figure 8A**) [13].

Analysis of the transcription start site by RNA ligase-mediated rapid amplification of cDNA ends (5′-RLM RACE) (**Figure 8B**) showed that the start site corresponded to the first intron of the HHV-1-TK gene (**Figure 8C**). This suggested that the second in frame ATG might have produced the 37 kDa band. Ellison and Bishop reported that HIV-1-LTR-driven HHV-1-TK ectopic expression was abolished by deleting the region between the multiple cloning site and the second ATG [41]. They suggested that removing this portion conferred DNA methylation-independent expression in the testis. Indeed, the corresponding region (144 bases) is GC-rich (67%) and contains 17 CpG sites. Currently, a HHV-1-TK vector free of the GC-rich region is available.

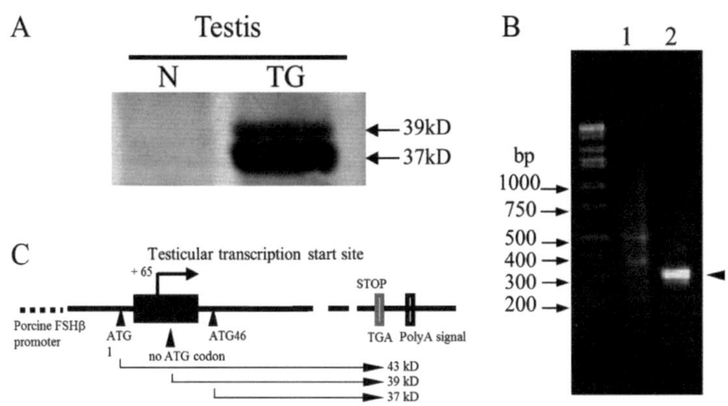

Figure 8. Identification of HHV-1-TK isoforms and transcription initiation sites in Tg rat testis. (A) Detection of HHV-1-TK in Tg rat testis by western blot analysis reveals two truncated isoforms (37 and 39 kDa) that do not correspond to the canonical form (43 kDa). (B) 5′-RLM-RACE analysis. Lane 1, PCR using a 5′-RACE outer primer set; lane 2, PCR with a 5′-RACE inner primer set. Products (approximately 300 bp) are indicated with an arrowhead. (C) Diagram showing the HHV-1-TK transcription initiation site (arrow), translation start sites (arrowheads and ATG with residue number), stop codon (grey box) and poly A signal (solid box). The closed box indicates a putative testis-specific promoter region within HHV-1-TK. Reproduced and modified from [13] with permission from the European Teratology Society.

Ectopic, testis-specific, expression of HHV-1-TK in Tg rats and mice raises the possibility that the same mechanism could also affect humans carrying HHV-1. Therefore, the transcriptional regulation exhibited by ectopic expression of HHV-1-TK in Tg rats and the effects of HHV-1-TK accumulation on spermatogenesis may be revelatory of the same mechanisms in humans.

6. HHV-1-TK accumulation disrupts spermatogenesis and causes male infertility

6.1. Ultrastructural abnormalities of spermatozoa in Tg rat testis

Scanning electron microscopy revealed abnormal ultrastructure of epididymal spermatozoa in 10-week-old Tg rats [13]. We observed that the head and tail regions of spermatozoa from 10-week-old normal rats exhibited smooth surface and a regular morphological conformation

(**Figure 9A**). Indeed, the morphology of these spermatozoa was different from those of Tg rats (**Figure 9B–F**). Spermatozoa with malformed heads, the consequence of a defective acrosome or reduced genome, were observed at high frequency among Tg rats (**Figure 9B–F**). Transmission electron microscopy (TEM) revealed that the cell membrane was missing from segments of the head (**Figure 9C**), midpiece (**Figure 9D**), and flagellum (**Figure 9F**). There were spermatozoa with looped tails (**Figure 9D**).

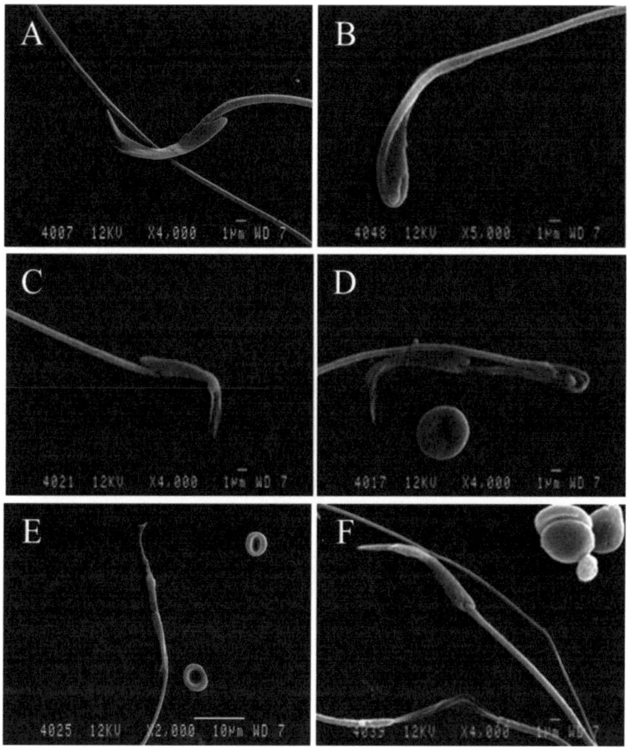

Figure 9. Scanning electron microscopy of Tg rat spermatozoa. Spermatozoa from caudal epididymis of 10-week-old rats visualized by scanning electron microscopy. (A) Normal rat sperm shows smooth head and tail. B–F. Tg rats present a deformed head (B), a microhead and absence of cell membrane (C), looped flagella and absence of cell membrane (D), defective acrosome and reduced genome (E), and absence of cell membrane in the flagellum (F). Reproduced and modified from [13] with permission from the European Teratology Society.

TEM of 3-month-old rat testis showed that in contrast with normal rats (**Figure 10A–C**), Tg rats displayed massive vacuoles within the seminiferous epithelium (**Figure 10D–E**, asterisks). These frequently presented degenerated spermatocytes in the seminiferous tubules (**Figure 10E–F**, arrowheads), in spite of confirmed spermatocytogenesis and meiosis. Moreover, TEM also showed elongated spermatids with disorganized heads partially devoid of cell membrane (**Figure 10G**, arrowhead), multiple flagella (**Figure 10H**, arrow), and absence of the inner arms of flagellar axonemes (**Figure 10I**, arrowheads) in the lumen of seminiferous tubules. In addition, vacuolization was also observed in the cytoplasm of spermatocytes (**Figure 10F**).

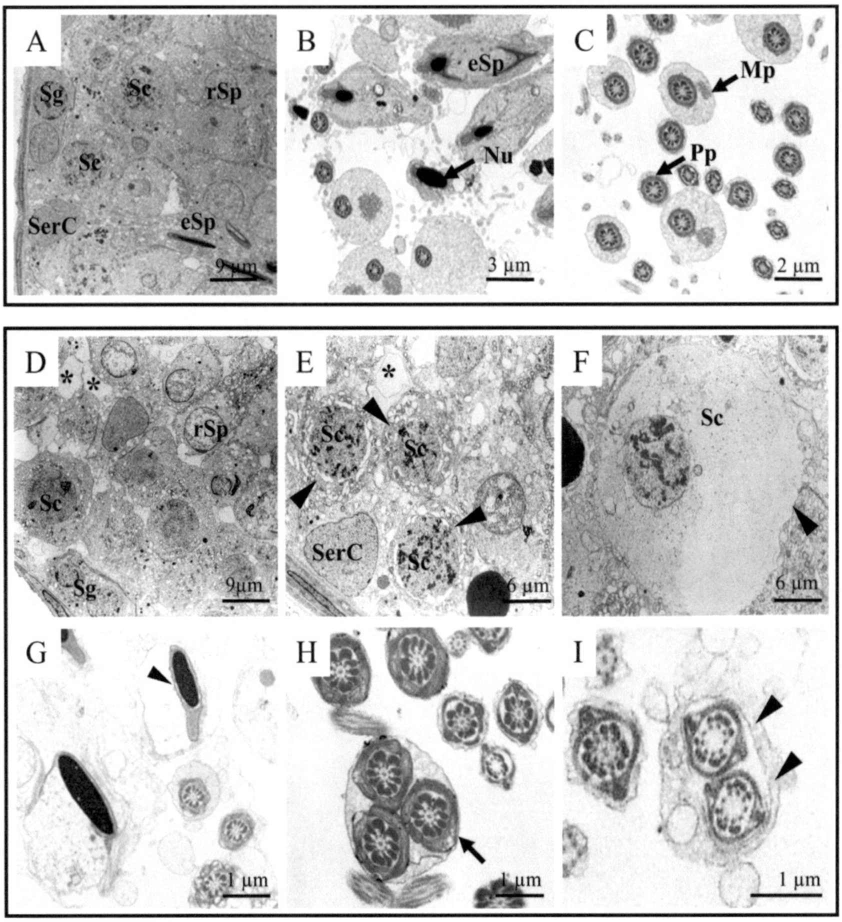

Figure 10. TEM of rat germ cells. Sections of 3-month-old normal (A–C) and Tg (D–I) rats analyzed by TEM. (A–C) Normal condensed nuclear, midpiece, and principle piece are indicated by arrows. (D–F) Numerous phagocytic vacuole compartments and massive vacuoles are present within the cytoplasm of Sertoli cells (D–E, asterisks), together with degeneration of spermatocytes (E–F, arrowheads). (G–I) Spermatozoa within the lumen of seminiferous tubules show various ultrastructural abnormalities, such as disorganized heads with a disrupted cell membrane (G, arrowhead), multiple flagella (H–I, arrow), and absence of inner arms of flagellar axonemes (I, arrowheads). Abbreviations: normal condensed nuclear (Nu), midpiece (Mp), principle piece (Pp), spermatogonium (Sg), spermatocyte (Sc), Sertoli cell (SerC), round spermatid (rSp), elongated spermatid (eSp). Reproduced and modified from [42] with permission from the Society for Reproduction and Development.

TEM also revealed the low number of spermatozoa in the epididymis of Tg rats (**Figure 11B**) as compared to normal rats (**Figure 11A**). Spermatozoa from normal rats displayed intact cell membranes and normal-shaped heads with complete chromatin condensation (**Figure 11A1**). Instead, those of Tg rats presented a number of defects: several immature spermatids detaching from Sertoli cells and sloughing into the epididymis (**Figure 11B**), degenerated round spermatids (**Figure 11B1**) and many types of abnormal elongated spermatids (**Figure 11B2–B4**). In addition, whereas normal rats presented the typically assembled flagellar axonemes composed of nine outer doublet microtubules and a pair of central microtubules (**Figure 11A2**), most spermatozoa from Tg rats were dead and showed various ultrastructural defects, including breakage of the surface membrane (**Figure 11B5**) and a decline in the number of outer dense fibers (**Figure 11B6**).

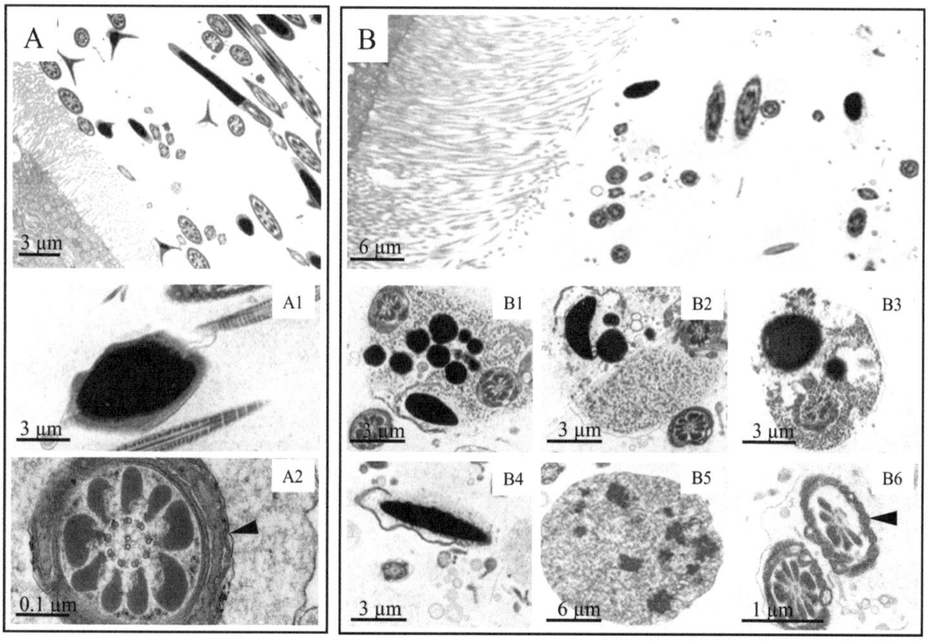

Figure 11. TEM of epididymal spermatozoa. TEM sections of epididymal spermatozoa from 3-month-old rats. (A) Spermatozoa from normal rats show intact acrosomes with condensed nuclear material (A1) as well as proper assembled flagellar axonemes displaying nine outer doublet microtubules and a pair of central microtubules (A2, arrowhead). (B) Spermatozoa in the epididymis of Tg rats appear dead, and display various ultrastructural defects, such as absence of acrosomes, disorganization of surface membranes, and degeneration of midpiece and tail (B1–B4). In addition, residual bodies of degenerated germ cells (B5) and missing outer doublet microtubules are frequently observed (B6, arrowhead). Reproduced and modified from [42] with permission from the Society for Reproduction and Development.

6.2. Disruption of Sertoli-germ junctions

Hematoxylin and eosin staining revealed various abnormal morphologies in Tg rat testis. Cytoplasmic vacuolation of Sertoli cells (**Figure 12A**, open arrowhead), disconnection between Sertoli and germ cells (**Figure 12B**, arrows), and disordered arrangement of elongated spermatids (**Figure 12C**, arrowhead) were present in many seminiferous tubules. In addition, immature spermatozoa falling off from the seminiferous epithelium were observed during all stages of spermatogenesis (**Figure 12D–H**, arrowheads). Furthermore, sperm development was disrupted and germ cells with different levels of maturity were observed simultaneously (**Figure 12D–H**). These results indicate that cell junctions between germ and Sertoli cells may have been affected. This hypothesis may be confirmed by analyzing gene expression profiles of Tg rat testis.

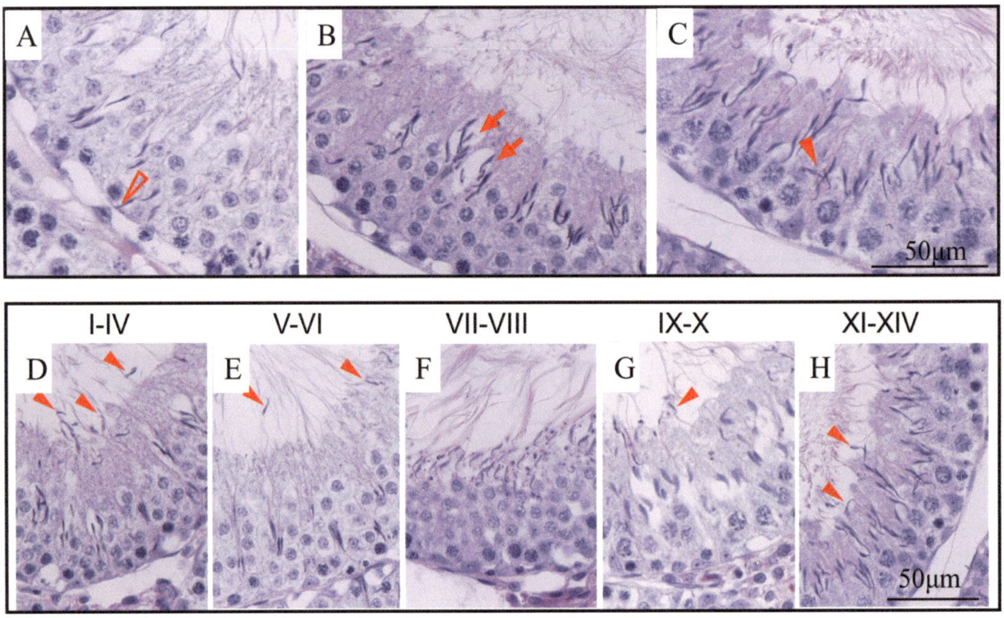

Figure 12. Histological analysis of Tg rat seminiferous tubules. Sections of 3-month-old Tg rat testis stained with hematoxylin and eosin. The following defects are observed: cytoplasmic vacuolation of Sertoli cells (A, open arrowhead), disconnection between Sertoli and germ cells (B, arrows), and disordered arrangement of elongated spermatids (C, solid arrowhead). (D–H) Immature spermatozoa falling off from the seminiferous epithelium (arrowheads) are observed at different maturation stages (I–XIV) and germ cell development is disrupted.

7. Alterations in gene expression profiles of Tg rat testis

Changes in gene expression evoked by HHV-1-TK accumulation in Tg rat testis were examined by cDNA microarray analysis. We found that 200 genes, 0.67% of all transcripts on DNA chips, were differently expressed between Tg and normal rats. We sorted the genes by their functional categories, such as apoptosis, cell cycle, development, oxidative stress, proteolysis, signal transduction, transcription, translation, transport, metabolism, immune response, and cell adhesion. The highest number of affected genes was linked to metabolism, with 8 genes up-regulated and 16 down-regulated by at least 1.5-fold in Tg rat testis (**Table 3**) [42].

RT-PCR was performed for 10 genes involved in cell adhesion, signal transduction, and transport: *Cnot7*, *Fgf7*, *Egfl6*, *Testin*, *Ostf1*, and *Atp2a2* (all up-regulated); and *Sh3bp4*, *Lamc2*, *Versican*, and *Mamdc1* (all down-regulated). As listed in **Table 4**, *Cnot7*, *Fgf7*, *Testin*, *Ostf1*, *Versican*, and *Mamdc1* were significantly up- or down-regulated, confirming microarray data. Testin is a signaling molecule responsible for monitoring Sertoli-germ cell adherens junctions. Increased secretion of testin by Sertoli cells causes disruption of these junctions [43, 44]. *Versican* is expressed in adult mouse brain, heart, lung, spleen, skeletal muscle, skin, tail, kidney, and

http://dx.doi.org/10.5772/64390

testis. It is suggested to play a role in cellular attachment, migration, and proliferation by interacting with cell surfaces and extracellular matrix molecules [45]. *Mamdc1*, a novel member of adhesion molecules of the immunoglobulin superfamily, is expressed in human Leydig cells of the testis. *Mamdc1* mRNA was shown to be up-regulated by pro-inflammatory cytokines, such as tumor necrosis factor-α and interferon-γ, involved in cell adhesion, migration, and recruitment to inflammatory sites [46]. However, the function of *versican* and *mamdc1* in spermatogenesis has not yet been established. Expression of *Fgf7*, *Ostf1*, and *Cnot7* [47] also increased significantly, indicating a stress response in Tg rat testis. The roles of these genes are listed in **Table 5**.

Biological process	Gene number of expression changed		
	Decreased	Increased	Total
Apoptosis	1	4	5
Cell cycle	2	4	6
Development	3	16	19
Oxidative stress	0	1	1
Proteolysis	3	7	10
Signal transduction	2	11	13
Transcription	6	6	12
Translation	1	1	2
Transport	12	11	23
Immune response	1	2	3
Metabolism	8	16	24
Cell adhesion	3	4	7
Others	54	21	75
Total	96	104	200

Note: The affected genes were classified into 12 functional categories according to "Gene ontology".

Gene ontology classification of genes whose expression changes by at least .5-fold in Tg with respect to normal rats, as revealed by cDNA microarray analysis. Reproduced and modified from [42] with permission from the Society for Reproduction and Development.

Table 3. Number of affected genes in testes of HHV-1-TK Tg rats revealed by cDNA microarray.

Notably, the contraceptive adjudin has been reported to induce morphological alterations in the seminiferous tubules similar to the ones we observed here, and target directly testin and actin-myosin [48]. However, the exact mechanism by which HHV-1-TK disrupts spermatogenesis and adherens junctions will require further work.

Gene product			Microarray analysis	Real-time PCR results	
Gene title	**Gene symbol**	**Category**	**Ratio of TG value/N value**	**Expression levels TG/N**	***p* value**
Up-regulated genes in TG rat testes					
CCR4-NOT transcription complex, subunit 7	Cnot7	Signal transduction	18.40	1.30	<0.05
Fibroblast growth factor 7	Fgf7	Development	6.10	2.00	<0.05
EGF-like-domain, multiple 6	Egfl6	Cell adhesion	3.70	0.91	NS
Testin gene	Testin	Cell adhesion	2.30	2.00	<0.05
Osteoclast stimulating factor 1	Ostf1	Transcription	1.68	1.30	<0.05
ATPase, Ca^{2+} transporting, cardiac muscle, slow twitch 2	Atp2a2	Transport	1.67	0.96	NS
Down-regulated genes in TG rat testes					
SH3-domain binding protein 4	Sh3bp4	Transport	0.06	0.91	NS
Lamimin, gamma 2	Lamc2	Cell adhesion	0.09	0.90	NS
Chondroitin sulfate proteoglycan 2	Versican	Cell adhesion	0.10	0.55	<0.05
MAM domain containing glycosylphosphatidylinositol anchor 2	Mamdc1	Cell adhesion	0.62	0.67	<0.05

Reproduced and modified from [42] with permission from the Society for Reproduction and Development.

Table 4. Expression level of genes assayed by microarray analysis and real-time PCR.

Gene name	Gene symbol	Category	Molecular function	Biological process
Up-regulated genes in TG rat testes				
CCR4-NOT transcription complex, subunit 7	Cnot7	Signal transduction	Has 3-5 poly(A) exoribonuclease activity, nucleic acid binding, transcription factor activity, catalytic component of the CCR4-NOT complex, cell proliferation factor, mRNA degradation, miRNA-mediated repression	spermatogenesis, tumor cell metastasis suppressor, bone metabolism, embryonic development, tumor suppressor

Gene name	Gene symbol	Category	Molecular function	Biological process
Up-regulated genes in TG rat testes				
Fibroblast growth factor 7	Fgf7	Development	chemoattractant activity, growth factor activity, mitogenic and cell survival activities activation of MAPKK activity actin cytoskeleton reorganization neurotrophin TRK receptor signaling pathway	embryonic development, cell growth, morphogenesis, tissue repair, tumor growth and invasion
Testin gene	Testin	Cell adhesion	regulation of cell motility, poly(A) RNA binding, zinc ion binding	cell adhesion, cell spreading, reorganization of the actin cytoskeleton, negative regulation of cell proliferation, tumor suppressor
Osteoclast stimulating factor 1	Ostf1	Transport	SH3 domain binding	induces bone resorption, enhancing osteoclast formation
Down-regulated genes in TG rat testes				
Chondroitin sulfate proteoglycan 2	Versican	Cell adhesion	interaction of integrins, anti-cell adhesion, regulation of cell motility, growth and differentiation, a key factor in inflammation hyaluronic acid binding,	embryonic development, embryonic cell migration important in the formation of the heart, neural crest cell migration, inhibit nervous system regeneration, axonal growth, tumor growth
MAM domain containing glycosyphosphatidylinositol anchor 2	Mamdc1	Cell adhesion	GPI-anchored protein, cell-cell interaction	neuron development and differentiation, neuronal migration, axon outgrowth, axon-target recognition

Table 5. The role of genes changed expression level significantly in Tg rats.

8. HHV-1-TK in human testis

Nested PCR for 4 types of HHVs was performed on 153 DNA samples prepared from human semen (**Figure 13**). Bands of 99, 150, 165, and 135 bp were observed for HHV-1, HHV-4, HHV-5, and HHV-6A/B (HHV-6A and 6B were detected together by common domains), respectively (**Figure 13A**). Samples showing positive bands by more than one PCR target indicated concomitant infection with multiple types of HHVs (**Figure 13A**). We identified nucleotide sequences corresponding to HHV-1, HHV-4, HHV-5, and HHV-6A/B (**Figure 13B**) in 39, 6, 33, and 3 patients, respectively, as summarized in **Table 6**. We observed double infection with HHV-1/HHV-5 (15 carriers), HHV-1/HHV-4 (1), HHV-1/HHV-6A/B (2) and HHV-4/HHV-5 (4). HHV-4 carriers presented a double infection 83% of the time, while for other HHVs it ranged from 46 to 66%.

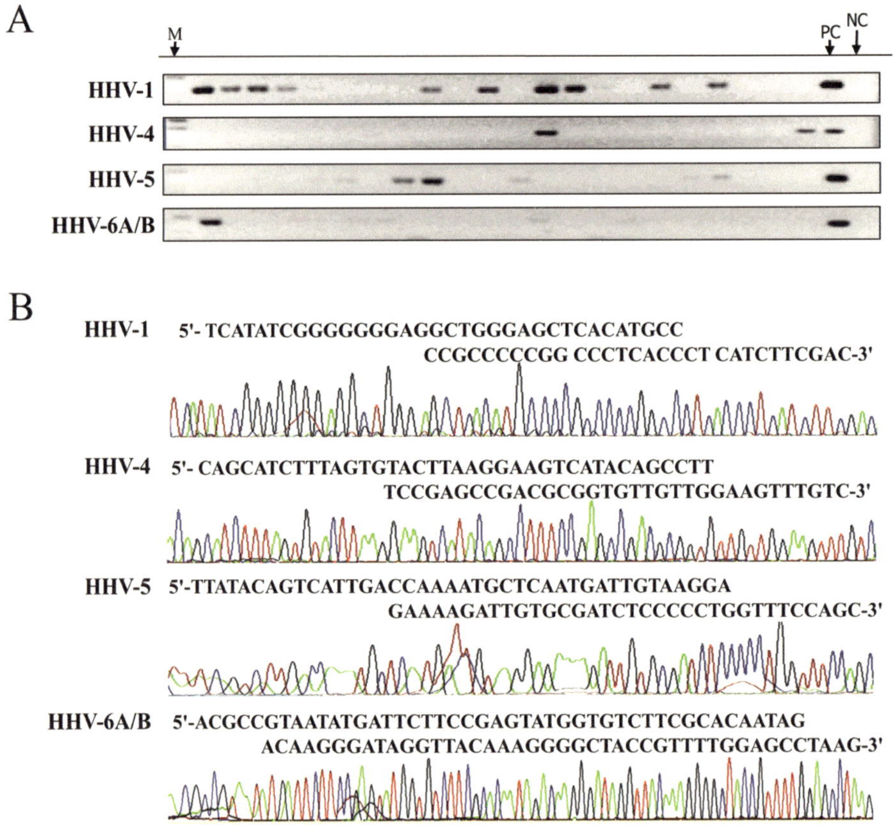

Figure 13. Detection of HHVs genomic DNA in human semen by PCR. (A) Agarose gel electrophoresis of PCR products using HHV-specific primers and human semen as template DNA. PC (positive control) and NC (negative control) indicate reactions with control viral fragments and without DNA template, respectively. M, size marker. (B) Sequence profiles of representative PCR products. Viral sequences are shown below the nucleotide sequence. Reproduced and modified from [21] with permission from the Society for Reproduction and Development.

Number of virus infection in patients (153)				
Type	**HHV-1**	**HHV-4**	**HHV-5**	**HHV-6A/B**
Total	39 (25%)	6 (4%)	33 (22%)	3 (2%)
Number of double virus infection				
Type	HHV-1	HHV-4	HHV-5	HHV-6A/B
HHV-1	–	1	15	2
HHV-4	1	–	4	0
HHV-5	15	4	–	0
HHV-6A/B	2	0	0	–
Total	18/39 (46%)	5/6 (83%)	19/33 (58%)	2/3 (66%)

HHV-6A and 6B were detected together by common domains.

Reproduced and modified from [21] with permission from the Society for Reproduction and Development.

Table 6. Number of cases with single and double viral infection.

The viral DNA-positive group showed a higher incidence of oligozoospermia compared with the viral DNA-negative group (38.5 vs. 16.7%, $P<0.05$; **Figure 14**). Therefore, to further confirm the relationship between HHVs infection and changes to semen parameters, large-scale analysis according to WHO Guidelines (5th edition) is strongly suggested.

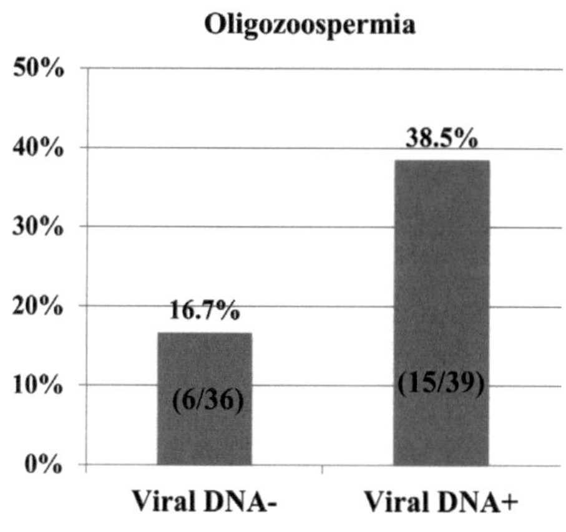

Figure 14. Comparison of oligozoospermia between viral DNA-negative and -positive groups. Analysis of oligozoospermia rates between viral DNA-negative (36 patients) and -positive (39 patients) according to WHO Guidelines (5th edition). Reproduced and modified from [21] with permission from the Society for Reproduction and Development.

9. Future perspectives

HHV-1 infection might strongly associate with human male infertility, possibly by testis-specific expression of the viral TK gene. However, conclusive evidence that HHV-1-TK causes male infertility is still missing.

As described above, HHV-1-TK is known as a suicide gene that kills target cells specifically in the presence of GCV. However, male infertility normally occurs in the presence of HHV-1 but absence of GCV. Degeneration of spermatogenesis was observed as early as 3 months in Tg rats ectopically expressing HHV-1-TK. With the exception of Sertoli cells, it later resulted in loss of germ cells, possibly by "bystander killing." In contrast, no abnormality in the pituitary gland of Tg rats was observed. This difference may indicate tissue-specific action of HHV-1-TK in the testis, which does not occur in the pituitary gland. At present, it is unclear why HHV-1-TK targets testis over other tissues and how it induces degeneration of spermatogenesis. Further work is required to elucidate this and other features of HHV-related infertility.

Expression of HHV-1-TK may be the main cause of infertility in HHV-1-infected human males. To firmly establish a causative link, several players require identification: (1) target molecule(s) of HHV-1-TK; (2) the HHV-1-TK-dependent mechanism responsible for failed spermatogenesis; and (3) the mechanism dictating postmeiotic spermatid-specific expression of HHV-1-TK. The identification of target molecule(s) is particularly important, since there is no evidence that enzymatically active HHV-1-TK is required, raising speculation it may only serve as a binding protein. Even if HHV-1-TK functioned as an enzyme, the substrate(s) might be testis-specific. Currently, the only known activity of HHV-1-TK is to catalyze the transfer of the γ-phosphate from ATP to substrate nucleotides and analogs. Recently, a stable-isotope substrate ($[\gamma\text{-}^{18}O_4]$ATP) for kinases has been developed [49]. Mass spectrometry could reveal the identity of $[\gamma\text{-}^{18}O_4]$ATP-labeled products obtained by incubating recombinant HHV-1-TK with testis homogenates. The identified HHV-1-TK target(s) may help elucidate the mechanisms determining failed spermatogenesis and postmeiotic spermatid-specific expression of HHV-1-TK. Moreover, knowing the target(s) molecular properties may help design appropriate analogs for pharmacological use. The significance of our results is particularly clear in view of expected novel male contraceptives and drugs for HHV-related male infertility.

Author details

Mo Chen[1,2], Li-yi Cai[3], Takako Kato[1,2] and Yukio Kato[3,4*]

*Address all correspondence to: yukato@isc.meiji.ac.jp

1 Organization for the Strategic Coordination of Research and Intellectual Property, Meiji University, Kawasaki, Kanagawa, Japan

2 Institute for Endocrinology, Meiji University, Kawasaki, Kanagawa, Japan

3 Center for Reproductive Medicine, Affiliated Wuxi Hospital for Maternal & Child Health Care of Nanjing Medical University, Wuxi, PR China

4 Department of Life Science, School of Agriculture, Meiji University, Kawasaki, Kanagawa, Japan

References

[1] Roizman B, Carmichael LE, Deinhardt F, de-The G, Nahmias AJ, Plowright W, Rapp F, Sheldrick P, Takahashi M, Wolf K. Herpesviridae. Definition, provisional nomenclature, and taxonomy. The Herpesvirus Study Group, the International Committee on Taxonomy of Viruses. Intervirology. 1981;16:201–17.

[2] Fishman JA. Overview: cytomegalovirus and the herpesviruses in transplantation. American Journal of Transplantation. 2013;13 Suppl 3:1–8. DOI: 10.1111/ajt.12002

[3] Grinde B. Herpesviruses: latency and reactivation – viral strategies and host response. Journal of Oral Microbiology. 2013;5:22766. DOI: 10.3402/jom.v5i0.22766

[4] Ochsendorf FR. Sexually transmitted infections: impact on male fertility. Andrologia. 2008;40:72–5. DOI: 10.1111/j.1439-0272.2007.00825.x

[5] el Borai N, Inoue M, Lefevre C, Naumova EN, Sato B, Yamamura M. Detection of herpes simplex DNA in semen and menstrual blood of individuals attending an infertility clinic. The Journal of Obstetrics and Gynaecology Research. 1997;23:17–24.

[6] Bezold G, Schuster-Grusser A, Lange M, Gall H, Wolff H, Peter RU. Prevalence of human herpesvirus types 1-8 in the semen of infertility patients and correlation with semen parameters. Fertility and Sterility. 2001;76:416–8.

[7] Garolla A, Pizzol D, Bertoldo A, Menegazzo M, Barzon L, Foresta C. Sperm viral infection and male infertility: focus on HBV, HCV, HIV, HPV, HSV, HCMV, and AAV. Journal of Reproductive Immunology. 2013;100:20–9. DOI: 10.1016/j.jri.2013.03.004

[8] Barton IG, Kinghorn GR, Najem S, Al-Omar LS, Potter CW. Incidence of herpes simplex virus types 1 and 2 isolated in patients with herpes genitalis in Sheffield. The British Journal of Venereal Diseases. 1982;58:44–7.

[9] Kapranos N, Petrakou E, Anastasiadou C, Kotronias D. Detection of herpes simplex virus, cytomegalovirus, and Epstein-Barr virus in the semen of men attending an infertility clinic. Fertility and Sterility. 2003;79 Suppl 3:1566–70.

[10] Bezold G, Politch JA, Kiviat NB, Kuypers JM, Wolff H, Anderson DJ. Prevalence of sexually transmissible pathogens in semen from asymptomatic male infertility patients with and without leukocytospermia. Fertility and Sterility. 2007;87:1087–97. DOI: 10.1016/j.fertnstert.2006.08.109

[11] Neofytou E, Sourvinos G, Asmarianaki M, Spandidos DA, Makrigiannakis A. Prevalence of human herpes virus types 1-7 in the semen of men attending an infertility clinic and correlation with semen parameters. Fertility and Sterility. 2009;91:2487–94. DOI: 10.1016/j.fertnstert.2008.03.074

[12] Cai LY, Kato T, Ito K, Nakayama M, Susa T, Aikawa S, Maeda K, Tsukamura H, Ohta A, Izumi S, Kato Y. Expression of porcine FSHbeta subunit promoter-driven herpes

simplex virus thymidine kinase gene in transgenic rats. Journal of Reproduction and Development. 2007;53:201–9.

[13] Cai LY, Kato T, Nakayama M, Susa T, Murakami S, Izumi S, Kato Y. HSV type 1 thymidine kinase protein accumulation in round spermatids induces male infertility by spermatogenesis disruption and apoptotic loss of germ cells. Reproductive Toxicology. 2009;27:14–21. DOI: 10.1016/j.reprotox.2008.11.052

[14] Himmel W, Ittner E, Kochen MM, Michelmann HW, Hinney B, Reuter M, Kallerhoff M, Ringert RH. Management of involuntary childlessness. British Journal of General Practice. 1997;47:111–8.

[15] Brugh VM 3rd, Lipshultz LI. Male factor infertility: evaluation and management. Medical Clinics of North America. 2004;88:367–85. DOI: 10.1016/S0025-7125(03)00150-0

[16] Hirsh A. Male subfertility. British Medical Journal. 2003;327:669–72. DOI: 10.1136/bmj.327.7416.669

[17] Gimenes F, Souza RP, Bento JC, Teixeira JJ, Maria-Engler SS, Bonini MG, Consolaro ME. Male infertility: a public health issue caused by sexually transmitted pathogens. Nature Reviews Urology. 2014;11:672–87. DOI: 10.1038/nrurol.2014.285

[18] Sethi S, Singh G, Samanta P, Sharma M. Mycoplasma genitalium: an emerging sexually transmitted pathogen. Indian Journal of Medical Research. 2012;136:942–55.

[19] Nwankwo EO, Sadiq MN. Prevalence of *Chlamydia trachomatis* infection among patients attending infertility and sexually transmitted diseases clinic (STD) in Kano, North Western Nigeria. African Health Sciences. 2014;14:672–8. DOI: 10.4314/ahs.v14i3.24

[20] Boitrelle F, Robin G, Lefebvre C, Bailly M, Selva J, Courcol R, Lornage J, Albert M. Bacteriospermia in assisted reproductive techniques: effects of bacteria on spermatozoa and seminal plasma, diagnosis and treatment. Gynécologie Obstétrique & Fertilité. 2012;40:226–34. DOI: 10.1016/j.gyobfe.2012.01.003

[21] Chen M, Cai LY, Kanno N, Kato T, Lu J, Jin F, Wang H, Sekita M, Higuchi M, Yoshida S, Yako H, Ueharu H, Izumi S, Kato Y. Detection of human herpesviruses (HHVs) in semen of human male infertile patients. Journal of Reproduction and Development. 2013;59:457–62. DOI: 10.1262/jrd.2013-023

[22] Monini P, de Lellis L, Fabris M, Rigolin F, Cassai E. Kaposi's sarcoma-associated herpesvirus DNA sequences in prostate tissue and human semen. The New England Journal of Medicine. 1996;334:1168–72.

[23] Eggert-Kruse W, Reuland M, Johannsen W, Strowitzki T, Schlehofer JR. Cytomegalovirus (CMV) infection-related to male and/or female infertility factors?. Fertility and Sterility. 2009;91:67–82. DOI: 10.1016/j.fertnstert.2007.11.014

[24] Michou V, Liarmakopoulou S, Thomas D, Tsimaratou K, Makarounis K, Constantoulakis P, Angelopoulou R, Tsilivakos V. Herpes virus infected spermatozoa following

density gradient centrifugation for IVF purposes. Andrologia. 2012;44:174–80. DOI: 10.1111/j.1439-0272.2010.01121.x

[25] Thomas R, Macsween KF, McAulay K, Clutterbuck D, Anderson R, Reid S, Higgins CD, Swerdlow AJ, Harrison N, Williams H, Crawford DH. Evidence of shared Epstein-Barr viral isolates between sexual partners, and low level EBV in genital secretions. Journal of Medical Virology. 2006;78:1204–9.

[26] Naumenko VA, Tyulenev YA, Yakovenko SA, Kurilo LF, Shileyko LV, Segal AS, Zavalishina LE, Klimova RR, Tsibizov AS, Alkhovskii SV, Kushch AA. Detection of human cytomegalovirus in motile spermatozoa and spermatogenic cells in testis organotypic culture. Herpesviridae. 2011;2:7. DOI: 10.1186/2042-4280-2-7

[27] Monavari SH, Vaziri MS, Khalili M, Shamsi-Shahrabadi M, Keyvani H, Mollaei H, Fazlalipour M. Asymptomatic seminal infection of herpes simplex virus: impact on male infertility. Journal of Biomedical Research. 2013;27:56–61. DOI: 10.7555/JBR.27.20110139

[28] Kaspersen MD, Larsen PB, Kofod-Olsen E, Fedder J, Bonde J, Hollsberg P. Human herpesvirus-6A/B binds to spermatozoa acrosome and is the most prevalent herpesvirus in semen from sperm donors. PLoS One. 2012;7:e48810. DOI: 10.1371/journal.pone.0048810

[29] Godet AN, Soignon G, Koubi H, Bonnafous P, Agut H, Poirot C, Gautheret-Dejean A. Presence of HHV-6 genome in spermatozoa in a context of couples with low fertility: what type of infection?. Andrologia. 2015;47:531–5. DOI: 10.1111/and.12299

[30] Naumenko V, Tyulenev Y, Kurilo L, Shileiko L, Sorokina T, Evdokimov V, Yakovleva V, Kovalyk V,Malolina E, Kulibin A, Gomberg M, Kushch A. Detection and quantification of human herpes viruses types 4-6 in sperm samples of patients with fertility disorders and chronic inflammatory urogenital tract diseases. Andrology. 2014;2:687–94. DOI: 10.1111/j.2047-2927.2014.00232.x

[31] Diafouka F, Foulongne V, Hauhouot-Attoungbre ML, Monnet D, Segondy M. Cytomegalovirus DNA in semen of men seeking fertility evaluation in Abidjan, Cote d'Ivoire. European Journal of Clinical Microbiology & Infectious Diseases. 2007;26:295–6. DOI: 10.1007/s10096-007-0271-y

[32] Greco O, Dachs GU. Gene directed enzyme/prodrug therapy of cancer: historical appraisal and future prospectives. Journal of Cellular Physiology. 2001;187:22–36. DOI: 10.1002/1097-4652(2001)9999:9999<::AID-JCP1060>3.0.CO;2-H

[33] Spencer DM. Developments in suicide genes for preclinical and clinical applications. Current Opinion in Molecular Therapeutics. 2000;2:433–40.

[34] Chen H, Beardsley GP, Coen DM. Mechanism of ganciclovir-induced chain termination revealed by resistant viral polymerase mutants with reduced exonuclease activity.

Proceedings of the National Academy of Sciences of the United States of America. 2014;111:17462–7. DOI: 10.1073/pnas.1405981111

[35] Smee DF, Martin JC, Verheyden JP, Matthews TR. Anti-herpesvirus activity of the acyclic nucleoside 9-(1,3-dihydroxy-2-propoxymethyl)guanine. Antimicrobial Agents and Chemotherapy. 1983;23:676–82.

[36] St Clair MH, Lambe CU, Furman PA. Inhibition by ganciclovir of cell growth and DNA synthesis of cells biochemically transformed with herpesvirus genetic information. Antimicrobial Agents and Chemotherapy. 1987;31:844–9.

[37] Moolten FL. Tumor chemosensitivity conferred by inserted herpes thymidine kinase genes: paradigm for a prospective cancer control strategy. Cancer Research. 1986;46:5276–81.

[38] Tomicic MT, Thust R, Kaina B. Ganciclovir-induced apoptosis in HSV-1 thymidine kinase expressing cells: critical role of DNA breaks, Bcl-2 decline and caspase-9 activation. Oncogene. 2002;21:2141–53. DOI: 10.1038/sj.onc.1205280

[39] Hamel W, Magnelli L, Chiarugi VP, Israel MA. Herpes simplex virus thymidine kinase/ganciclovir-mediated apoptotic death of bystander cells. Cancer Research. 1996;56:2697–702.

[40] al-Shawi R, Burke J, Wallace H, Jones C, Harrison S, Buxton D, Maley S, Chandley A, Bishop JO. The herpes simplex virus type 1 thymidine kinase is expressed in the testes of transgenic mice under the control of a cryptic promoter. Molecular and Cellular Biology. 1991;11:4207–16.

[41] Ellison AR, Bishop JO. Herpesvirus thymidine kinase transgenes that do not cause male sterility are aberrantly transcribed and translated in the testis. Biochimica et Biophysica Acta. 1998;1442:28–38.

[42] Cai LY, Kato T, Chen M, Wang H, Sekine E, Izumi S, Kato Y. Accumulated HSV1-TK proteins interfere with spermatogenesis through a disruption of integrity of sertoli-germ cell junctions. Journal of Reproduction and Development. 2012;58:544–51.

[43] Cheng CY, Silvestrini B, Grima J, Mo MY, Zhu LJ, Johansson E, Saso L, Leone MG, Palmery M, Mruk D. Two new male contraceptives exert their effects by depleting germ cells prematurely from the testis. Biology of Reproduction. 2001;65:449–61.

[44] Cheng CY, Mruk DD. Cell junction dynamics in the testis: Sertoli-germ cell interactions and male contraceptive development. Physiological Reviews. 2002;82:825–74. DOI: 10.1152/physrev.00009.2002

[45] Naso MF, Morgan JL, Buchberg AM, Siracusa LD, Iozzo RV. Expression pattern and mapping of the murine versican gene (Cspg2) to chromosome 13. Genomics. 1995;29:297–300. DOI: 10.1006/geno.1995.1251

[46] Hellquist A, Zucchelli M, Lindgren CM, Saarialho-Kere U, Jarvinen TM, Koskenmies S, Julkunen H, Onkamo P, Skoog T, Panelius J, Raisanen-Sokolowski A, Hasan T, Widen

E, Gunnarson I, Svenungsson E, Padyukov L, Assadi G, Berglind L, Makela VV, Kivinen K, Wong A, Cunningham Graham DS, Vyse TJ, D'Amato M, Kere J. Identification of MAMDC1 as a candidate susceptibility gene for systemic lupus erythematosus (SLE). PLoS One. 2009;4:e8037. DOI: 10.1371/journal.pone.0008037

[47] Aslam A, Mittal S, Koch F, Andrau JC, Winkler GS. The Ccr4-NOT deadenylase subunits CNOT7 and CNOT8 have overlapping roles and modulate cell proliferation. Molecular Biology of the Cell. 2009;(20):3840–50. DOI: 10.1091/mbc.E09-02-0146

[48] Mruk DD, Cheng CY. Testin and actin are key molecular targets of adjudin, an anti-spermatogenic agent, in the testis. Spermatogenesis. 2011;1:137–46. DOI: 10.4161/spmg.1.2.16449

[49] Molden RC, Goya J, Khan Z, Garcia BA. Stable isotope labeling of phosphoproteins for large-scale phosphorylation rate determination. Molecular & Cellular Proteomics. 2014;13:1106–18. DOI: 10.1074/mcp.O113.036145

Section 3

Viro-Immunological Background of Human Herpesvirus Pathogenesis

Chapter 5

Immune Evasion by Herpes Simplex Viruses

Angello R. Retamal-Díaz, Eduardo Tognarelli,
Alexis M. Kalergis, Susan M. Bueno and
Pablo A. González

Additional information is available at the end of the chapter

http://dx.doi.org/10.5772/64128

Abstract

Infection with herpes simplex viruses type 1 (HSV-1) and type 2 (HSV-2) is extremely frequent in the human population, as well as recurrent reactivations due to lifelong infection. Infection and persistence of HSVs within healthy individuals likely results as a consequence of numerous molecular determinants evolved by these pathogens to escape both immediate and long-term host antiviral mechanisms. Indeed, HSVs harbor an arsenal of proteins that confer them stealth by negatively modulating immune function. Consequently, these viruses perpetuate within the host, altogether silently shedding onto other individuals. In this chapter, we discuss HSV determinants that interfere with cellular antiviral factors, as well as viral determinants that hamper innate and adaptive immune components intended to control such microbes. The identification of HSV evasion molecules that modulate the immune system, as well as the understanding of their mechanisms of action, should facilitate the design of novel prophylactic and therapeutic strategies to overcome infection and disease elicited by these viruses. This chapter is intended to provide an overview of the evasion mechanisms evolved by herpes simplex viruses to escape numerous host antiviral mediators.

Keywords: immune evasion, innate immunity, adaptive immunity, antiviral response

1. Introduction

Herpes simplex viruses (HSVs, HSV-1 and HSV-2) are extremely prevalent in the human population with virtually half of the world inhabitants infected with HSV-1 [1] and nearly 500 million with HSV-2 [2]. Novel infections with HSVs are estimated at a rate of dozens of millions individuals per year [3]. Importantly, the prevalence of HSV infection significantly varies depending on the geographical location of individuals, sex, and ethnicity [3–7]. While primary HSV-1 infection is well known for its pathological effects in the oro-facial area, where it mainly produces lesions in the mouth, it is also responsible for most cases of infectious blindness in developed countries [8–21]. On the other hand, HSV-2 is widely recognized as an important contributor to neonatal encephalitis and, most importantly, the main cause of genital ulcers in the world [8–21]. Nevertheless, despite this latter association between HSV-2 and genital infection, HSV-1 is at present the main cause of primary genital infection [9, 12]. This apparent paradox may be explained by the fact that HSV-2 recurs significantly more frequently in the genitalia than HSV-1, while the opposite occurs for the oro-facial area [22]. Such differences may be accounted by disparities in the capacity of each of these viruses to establish latency in the sacral and trigeminal ganglia [23], although another study proposes that this is not the case [24]. Regardless of differences in neuron infection or reactivation capacity from these sites, overall HSV-2 is isolated more frequently than HSV-1 in the genitalia during the lifespan of an individual [23]. Importantly, HSV-2 is considered at present a meaningful contributor to the fueling of human immunodeficiency virus (HIV) infection in the world, and is discussed in detail below [22, 25–27].

Besides viral encephalitis in neonates, as well as oro-facial and genital lesions, HSV-1 and HSV-2 are also responsible for numerous other diseases in humans, such as adult encephalitis, herpetic keratitis, conjunctivitis, and skin lesions, within many other clinical manifestations [4]. The variety of pathologies produced by HSVs and tissues affected may be due, at least partially, to the wide distribution of their receptors, which are virtually present on all cells of the body [28]. Noteworthy, such clinical outcomes can occur indistinguishably both in immunocompetent and immunocompromised individuals and are likely a result of the evolution and selection of HSV determinants that interfere with early antiviral cellular mechanisms, innate- and adaptive-immune components. Noteworthy, HSV genomes encode numerous gene products (at least 70), which likely warrants these microbes a collection of proteins with immune evasion properties [29]. Below, we discuss several of these viral determinants, as well as how they interfere with host antiviral processes.

2. Herpes simplex viruses escape early antiviral responses

2.1. Interference with host pathogen recognition receptors

Upon encounter with foreign molecules or danger elements, host immune and nonimmune cells may sense such stimuli and initiate intracellular-activating signaling pathways that lead to their alertness and that of surrounding cells. Importantly, complex host organisms have evolved as specialized receptors for recognizing these microbial elements or self-induced danger molecules during abnormal processes elicited by these microbes. Such receptors are usually termed pattern recognition receptors (PRRs) [30]. PRRs can recognize pathogen-associated molecular patterns (PAMPs), which consist on a diverse collection of biomolecules derived from microbial elements, such as proteins, lipids, carbohydrates, or particular arrangements or sequences of nucleic acids, within others [31]. Alternatively, these receptors

http://dx.doi.org/10.5772/64128

can also detect danger signals released by host cells undergoing stress circumstances, such as those that might be elicited by virus replication. These latter danger signals are termed damage-associated molecular patterns (DAMPs) [32]. Upon engaging PAMPs and DAMPs, PRRs elicit intracellular signals that result in the transcription and translation of antiviral genes, as well as the expression of soluble and membrane-bound molecules. Timely and robust detection of PAMPs and DAMPs by the host after viral infection can lead to effective microbe control and promote the establishment of protective immunity [31, 33].

Upon exposure to HSVs, the main host cells susceptible to infection are likely live epithelial cells. These cells are largely present at the interphase with the exterior world and abundantly present in the mucosae and to a lesser extent, in microscopic skin lesions. As most nonimmune cells in the organism, these cells express the main HSV receptor, nectin-1 [28]. After attaching and binding to their receptors, the membranes of these viruses undergo a fusion process with that of the host cell to release the viral capsid and surrounding tegument proteins within the cytoplasm [34]. While the tegument proteins remain in the cytoplasm, where they exert numerous cellular modulatory effects, the capsid associates to microtubules and travels to the outer nuclear membrane, where it binds to host nuclear pore proteins and releases the viral DNA into the nucleus [35]. It has been described that at this stage host molecular sensors can sense HSV-2 determinants (**Table 1**). Interferon-gamma inducible-16 (IFI-16) detects the HSV genome and subsequently induce IL-6 and IFN-α production in primary vaginal epithelial cells [36–38]. On the other hand, the cyclic guanosine monophosphate-adenosine monophosphate (cGAMP) synthase (cGAS), a recently described DNA sensor, has also been reported to detect HSV-derived nucleic acids and lead to IFN-α and IFN-β secretion by both immune cells, such as macrophages and dendritic cells (DCs), and nonimmune cells, such as fibroblasts [39]. Importantly, animals that lack cGAS are vulnerable to HSV, while functional cGAS leads to T-cell activation and antibody production by B cells [40]. Although HSVs seem to be unable to interfere with cGAS sensing, other herpesviruses (gammaherpesviruses) have been recently described to encode viral determinants that impair the function of this molecule, namely, ORF52 of Kaposi's sarcoma herpesvirus [41]. Interestingly, a recent study suggests that IFI16 and cGAS work cooperatively to sense HSV, as silencing one or both proteins significantly decreases virus detection. More specifically, cGAS was shown to directly interact with IFI-16 in fibroblasts and to promote the stability of the latter [39]. Noteworthy, both sensors IFI-16 and cGAS signal intracellularly through interferon regulatory factor-3 (IRF3) and again silencing either sensor inhibits the activation of IRF3 in response to HSV DNA [42]. Further, the importance of IFI-16 in limiting HSV infection has been recently shown *in vivo*. Knocking down IFI-16 led to the loss of IFN-α production, as well as reduced viral control in the corneal epithelium [38]. While the mechanism by which IFI-16 recognizes HSV DNA remains somewhat unclear, a recent study using chromatin immunoprecipitation (ChIP) found that IFI-16 binds to HSV promoter sequences and that reducing the levels of IFI-16 expression resulted in host proteins binding to these elements, ultimately favoring viral gene transcription [43].

Host sensor	Viral determinant involved	Outcome	Mechanism	References
IFI-16	Nuclear virus DNA	HSV sensed. IL-6, IFN-α secretion	IFI-16 binds to viral promoters	[36–38, 43]
cGAS	Nuclear virus DNA	HSV sensed. IFN-α, IFN-β secretion	cGAS binds directly to B-DNA	[39]
DAI	Cytosolic virus DNA	HSV sensed. IL-6, IFN-β secretion	DAI binds directly to B-DNA	[36]
MDA5	vhs	Unable to sense viral nucleic acids	vhs protein reduces host protein expression	[44, 45]
RIG-1	vhs	Unable to sense viral nucleic acids	vhs protein reduces host protein expression	[44, 45]
TLR-9	Cytosolic virus DNA	HSV sensed. IL-6, IL-12, type-I IFN secretion	Undetermined	[36, 46]
PKR	γ34.5 and U_S11	Impaired viral dsRNA recognition	Viral proteins block eIF2-α phosphorylation	[53–57]
TLR7	Undetermined	HSV sensed	Undetermined	[58]
TLR3	Virus or virus-induced host nucleic acids	HSV sensed. IL-6, TNF-α secretion	TLR-3 signals through IRF3	[63–65]
$\alpha v\beta 3$	ICP0	Inhibited detection of viral proteins	ICP0 blocks type-I IFN transcription and virus targeting to degradation	[74–76]
TLR2	dUTPase	HSV sensed. IL-6, IL-8, IL-10, IL-12, and TNF-α secretion	Undetermined	[77]
Inflamm–asome	ICP0	ICP0 reduces IL-1β secretion	Inflammasome directed to proteasome degradation in timely manner	[32, 43]

IFI-16 (gamma-interferon-inducible protein); cGAS (cyclic GMP-AMP synthase); DAI (DNA-dependent activator of Interferon-regulatory factor); MDA5 (melanoma differentiation-associated protein 5); vhs (virion host shutoff protein); RIG-1 (retinoic acid-inducible gene 1); TLR-2, -7, -9 (Toll-like receptor-2, -7 and -9); PKR (protein kinase RNA-activated); $\alpha v\beta 3$ (integrin alphaVbeta3); γ34.5 (late gene gamma 34.5, ICP34.5); U_S11 (short unique region 11); IRF3 (interferon regulatory factor 3); ICP0 (infected cell protein 0); IL-1β, -6, -8, -10,-12 (interleukin-1β, -6, -8, -10, and, -12); IFN-α/β (interferon alpha and beta); TNF-α (tumor necrosis factor-alpha).

Table 1. HSV evasion of host virus sensing.

Another host DNA sensor capable of detecting HSV genetic material is DNA-dependent activator of interferon (DAI), which is expressed in primary vaginal epithelial cells and leads to cytokine expression by these cells, such as IL-6 and IFN-β after virus exposure (**Table 1**) [36]. Surprisingly, DAI is expressed in the cytoplasm, suggesting that HSV DNA likely escapes or leaks from the nucleus, or capsids into the cytoplasm where it reaches this sensor.

Other nucleic acid detectors intended to perceive microbe-derived genetic material are retinoic acid-inducible gene-1 (RIG-I) and melanoma differentiation-associated protein-5 (MDA5) (**Table 1**) [44]. Unlike the other DNA sensors discussed above, the functions of RIG-I and MDA5 are hampered by HSV, namely, by the viral protein designated virion host shutoff protein (vhs). The vhs has been shown to specifically reduce the expression RIG-I and MDA5, as a mechanism to interfere with downstream signaling events carried out by these detectors, which are intended to alert neighboring and immune cells when viral elements are present (**Table 1**) [45]. Similar to DAI, RIG-I and MDA5 are also present in the cytoplasm of cells, which indicates that HSV DNA likely reaches this compartment during the infectious cycle [36].

Another PRR that also recognizes viral DNA is Toll-like receptor-9 (TLR9), which is mainly known for its role in sensing bacterial-derived nucleic acids, namely, CpG-oligodeoxynucleotides (CpG ODNs). TLR9, which is expressed both by immune and nonimmune cells, has been shown to detect HSV elements and produce IL-6, IL-12, and type-I IFN, within others (**Table 1**) [36, 46]. Although TLR9 is capable of sensing HSV, its function seems nonessential for animal survival upon viral challenge. Indeed, TLR9 knockout mice survive central nervous system (CNS) infection, although they do display increased viral loads in the brain, when compared to wild-type mice [47]. Remarkably, animals treated with TLR9 agonists, such as CpG ODNs previous to infection, display significantly reduced viral loads and inflammatory cytokines in the brain (CCL2, IL-6, and CCL5) [48]. A similar protective effect has been observed for CpG ODNs in mice that were treated locally with such stimulators and then challenged in the genitalia with HSV [49–52]. These results suggest that engaging TLR9 receptors, or promoting their signaling pathways may be a promising strategy for preventing HSV burden in the host.

Although the genomes of HSVs are composed of DNA, these viruses produce viral RNA molecules during their infectious cycles that are generated as a consequence of transcription. These RNA molecules are then processed into mRNAs and miRNAs that may form tridimensional structures, which could be recognized by host sensors. One such sensor is host protein kinase R (PKR), which can detect double-stranded RNA molecules and mediate downstream signaling events that lead to limited virus replication by favoring NF-kB activation and cytokine release, while altogether inhibiting protein synthesis through the phosphorylation of the host translation initiation factor 2-alpha (eIF2α), which ultimately can promote cell death (apoptosis) [53]. To date, numerous studies have demonstrated that HSV can indeed interfere with PKR function both *in vitro* and *in vivo* in such a way to promote their infectious cycles (**Table 1**) [54, 55]. Furthermore, interference with the capacity of PKR to phosphorylate eIF2α has been shown to be mediated by the HSV proteins γ34.5 and U_S11, which allows viral protein synthesis to occur efficiently within infected cells [56, 57].

Another nucleic acid-sensing molecule capable of recognizing double-stranded RNA species produced during viral infection is TLR7, although to date this particular receptor has not been described to sense any particular form of nucleic acid generated during HSV infection (**Table 1**). Nevertheless, some studies report that the application of TLR7 agonists, such as imiquimod to experimental animals can significantly decrease HSV infection and disease after virus challenge [58]. Such findings have led to the assessment of imiquimod as a therapeutic approach to treat HSV infection in humans, particularly for combating HSV isolates that are resistant to acyclovir, which are commonly found in immunocompromised patients [59–61]. For example, a recent report described successful treatment of hypertrophic genital herpes in a HIV-positive patient after using 5% imiquimod applied in a topical manner after repeated failure to resolve the symptoms in the patient with oral and intravenous antivirals [62]. Although the results obtained till date on this type of approach have been promising, the mechanism of action of imiquimod over HSV remains unclear, as both interferon-dependent and interferon-independent mechanisms seem to play favorable roles against viral infection, which may further be mediated by processes that are independent of TLR engagement [60].

Lastly, another host nucleic acid sensor is TLR3, which is mainly known to recognize double-stranded RNA [63]. Importantly, TLR3 has been reported to play relevant roles in HSV disease, although its participation during infection has mainly been inferred by its deficiency (**Table 1**). For instance, $TLR3^{-/-}$ mice display severe HSV burden within the CNS after infection, which is thought to be mediated by astrocyte infection. Indeed, the expression of TLR3 in such cells increases the control of HSV infection early after virus entry into the CNS, seemingly by inducing type-I IFN responses [64]. Such interferon response would be mediated by TLR3-induced NF-kB activation in astrocytes and a posterior increase in the expression of IL-6 and TNF-α, which likely play antiviral functions in this tissue [65]. A relevant role for TLR3 in humans was initially proposed for infants, but has now extended onto adults thanks to recent studies performed on individuals that carry mutations in this receptor that negatively modulate its function. For instance, individuals harboring mutations in TLR3 have been reported to display a history of HSV encephalitis [66–69]. Additionally, a direct relationship between downstream TLR3 signaling, TLR3 defects, and virus burden in astrocytes has been shown with *ex vivo* differentiated neurons, astrocytes, and oligodendrocytes obtained from patients that display TLR3 deficiencies. Cell cultures derived from these individuals and infected with HSV show reduced virus control *in vitro*, as compared to cells obtained from controls, which secreted more interferon [70]. Furthermore, HSV-susceptible individuals have also been reported to display mutations in proteins that are involved in the downstream signaling of TLR3, such as in IRF3 [69, 71, 72]. As with TLR9 and TLR7, agonists for TLR3 such as polyI:C have also been shown to reduce viral burden when applied in the genitalia or intraperitoneally previous to a genital challenge with HSV [73]. Overall, these results highlight an important role for TLR3 in HSV encephalitis, altogether proposing potential new treatment alternatives for reducing HSV burden in the brain and other tissues.

While HSV-derived nucleic acids are perceived by numerous host sensors in infected cells, relatively few HSV proteins have been described to be detected by the host (**Table 1**). Integrin $\alpha v\beta 3$, which has seldom been recognized as a PRR was recently described as a sensor for HSV, which is negatively modulated by these viruses. Furthermore, the HSV protein ICP0 has been proposed to be responsible for blocking the signaling events triggered by integrin $\alpha v\beta 3$ within infected cells, which otherwise would lead to NF-kB activation, type-I IFN transcription, and the direction of virus particles to cholesterol-rich microdomains that are targeted for degradation [74–76].

An HSV protein that is successfully detected by host sensors is the viral dUTPase, which has been shown to be sensed by TLR2 in DCs and leads to IL-6, IL-8, IL-10, IL-12, and TNF-α

secretion (**Table 1**) [77]. Interestingly, TLR2 has also been reported to recognize other HSV elements, with partial modulation by TLR9 [78]. Noteworthy, experiments performed with TLR2$^{-/-}$ knockout mice showed that these animals displayed increased survival rates, as compared to wild-type animals after challenge with HSV, which suggests a potentially negative role for this receptor in disease severity. Yet the knockout animals had similar levels of viral loads in their tissues, as control animals [79]. Remarkably, microglia cells obtained from TLR2$^{-/-}$ mice have been shown to produce reduced levels of reactive oxygen species (ROS) after HSV infection, when compared to control cultures, which might result in decreased cellular oxidative toxicity to neurons and positively impact on their viability [80].

The inflammasome is a host multiprotein complex harboring the cytoplasmatic sensors NLRP3, AIM2, and IFI-16, which has been described to sense HSV constituents, although its activation is negatively modulated during infection (**Table 1**) [32]. While IFI-16 and NLRP3 are activated early after HSV infection with consequent IL-1β release, at later time points IFI-16 has been reported to be directed to the proteasome by the viral protein ICP0 [32, 43]. This observation implies that the overall function of this sensor complex is likely hampered by HSV and thus limited at properly alerting other cells of an ongoing viral infection.

Taken together, HSVs seem to be sensed by host cells mainly at the nucleic acid level rather than protein level. This observation is quite surprising considering that HSVs encode numerous gene products within their genomes (>70 ORFs) and at least 11 surface glycoproteins. This stealth attribute might be explained within others by the ability of these viruses to interfere with downstream signaling events mediated by PRRs, as discussed in detail below. Additionally, their apparent invisibility might also be a consequence of the viruses' capacity to interfere with host translation of mRNA transcripts that encode soluble and membrane-bound mediators required for cell alertness after infection and also communicating infection onto other cells. Indeed, the HSV-1 and HSV-2 vhs proteins efficiently inhibit the translation of host mRNAs by promoting their degradation directly through their ribonuclease activity [81]. Importantly, increased degradation of host transcripts over viral mRNAs would be mediated by the spatial-temporal regulation of vhs expression in infected cells, as vhs proteins are delivered together with the tegument immediately after infection, then poorly expressed during viral replication and then abundantly produced immediately before virus packaging and exit [82]. More recently, vhs proteins have been reported to interfere with stress granule formation within infected cells, thus counteracting host antiviral stress responses that are usually elicited early after infection [83].

2.2. Negative modulation of interferon pathways

An effective mechanism by which host cells restrict viral replication is due to interferons, soluble proteins, that induce antiviral responses both in cells that secrete these mediators as well as neighboring cells [84]. While type-I interferons (IFN-α, IFN-β, and IFN-ε, within others) are usually secreted early after microbe infection by diverse cell types, type-II interferons (IFN-γ) are secreted by specific subsets of immune cells at later stages of infection. On the other hand, type-III interferons (IFN-λ1, IFN-λ2, and IFN-λ3) have similar effects and kinetics than type-I IFNs, although they are mostly restricted to epithelial cells [63, 85–89]. While type-I and type-III IFNs induce multiple antiviral effects in most host cells, type-II IFNs play more regulatory roles, mainly in immune cells.

Target host molecule	Viral determinant	Outcome	Mechanism	References
IRF3 function	ICP0	Inhibits type-I IFN expression	ICP0 RING finger motif inhibits IRF3-mediated transcription of interferon stimulating genes	[90, 91]
	U_s3	Decreases IFN-β production	Viral Ser/Thr kinase activity hyperphosphorylates IRF3, blocking its dimerization and nuclear translocation	[92]
	U_L36	Inhibits IFN-β transcription	U_L36 de-ubiquitinates TRAF3, which inhibits stimuli induced dimerization of IRF3	[94]
IRF3, NF-kB	VP16	Inhibits IFN-β expression	Inhibits NF-kB activation and blocks the recruitment of IRF3 co-activator CBP	[93]
STAT-1 function	ICP27	Neutralizes expression of IFN-I	Interferes with nuclear accumulation of STAT-1, impairing with the activity of this transcription factor	[96]
STAT-2 function	Undetermined, vhs (partially)	Interferes with IFN-I signaling	Partially attributed to vhs-mediated reduction of transcription factor activity	[97, 98]
Jak-1 function	Undetermined, vhs (partially)	Interferes with IFN-I signaling	Partially attributed to vhs-mediated reduction of transcription factor activity	[97, 98]
IFN-ε, IFN-α	Undetermined	Reduces viral dissemination and reactivation	Activates TLR signaling through unknown viral agonist	[99–102]
IL-29 function	Undetermined	Induces IFN-β expression. Prevents keratinocyte and neural infection	Unknown viral antigen activation of TLR3 and Jak-STAT signaling	[104]
IL-28A function	Undetermined	Prevents neural infection	Unknown viral antigen. TLR-mediated activation of IRF7	[105]

IRF3 (interferon regulatory factor 3); NF-kB (nuclear factor kappa-light-chain-enhancer of activated B cells); STAT-1, -2 (signal transducer and activator of transcription-1, -2); Jak-1 (Janus kinase 1); IFN-ε, IFN-α (interferon-epsilon, -alpha); IL-28A, -29 (interleukin-28A, -29); U_L36 (long unique region 36); VP16 (viral protein 16); ICP27 (infected cell protein 27); TRAF3 (TNF receptor-associated factor 3); CBP (CREB-binding protein).

Table 2. HSV interference with host intracellular signaling.

HSVs encode numerous virulence factors that negatively modulate the induction of host interferon responses and their effects, some of which were briefly discussed above (**Table 2**).

For instance, HSVs interfere with PRR-mediated intracellular signaling events that otherwise would lead to the transcription of IFN-I. Such effect has been reported to be mediated by HSV proteins such as ICP0, which interferes with IRF3 to block the transcription of target genes, namely, type-I IFNs [90, 91]. On the other hand, the HSV Ser/Thr kinase U_S3 has also been shown to interfere with signaling mediated by this transcription factor by carrying out its hyperphosphorylation, which blocks its dimerization, nuclear translocation, and hampers IFN-β production [92]. Additionally, the tegument protein VP16 has also been described to abrogate IFN-β expression by inhibiting IRF3 and NF-kB activation, specifically by impairing the recruitment of the coactivator CBP (CREB binding protein) and not necessarily through a mechanism that affects IRF3 dimerization, nuclear translocation, or its DNA binding activity [93]. Finally, IFN-β transcription has also been reported to be inhibited by the viral ubiquitin-specific protease U_L36, which de-ubiquitinates TRAF3 (TNF receptor-associated factor-3) and consequently inhibits stimuli-induced IRF3 dimerization [94]. Interference with signaling events that lead to type-I IFN secretion has also been evidenced *in vivo* by the observation that only reduced amounts of IFN-*α* and IFN-β are produced in the genital tract after HSV infection [90, 95]. Negative modulation of the interferon pathway is summarized in **Table 2**.

Although small amounts of type-I IFNs are produced during HSV infection, the effects of these meager amounts of interferons are neutralized by HSVs, thanks to the activity of the viral protein ICP27, which interferes with STAT signaling (signal transducer and activator of transcription), which is located downstream of IFN-I receptors. Indeed, HSV ICP27 interfere with nuclear accumulation of STAT-1 and impair the function of this transcription factor [96]. Additionally, other transducers of IFN-I signaling, such as STAT-2 and JAK1 (Janus Kinase), have also been reported to be reduced in HSV-infected cells and experiments with mutant viruses suggest that these effects would be mediated, at least partially by virally encoded vhs [97]. Additional viral and nonviral determinants released by HSV-infected cells have been suggested to interfere with IFN-I signaling, although their nature has not been fully characterized [98]. Although IFN-ε signals through similar receptors than IFN-α and IFN-β, this recently described mediator is constitutively expressed by epithelial cells in the genitalia and would likely play a role against HSV burden [99–101]. However, the mechanism by which IFN-ε would limit HSV infection remains to be determined. Consistent with an important role for type-I IFNs in response to HSV infection, treatments with TLR agonists, such as imiquimod, poly(I:C), or CpG-ODNs, discussed above all induce strong interferon responses [51, 52, 58–61, 73]. Additionally, application of topical IFN-*α* has been shown to significantly reduce viral dissemination, as well as the frequency of viral recurrences in HSV-infected patients that manifest frequent genital viral reactivations [102]. The role of IFN-I in HSV infection is also evidenced in experiments assessing mice that lack the receptor for this molecule (IFNAR1 and IFNAR2c), which were inoculated in the footpads with the virus. These animals displayed reduced HSV control and systemic infection that affected multiple organs, although the disease was nonlethal [103].

At present, several studies seem to have identified a favorable role for type-II IFNs in HSV infection, as discussed in the following sections. Yet surprisingly, one study that evaluated infection in mice that had the IFN-II receptor deleted (IFNGR1 and IFNGR2) showed that these animals had comparable levels of virus than wild-type controls [103].

Unlike type-I IFNs, relatively few reports have documented a role for type-III IFNs in HSV infection. One such study has reported that IFN-λ1 (IL-29) induces the expression of several antiviral proteins in human keratinocytes. Furthermore, administration of this cytokine, previous to HSV infection induced IFN-β and prevented keratinocyte infection upon HSV challenge. Notably, the effect of this interferon depended on TLR3 expression, which was upregulated, and JAK-STAT activation [104]. Additionally, IFN-λ1 and IFN-λ2 (IL-28A) have also been reported to suppress HSV infection in human neurons (**Table 2**). Again, IFN-III was shown to induce TLR expression and elicit TLR-mediated antiviral pathways that involved IRF7 [105]. Noteworthy, the secretion of type-III IFNs in the vaginal mucosa has been suggested to be mainly mediated by DCs, although this has not been evaluated yet in the context of an HSV infection [106].

Taken together, HSVs have evolved multiple mechanisms to interfere with host interferon responses, from IFN transcription to IFN signaling. These evasion mechanisms, largely redundant, highlight the importance of this type of response in limiting HSV infection. Indeed, novel therapeutic strategies seem to share in common the induction of type-I IFNs, which should facilitate the identification of novel formulations that provide beneficial effects against these viruses.

2.3. HSV modulation of cell viability

Viruses utilize cells as substrates for replication and require, within others their translation machinery for synthesizing their proteins. Maximization of virion production is favored by extended cell survival and thus viruses have evolved molecular mechanisms to inhibit cell apoptosis. As discussed above, interference with programed cell death is achieved in part by the blockage of virus detection, but also thanks to viral determinants that directly hamper this cellular antiviral function. Cellular apoptosis can be mediated by two major pathways triggered either by intrinsic or extrinsic stimuli [107]. While the intrinsic pathway can be initiated by intracellular events that alter the redox state of the cells, damage the host DNA, or compromise mitochondrial integrity, within others, the extrinsic pathway can be elicited by the engagement of surface receptors, such as Fas [107]. HSVs have evolved molecular determinants that block both, intrinsic and extrinsic apoptosis signaling pathways in infected cells (**Table 3**). For instance, inhibition of apoptosis has been described to be mediated by the viral proteins U_S3, U_S5, and U_S12, each with unique inhibitory effects over the viability of the infected cells, either confronted or not to cytotoxic T cells [108]. More specifically, the HSV protein U_S3 has recently been described to mediate its antiapoptotic effects in epithelial cells, by interacting with programmed cell death protein 4 (PDCD4) and retaining it within the nucleus of infected cells [109]. HSV ICP10PK and U_L14 would also harbor antiapoptotic effects in neurons and epithelial cells, although the mechanisms mediating these effects remain unknown [110, 111].

On the other hand, inhibition of apoptosis in HSV-infected cells by the extrinsic pathway has been suggested to occur by the sequestering of Fas ligand, which consequently would hamper Fas/FasL (CD95/CD95L) engagement, and thus block the capacity of T cells to mediate the killing of target cells [112]. Additionally, a recent study found that although some HSV-infected cells express Fas on their surface, HSVs can block Fas-mediated apoptosis by a mechanism that is independent of viral activation of NF-kB, as this transcription factor could be detected within the nucleus of infected cells [113]. Consistent with altered Fas/FasL function in HSV-infected cells, therapeutic application of soluble Fas ligand has been reported to ameliorate acute and recurrent herpetic stromal keratitis (HSK) in mice, by reducing inflammatory infiltration into the eye and decreasing eye neovascularization in primary and recurrent forms of HSK [114]. Interestingly, HSV glycoproteins gJ and gD have been proposed to mediate, at least partially the inhibition of Fas-mediated apoptosis [115, 116]. Paradoxically, gJ induces ROS within cells, which could trigger intrinsic pro-apoptotic stimuli. On the other hand, HSVs have been recently described to be able to suppress necroptosis in human cells as a mechanism to extend cell viability [117]. The viral proteins ICP6 and ICP10 have been recently described as the viral determinants that block necroptosis elicited by TNF in human cells [117]. The effects of HSV determinants over cell viability are summarized in **Table 3**.

Cell type	Viral determinant	Outcome	Mechanism	References
Epithelial	U_S3	Prevents apoptosis	Acts retaining PDCD4 within the nucleus	[108, 109]
Fibroblast	U_s5	Prevents apoptosis	Unclear. Inhibition of caspase 3 activation	[108]
Fibroblast	U_s12	Prevents physiologic and CTL-induced apoptosis	Unclear. Inhibition of caspase 3 activation	[108]
Epithelial and neuronal	ICP10PK and U_L14	Prevents apoptosis	Unknown	[110, 111]
Neuronal	gD and gJ	Prevents apoptosis	Inhibits Fas-mediated pathway	[115, 116]
Neuronal	LAT	Prevents cold shock-induced apoptosis	Maintains high levels of phosphorylated AKT in cells	[125]
Epithelial	ICP6 and ICP10PK	Prevents necroptosis	Blocks cell death elicited by TNF	[117]
Dendritic cell	Undetermined	Induces cell death-related processes	Unclear	[118–120]
Natural killer	Undetermined	Induces apoptosis	Induction of Fas/FasL through infected macrophage expression	[121]
Fibroblast	ICP6	Induces necroptosis	Interacts with host RIP-3	[122]

U_S3, 5, 12 (short unique region 3, 5, 12); ICP10PK (ICP10 serine-threonine protein kinase); U_L14 (long unique region 14); gD, gJ (glycoprotein D, J); LAT (latency-associated transcript); AKT (protein kinase B); ICP6, 10 (infected cell protein 6, 10); CTL (cytotoxic T lymphocyte); PDCD4 (programmed cell death protein 4); RIP-3 (receptor-interacting protein kinase 3); TNF-α (tumor necrosis factor-alpha).

Table 3. HSV modulation of cell death.

Contrarily to the observations discussed above, other studies have reported proapoptotic effects for HSV proteins, as well as pronecrotic effects. For instance, infection of murine and human dendritic cells with HSV induces apoptosis, but after the virus has negatively modulated some of their properties ([118–120] and below). Additionally, HSV has also been described to induce apoptosis in natural killer cell (NK cells) upon their interaction with infected macrophages that express Fas/FasL [121]. On the other hand, HSVs have been described to induce necroptosis in mouse fibroblasts through the direct interaction of viral ICP6 with host RIP3 (receptor-interacting kinase 3) [122]. Importantly, an HSV virus with ICP6 deleted was unable to produce necrosis in HSV-infected cells and $RIP3^{-/-}$ mice displayed compromised control of HSV pathogenesis and replication [123].

Importantly, several reports have described that neuron infection with HSV does not lead to cell death, but rather extends their life. Indeed, lower levels of caspase-3 transcripts have been found in HSV-positive, rather than HSV-negative trigeminal ganglia and neurons [124]. Furthermore, HSV determinants such as the latency-associated transcript (LAT), which is mainly expressed within infected neurons has been reported to protect cells from cold-shock-induced apoptosis by maintaining high levels of phosphorylated protein kinase AKT within the cells [125].

Taken together, these studies highlight unique properties of HSV in their capacity to modulate cell viability in a cell-specific manner. While the viability of nonimmune cells that serve as a substrate for virus replication is extended by antiapoptotic viral determinants, immune cells are targeted for death in such a way to evade the immune system. Noteworthy, neurons which act as reservoirs for the virus are maintained viable during infection.

2.4. Soluble mediators secreted shortly after HSV infection

Despite the capacity of HSV to limit the cell's capacity to sense viral components or transduce activating signals after virus detection, which otherwise could lead to optimal antiviral responses, cells infected with HSV nevertheless secrete numerous cytokines upon infection. Secretion of these cytokines might be promoted by host sensors that effectively detect HSV determinants or alternatively might result from virus-oriented immune modulation intended to promote infection and persistence [32]. Thus, to date it is unclear whether soluble mediators secreted by HSV-infected cells either contributes to virus control and spread or promotes the virus' life cycle within the host.

Signaling events that lead to the secretion of soluble mediators after microbe or danger signal detection is frequently mediated by the nuclear factor NF-kB, which translocates from the cytoplasm to the nucleus to promote gene transcription [126]. Because of the importance of NF-kB in this process, HSV encode several determinants to dampen the activity of this transcription factor. For instance, the HSV U_S3 kinase has been reported to hyperphosphorylate NF-kB (p65) and impairs its translocation to the nucleus, interfering with IL-8 secretion [127]. On the other hand, the HSV U_L42 protein, which encodes for a DNA polymerase processivity factor, also binds to p65/RelA and to p50/NF-kB1 (NF-kB1 forms) to negatively modulate their migration into the nucleus after stimulation with TNF-α [128]. HSV ICP0 has also been described to inhibit NF-kB activation mediated by TNF-α, by interacting similarly with p65/

http://dx.doi.org/10.5772/64128

RelA and p50/NF-kB1 [129]. HSV VP16 similarly has been shown to interfere with NF-kB activation in human endothelial kidney cells [93]. Paradoxically, other studies have proposed that HSV infection can induce persistent NF-kB nuclear translocation, although without concomitant transactivation activity and in epithelial cells from the retina (retinoblastoma) [130, 131]. Importantly, blocking NF-kB nuclear translocation in these cells significantly reduced virus yield. Altogether, these studies demonstrate significant modulation of this important transcription factor by HSV determinants, which may result in different cellular outcomes depending on the cell type infected.

Although HSV negatively modulates NF-kB activation, HSV-infected cells can produce numerous soluble mediators. For instance, primary endometrial genital epithelial cells infected with HSV produce CCL2, IL-8, IL-6, and TNF-α [132]. On the other hand, samples from the cervical mucus of women infected with HSV show elevated amounts of CXCL9 [133]. The latter chemokine together with CXCL10 have been shown to participate in antiviral responses against HSV in CNS infection in the mouse model by recruiting NK and cytotoxic T cells to the infected tissue [134]. Other chemokines, such as CCL2, which are promoted by HSV infection, may play positive roles against the virus in ocular infection, as shown in mice; CCL2 knockout mice displayed significant viral infection and reduced inflammatory monocyte recruitment into the affected tissue [135]. On the contrary, blocking specific chemokines such as CXCL2 which is released by monocytes in response to HSV is thought to bring neutrophils into the infection site, which would promote unwanted damaging responses to the host, particularly neurons [136].

HSV also induces IL-6 in numerous cell types after infection, such as microglia, mast cells, and dendritic cells. Importantly, this cytokine shows protective effects in microglia, which seems to be mediated by STAT3; however, the details of the processes that converge toward its protective effects remain unresolved [137, 138]. Mast cells secrete IL-6 early after HSV infection, as well as TNF-α. Interestingly, these soluble mediators are not promoted by HSV directly in this case, but by soluble molecules secreted by keratinocytes infected with HSV [139]. Importantly, animals that lack IL-6 or TNF-α succumb to death after HSV infection, which indicates that these soluble molecules play positive antiviral effects for the host [139]. Nevertheless, other studies propose that this latter cytokine might play a negative role for the host, as treating animals with an anti-TNF-α antibody in combination with the antiviral valacyclovir significantly ameliorated the prognosis of HSV encephalitis [140]. On the other hand, before DCs are killed by HSV, these cells secrete IL-6 and numerous other cytokines [119].

Noteworthy, HSV has also been described to induce the secretion of cytokines and chemokines that could favor host infection by other sexually transmitted microbes, such as the human immunodeficiency virus [141]. Accumulating evidence indicates that infection with HSV-2 can increase host susceptibility up to fourfold to acquiring HIV [142–145]. Additionally, coinfection with these pathogens augments the shedding of both viruses, likely worsening patient prognosis. Importantly, similar findings have been observed in the mouse model with HIV/HSV coinfections [146]. Such increase in the susceptibility of acquiring HIV in HSV-infected individuals would be mediated by numerous factors, such as the increased recruitment, to the infection site of cells that are targeted by HIV [147–149]. Furthermore, cells infected with HSV secrete cytokines that reactivate latent HIV from infected cells [119, 150] and may augment the expression of surface ligands that promote HIV infection [151, 152]. Finally, HSV infection can downmodulate the expression of molecules that favor the neutralization and destruction of HIV [153].

A soluble mediator frequently associated with virus control and clearance is IFN-γ. This innate and adaptive immune cytokine is recurrently associated with increased protection against HSV in numerous HSV infection models and considered an important mediator in the mechanism of action of different prophylactic formulations [154–157]. Importantly, in the absence of IFN-γ, T cells directed against HSV secrete alternative cytokines that are known to possess antiviral functions, yet they are not protective against genital infection [158]. Thus, IFN-γ seemingly plays an important role in eliciting protective immunity against HSV.

Taken together, HSVs elicit the secretion of cytokines and chemokines both by immune and nonimmune cells. Yet, whether these soluble mediators play favorable roles for the host or these viruses remains somewhat unknown and requires further examination. To date, only type-I IFNs and IFN-γ seem to play evident favorable roles against HSV.

3. Herpes simplex viruses interfere with innate immunity

3.1. Interference with complement function

Complement is an acellular component of innate immunity that recognizes foreign elements and subsequently undergoes a series of controlled molecular chain reactions that either culminate with the establishment of a protein pore-forming complex that attacks bilipid membranes or induce receptor-mediated engulfment by cells [159]. Importantly, formation of the pore complex can be promoted either directly by the recognition of microbial molecular patterns on the surface of the virus by complement components, or induced by the Fc portion of antibodies that bind to foreign elements.

To counteract the effect of the complement, HSVs utilize glycoprotein gC, which binds to C3b and blocks its activity by impairing antibody-induced complement activation (**Table 4**) [160, 161]. Inhibition of C3 impairs complement-mediated virus inactivation and the lysis of virus-infected cells. Furthermore, gC also binds to complement component C5 to block its downstream activities, such as immune cell chemoattraction and membrane attack complex formation (**Table 4**) [162, 163].

HSVs have also evolved molecular determinants that bind to complement components required for antibody-mediated complement activation, as discussed below. Thus, by interfering with complement components HSVs increase their viability in the mucosae and sera of infected patients, which favors the infection of target cells.

Innate immune process altered	Viral determinant	Outcome	Mechanism	References
Complement	gC	Inhibits antibody-mediated complement activation	Acts as a receptor for complement component C3b	[160, 161]
Complement	gC	Impairs chemoattraction and membrane attack complex formation	Binds to complement component C5 hampering its catalytic activity and inhibiting downstream events	[162, 163]
Natural killer	gD	Suppresses NK degranulation and cell-mediated lysis of infected cells	CD112 downregulation leading to reduced DNAM-1 activity	[168]
Natural killer	Undetermined	Decreases NK activation	Reduces the surface expression of MICA, ULBP1, ULBP2 and ULBP3	[169–171]
Natural killer	Undetermined	Induces cell apoptosis	Induces Fas/FasL interactions through infected macrophages	[121]
Natural killer T cells	U_S3	Inhibition of antigen presentation to NKT cells	Phosphorylation of KIF3A produces CD1d downregulation in infected cells	[175–177]

gC, gD (glycoprotein C, D); U_S3 (short unique region 3); C3b, C5 (complement component 3b, 5); NK (natural killer cell); CD112 (nectin-2); DNAM-1 (DNAX accessory molecule-1); MICA (MHC class I polypeptide-related sequence A); ULBP1, 2, and 3 (UL16 binding protein 1, 2 and 3); KIF3A (kinesin family member 3); CD1d (antigen-presenting glycoprotein CD1d).

Table 4. Evasion of innate immunity.

3.2. Negative modulation of NK and NKT function

Besides complement, innate immunity is also composed of numerous cells, such as macrophages, neutrophils, mast cells, basophils, eosinophils, and innate lymphoid cells (ILCs), within others. Importantly, HSV modulates the function of some of these cells, notably NK (**Table 4**). NK cells usually play important roles in eliminating infected cells that have lost class I major histocompatibility complex molecules (MHC-I) on their surface, because of microbe interference. Although NK cells can directly sense HSV through TLR2 and have been reported to be activated by plasmacytoid dendritic cells that have contacted HSV, their function is nevertheless dampened by the virus [164–167]. Indeed, gD has been shown to suppress DNAM-1-dependent NK-cell-mediated lysis of HSV-infected cells [168]. Furthermore, HSVs can dampen the surface expression of the NK-activating ligand MICA (MHC class I polypeptide-related sequence A) in infected cells, by retaining this molecule intracellularly [169, 170]. More recent studies have revealed that HSV can also interfere with the expression of additional NK-activating ligands, such as ULBP1, ULBP2, and ULBP3 [171]. Importantly, HSVs can induce apoptosis in NK cells through Fas/FasL interaction between NK cells and HSV-infected macrophages, thus eliciting their deletion upon infection [121]. Although there is abundant evidence for negative modulation of NK cells by HSV, the contribution of these cells to HSV pathology remains somewhat controversial as both, negative and positive roles have been described for this cell population during HSV infection [172, 173].

Another innate immune cell type directly affected by HSV is natural killer T cells (NKT cells) (**Table 4**). These cells recognize glycolipid antigens presented on CD1d molecules [174]. Importantly, cells infected with HSV display reduced expression of CD1d on their surface, as they are redirected by viral determinants to intracellular compartments [175, 176]. Redirection of CD1d from the cell surface is mediated by the phosphorylation of host KIF3A by the viral kinase U_S3 [177]. Interestingly, vaginal application of α-galactosyl-ceramide an NKT ligand is shown to activate and recruit NKT cells to the genital tissue and decrease the susceptibility to HSV infection [178]. Remarkably, a recent report showed that NKT cells can contribute at determining the magnitude and profile of HSV-specific IgG antibodies upon HSV infection. HSV-infected NKT-cell-deficient mice displayed reduced amounts of antiviral IgM and IgG antibodies, as compared to wild-type mice [179]. These results suggest that NKT cells play an important role against HSV and that these viruses have evolved molecular mechanisms to interfere with their function. Furthermore, activating NKT cells with glycolipids may serve as a strategy to promote robust antibody responses against these viruses.

3.3. HSV interfere with dendritic cell function

Dendritic cells are immune cells strategically positioned at the interphase of innate and adaptive immunity. They are specialized in sensing microbes and danger signals, and also in integrating these signals and transducing them onto other cells for modulating the immune response to antigens [180–183]. Because DCs are key at connecting innate and adaptive immunity and clearing microbes, pathogens have evolved numerous immune evasion mechanisms to overcome their function [181, 184–189]. Importantly, HSV has been shown to infect DCs and to modulate their function by altering their maturation and capacity to activate T cells (**Table 5**) [118, 119, 190]. Furthermore, HSV can negatively modulate the autophagosome within DCs and interfere with their antigen processing capacity. This process is mediated by the viral protein γ34.5, which blocks autophagosome maturation [191, 192]. On the other hand, HSV-2 protein ICP47 has been shown to specifically block the expression of particular alleles of MHC-I on the surface of human DCs, namely, HLA-C, potentially rendering these cells more susceptible to NK killing and reducing the spectrum of HSV-derived antigens presented by these cells [193]. Remarkably, HSV has been shown to suppress many functions of DCs via caveolin-1 (Cav-1) by studying these cells in the lungs. HSV-induced Cav-1 was shown to downregulate the expression of inducible nitric oxide synthase; indeed, Cav-1-deficient mice or enhancement of nitric oxide production in wild-type mice ameliorated virus elimination and reduced pathology after HSV infection [194]. Furthermore, such crosstalk may occur between nonvirally infected dermal dendritic cells phagocytizing HSV-infected epidermal Langerhans cells, which are the first dendritic cells to encounter HSV in the skin [195].

http://dx.doi.org/10.5772/64128

Adaptive immune cell affected	Viral determinant	Outcome	Mechanism	References
Dendritic cell	Undetermined	Altered DC maturation and capacity to activate T cells	Undetermined	[118, 119, 190]
Dendritic cell	γ34.5	Interference with autophagosome function and hence antigen processing	Blocks autophagosome maturation	[191, 192]
Dendritic cell	ICP47	Increased susceptibility to NK attack	Blocks MCH expression (HLA-C allele)	[193]
Dendritic cell	HSV-induced Cav-1	Reduced virus elimination and increased pathology	Downregulates the expression of inducible nitric oxide synthase	[194]
Dendritic cell	Undetermined	Induces DC cell death	Undetermined	[118–120]
Humoral	gE	Blocks antibody function related to complement activation and antigen phagocytosis	Binding to the Fc portion of antibodies. Competes with C1q and FcγRs	[201, 202]
T cell	ICP47 and U_S3	Reduced CTL recognition of infected cells and decreased naïve T cell activation	Interferes with host TAP protein, impairing peptide-MHC complex presentation	[205, 206]
T cell	gD, gB, gH, gI, and gL	Reduction in T cell activation and function. Decreases IL-2 secretion	Signals through HVEM. Alters CD3-dependent intracellular calcium signaling	[208]
T cell	U_S3	Impairs T-cell activation	Interferes with TCR signaling. Blocks TRAF6 activity, altering LAT function	[209]
T cell	gD	Promotes Treg cell function with increased IL-10 secretion. Likely to alter CTL activity	Induces proliferation of T $CD4^+$ $FoxP3^+(CD25^+)$ cell subsets	[213–217]

γ34.5 (late gene gamma 34.5, ICP34.5); ICP47 (infected cell protein 47); Cav-1 (caveolin-1); gB, gD, gE, gH, gI, gL (glycoproteins B, D, E, H, I, L); U_S3 (short unique region 3); DC (dendritic cell); NK (natural killer cell); Treg (regulatory T cell); MHC (major histocompatibility complex); HLA-C (human major histocompatibility complex chain C); C1q (subcomponent of the C1 complex of the classical pathway of complement activation); FcγR (Fc gamma receptor); TAP (transporter associated with antigen processing); HVEM (herpesvirus entry mediator); IL-2 (interleukin 2); CD3 (cluster of differentiation 3); TCR (T-cell receptor); TRAF3 (TNF receptor-associated factor 3); LAT1 (linker for activation of T cells); FoxP3 (forkhead box P3 protein).

Table 5. Evasion of adaptive immunity.

Importantly, experiments with animals depleted of DCs have shown that these cells are involved in neuron infection, as up to fivefold less latent virus can be found in the trigeminal ganglia of animals devoid of these cells [196]. Consistent with this notion, another study found that depletion of $CD11c^+$ $CD8\alpha^+$ DCs reduced HSV latency in neurons after ocular infection and that Flt3L treatment, which increases the number of DCs in the tissues, enhanced virus infection of neurons [197]. These studies suggest that DCs may be used as Trojan horses by HSV to reach neurons or that the virus might manipulate these cells in such a way to gain access to the former. However, another study that assessed HSV infection through the footpad in the mouse model found that depletion of DCs was associated with increased viral loads in neurons [198].

Taken together, these studies evidence numerous evasion strategies evolved by HSV to alter the function of DCs and consequently innate and adaptive immunity (discussed below). Additionally, these viruses seem to have harnessed the mobile properties of DCs to spread onto other host cells and tissues, namely, neurons. The fact that HSVs ultimately induce DC apoptosis will likely interrupt the establishment of effective and robust immune responses against these viruses.

4. Herpes simplex viruses evade adaptive immunity

4.1. Interference with humoral immunity

Although natural infection with HSV elicits antiviral antibodies with *in vitro* neutralizing capacities, these responses seem largely insufficient in most individuals when it comes to limit HSV symptoms and virus shedding. This host antibody response is mostly directed to few surface viral antigens, mainly gD, gB, and, to a lesser extent, gC all of which are essential for virus entry, except for gC in HSV-2 [199]. For antibodies to exert effective antiviral activities they need not to be necessarily neutralizing, as antibodies can also elicit complement activation and immune complex-induced phagocytosis, thanks to their Fc portion [200]. However, HSVs have evolved molecular mechanisms to evade these antibody functions (**Table 5**). Notably, the HSV-encoded glycoprotein E (gE) can interfere with complement activation by directly binding to the Fc portion of antibodies and competing with complement component C1q [201, 202]. Indeed, gE functions as an IgG Fc receptor (FcγR) that binds the Fc domain of IgG antibodies and thus blocks their capacity to promote complement activation, altogether impeding phagocytosis by immune cells [202–204]. Importantly, specific interference with anti-HSV antibodies and not other circulating antibodies is achieved, thanks to the relatively low affinity of gE for the Fc portion of antibodies; antibodies are stabilized on the virus surface only if the Fab portion of the antibody is also bound to a viral antigen by its antigen-binding region. Hence, HSV has evolved molecular determinants to persist within the host and shed onto others, despite the existence of virus-neutralizing antibodies. Such evasion mechanisms have led to difficulties in the development of prophylactic formulations against HSV, and is further discussed below.

4.2. Evasion of T cell immunity

T cells can recognize microbe-derived protein fragments presented on the surface of infected cells and destroy these cells to limit virus replication and shedding onto other tissues and organisms. However, HSV encode molecular determinants that interfere with viral antigen presentation to T cells, namely, with MHC-I presentation, and thus the virus can hamper T-cell recognition of infected cells. HSVs interfere with the presentation of viral antigens by blocking the function of host TAP protein (transporter associated with antigen processing), which translocates self- and foreign peptides from the cytoplasm into the rough endoplasmatic reticulum for peptide loading onto MHC-I molecules (**Table 5**); TAP inhibition is mediated by the HSV protein ICP47 [205] and the U_S3 kinase [206]. Reduced peptide/MHC (pMHC) complexes on the surface of infected cells dramatically reduces the chances of cytotoxic T cells detecting HSV-infected cells, as well as the capacity of HSV-infected professional antigen presenting cells to activate naïve T cells.

Furthermore, additional mechanisms exist by which HSVs can negatively modulate the activation and proliferation of T cells (**Table 5**). For instance, the viral glycoprotein D binds to HVEM (herpesvirus entry mediator) on the surface of immune cells, which is a receptor belonging to the TNF-receptor superfamily and whose intracellular signaling mechanisms depends within others on the engagement of its different ligands and their orientation (*cis vs. trans*) [207]. gD binding to the cell surface of T cells has shown to alter calcium signaling within T cells after CD3 engagement, likely by interfering with the capacity of T-cell receptor to appropriately transduce intracellular signals that lead to suitable activation and function of these cells [208]. For instance, Jurkat T cells cultured with HSV and an activating CD3 antibody exhibit hampered IL-2 secretion [208]. A similar effect was observed with other HSV glycoproteins, namely, gB, gH, gI, and gL in the same study [208]. A recent report suggests that impaired T-cell activation would also be mediated by HSV U_s3 protein interference with T-cell receptor signaling, specifically by altering linker for activation of T cells (LAT1) within these cells [209]. Importantly, infection of T cells (other than Jurkat cells) requires the presence of antigen-presenting cells for efficient virus transfer, a process termed virological synapse. Indeed, primary cultures of T cells incubated with HSV alone are only infected at very low frequencies, while adding fibroblasts significantly enhances the formation of virological synapses that culminate in a substantial increase in the number of T cells infected with these viruses [210]. Importantly, HSV has been described to lead to T-cell apoptosis [211].

T cells can carry out numerous functions depending on their phenotype. While cytotoxic T cells are specialized in killing microbe-infected cells, regulatory T cells (Tregs) are specialized within others in controlling the magnitude of the immune response to antigens [212]. In this regard, HSV seems to promote the proliferation of regulatory T cells through the binding of gD to HVEM receptors on the cell surface to promote the secretion of signature cytokines attributed to these cells, such as IL-10 (**Table 5**) [213–216]. The promotion of Tregs might alter the activity of cytotoxic T cells intended to control the virus [213, 217]. Consistent with a negative role for Tregs in HSV infection, protection elicited against this virus in an animal model with previous immunization correlates with relatively low numbers of Tregs [218]. Nevertheless, another study proposes that deletion of Tregs in HSV-infected animals interferes with the migration of immune cells to the site of infection, negatively affecting the survival of infected animals [219]. Thus, further studies are needed to determine the contribution of Tregs in HSV infection.

4.3. Past and present vaccine attempts

Availability of an effective vaccine against HSV would be an important public health advance, mainly because individuals with genital herpes display increased susceptibility to acquire HIV [141–145]. Importantly, previous efforts invested on the development of vaccines against HSV have concentrated on subunit approaches consisting mainly on one viral glycoprotein, namely, gD (**Table 6**) ([220], http://clinicaltrials.gov). Glycoprotein gD is conserved within HSV serotypes and plays a key role during cell infection [221]. Furthermore, this viral protein harbors epitopes for $CD4^+$ T cells [222], $CD8^+$ T cells [223], and neutralizing antibodies [224] and is immunodominant as evidenced by clinical data showing that the majority of HSV-infected individuals have neutralizing antibodies against this protein [199]. Regretfully, this insisted strategy, which combines gD with adjuvants, recently failed in a phase 3 clinical trial; indeed, the formulation failed at reducing both HSV-2 infection and minimizing the shedding of the virus [225, 226]. Remarkably, the formulation tested in this and previous clinical trials induced anti-gD neutralizing antibodies in the vaccinated, as well as T $CD4^+$ cells [220, 227–230]. However, the magnitude of these responses may have been too weak for significant protection against HSV-2 after exposure [199, 228, 231, 232]. Unexpectedly, the vaccine provided 35% cross-protection against HSV-1 infection and 58% cross-protection against HSV-1 disease [227]. An important concern that arose from these results was whether the current animal models used to assess the efficacy of new HSV vaccines satisfactorily recapitulate what occurs in humans. It is also unclear whether the amount and/or quality of neutralizing antibodies elicited against HSV and T cells produced by vaccine formulations, such as the glycoprotein D/AS04 vaccine, play any relevant role in protection against HSV-2; furthermore, whether previously considered correlates of protection as anti-gD antibodies play any relevant role against this virus.

Importantly, a recent study suggests that anti-HSV antibodies, different from those directed against gD, might account for effective protection against HSV-2 after immunization with a discontinuous virus (**Table 6**). Indeed, animals immunized subcutaneously with a genotypically deleted gD virus elicited remarkable protection against genital and skin challenge with HSV-1 and HSV-2, which was mediated by antibodies. Noteworthy, the antibodies elicited by this attenuated HSV strain were poorly neutralizing and were mainly directed against gB [233]. A somewhat similar result was found in another study with an 0ΔNLS-attenuated HSV strain, which elicits antibodies against numerous virus-infected cell proteins (ICP) and gB, within others (**Table 6**) [234–236]. Other attenuated HSV strains have also provided promising results in numerous mouse models and should move onto clinical trials, such as the HSV-2 dl5-29 strain, which has U_L5 and U_L29 deleted from its genome (**Table 6**) [237–239]. Additional attenuated viral strains that confer significant protection against viral challenge are HSV strains that are impaired at infecting neurons, such as a gD mutant virus [240], HSV deleted at U_L39 (ICP10ΔPK) [241], and HSV deleted at *gE* (**Table 6**) [242]. Regretfully, an HSV strain

http://dx.doi.org/10.5772/64128

deleted at *gH*, which showed early promising results in animal models, was later shown to be ineffective in humans in a clinical trial [243]. Although most of these strategies elicit both anti-HSV antibodies and antiviral T cells, the main immune components involved in protection against HSV challenge remain unknown. Importantly, a recent study suggests that other animal models different from the guinea pig and the mouse infection model might be better suited for testing anti-HSV vaccine formulations. For instance, the cotton rat *Sigmodon hispidus* parallels well the results obtained with the D/AS04 vaccine in humans, both for HSV-1 and HSV-2 [244].

Formulation type	Outcome	Development stage	References
Subunit protein gD plus adjuvant Alum and MPL (gD/AS04)	Induces T $CD4^+$ and antibody response. No clinical protection for shedding and infection.	Clinical phase 3 (completed)	[199, 220, 225–233]
Live attenuated, HSV-2 virus with gH deletion (HSV-2 ΔgH)	Safe and immunogenic, yet did not confer protection to HSV infection.	Clinical phase 2 (completed)	[243]
Live attenuated, HSV-2 virus with U_L39 deletion (ICP10ΔPK)	Induction of Th1 immunity	Clinical phase 2 (completed)	[241]
Live attenuated, HSV-2 virus with U_L5 and U_L29 deletions (ACAM529)	Reduced disease, shedding, seroconversion, and latency	Preclinical stage	[237–239]
Live attenuated HSV-2 virus with gD mutation (HSV-2-gD27)	Protects from challenge and reduces viral load in neurons	Preclinical stage	[240]
Live attenuated HSV-2 virus with gD deletion (HSV-2 $\Delta gD^{-/+}$)	Protects from genital and skin challenge and blocks neuronal infection. Antibody-mediated protection	Preclinical stage	[233]
Live attenuated, HSV-2 virus with gE deletion (HSV-2 ΔgE2)	Reduced infection and recurrence	Preclinical stage	[242]
Live attenuated HSV- 2 virus with ICP0 deletion (0ΔNLS)	Antibody response against gB and ICP viral proteins	Preclinical stage	[234–236]

AS04 (adjuvant system 04); MPL (monophosphoryl lipid A); gD, gE, gH (glycoprotein D, E, H); ICP10ΔPK (infected cell protein 10 lacking the PK domain); Th1 (T helper-1); U_L5, U_L29, U_L39 (short unique region 5, 29, and 39); ICP0 (infected cell protein 0).

Table 6. Past and present vaccine attempts against HSV.

On the contrary to the evidence that suggests a role for antibodies in protection against HSV infection, a recent study proposes that effective protection against ocular HSV may be achieved by eliciting a robust T cell response alone. Indeed, humanized HLA transgenic animals vaccinated with T cell epitopes from different viral proteins identified in asymptomatic individuals and combined with adjuvant was shown to confer protection against ocular herpes [245–247]. However, whether such results relate specifically to this type of herpetic disease or whether these T cells ultimately elicit an antibody response against HSV upon virus challenge remains unknown. Noteworthy, an important limitation of vaccine approaches that are based on one or few viral proteins is that only an oligoclonal set of T cells will be elicited, which may limit the effectiveness of formulation to a narrow set of individuals [248, 249].

Taken together, the HSV vaccine field has suffered an important failure and will need to revisit the immunobiology of its diseases. Importantly, the race for the development of novel prophylactic formulations against these viruses is reopened. While numerous groups aim at vaccine strategies that are based on defined viral proteins or viral epitopes, others propose attenuated HSV strains as an alternative for eliciting multiantigenic immune responses against these viruses. Regardless of the methods, a novel vaccine against HSV must guarantee safety for the immunocompetent and notably immunocompromised individuals. Remarkably, the lack of vaccines against HSV has encouraged considerable research in the field of microbicides, which might provide a strategy to prevent infection with these viruses [4].

5. Concluding remarks

Herpes simplex viruses have proven to be masters of immune evasion as they encode numerous molecular determinants that promote evasion of host sensing, signal transduction, cytokine secretion by immune and nonimmune cells, and, most importantly, interference with innate and adaptive immunity. These attributes likely explain the coexistence of HSV and humans since time immemorial and facilitates their high prevalence in the population [250]. Although HSV are seldom life threatening, the important economic burden they elicit with the diseases they produce and their association with HIV infection calls for the implementation of novel vaccines and improved treatments to stop their effects. Hopefully, lessons learned from past failed clinical trials will lead to novel strategies that will ultimately limit the impact of these viruses.

Acknowledgements

Authors are supported by the Millennium Institute on Immunology and Immunotherapy (n° P09/016-F) from the Iniciativa Científica Milenio (ICM, Millennium Scientific Initiative), as well as grants CRP-ICGEB CRP/CHI14-01, FONDECYT 1140011, FONDECYT 1140010, FONDECYT 11075060, FONDECYT 1100926, FONDECYT 1110518, FONDECYT 1110397. A.R.D. is a CONICYT fellow. A.M.K. is Chaire De La Région Pays De La Loire, Chercheur Etranger d'Excellence and a CDD-DR INSERM.

Author details

Angello R. Retamal-Díaz[1], Eduardo Tognarelli[1], Alexis M. Kalergis[1,2,3], Susan M. Bueno[1,3] and Pablo A. González[1*]

*Address all correspondence to: pagonzalez@bio.puc.cl

1 Millennium Institute on Immunology and Immunotherapy, Departamento de Genética Molecular y Microbiología, Facultad de Ciencias Biológicas, Pontificia Universidad Católica de Chile, Santiago, Chile

2 Departamento de Endocrinología, Facultad de Medicina, Pontificia Universidad Católica de Chile, Santiago, Chile

3 INSERM U1064, Nantes, France

References

[1] Looker, K.J., et al. Global and regional estimates of prevalent and incident herpes simplex virus type 1 infections in 2012. PLoS ONE. 2015; 10: p. e0140765. DOI:10.1371/journal.pone.0140765.

[2] Looker, K.J., et al. Global estimates of prevalent and incident herpes simplex virus type 2 infections in 2012. PLoS ONE. 2015; 10: p. e114989. DOI: 10.1371/journal.pone.0114989.

[3] Looker, K.J., G.P. Garnett, and G.P. Schmid. Bulletin of the World Health Organization. 2008; 86: Pp. 805–812, A.

[4] Suazo, P.A., et al. Herpes simplex virus 2 infection: molecular association with HIV and novel microbicides to prevent disease. Med Microbiol and Immunol. 2015; 204: p. 161–176. DOI: 10.1007/s00430-014-0358-x.

[5] Yawn, B.P. and D. Gilden. The global epidemiology of herpes zoster. Neurology. 2013; 81: p. 928–930. DOI:10.1212/WNL.0b013e3182a3516e 10.1212.

[6] Centers for Disease, C. and Prevention. Seroprevalence of herpes simplex virus type 2 among persons aged 14-49 years--United States, 2005–2008. Morb and Mortal Wkly Rep. 2010; 59: p. 456–459.

[7] Dickson, N., et al. HSV-2 incidence by sex over four age periods to age 38 in a birth cohort. Sex Transm Infect. 2014; 90: p. 243–245. DOI:10.1136/sextrans-2013-051235 10.1136.

[8] Roberts, C.M., J.R. Pfister, and S.J. Spear. Increasing proportion of herpes simplex virus type 1 as a cause of genital herpes infection in college students. Sex Transm Dis. 2003; 30: p. 797–800. DOI: 10.1097/01.OLQ.0000092387.58746.C7.

[9] Buxbaum, S., et al. Epidemiology of herpes simplex virus types 1 and 2 in Germany: what has changed? Med Microbiol Immunol. 2003; 192: p. 177–181. DOI:10.1007/s00430-003-0183.

[10] Coyle, P.V., et al. Emergence of herpes simplex type 1 as the main cause of recurrent genital ulcerative disease in women in Northern Ireland. J Clin Virol. 2003; 27: p. 22–29.

[11] Pereira, V.S., et al. Herpes simplex virus type 1 is the main cause of genital herpes in women of Natal, Brazil. Eur J Obstetrics Gynecol Reproductive Biol. 2012; 161: p. 190–193. DOI:10.1016/j.ejogrb.2011.12.006.

[12] Xu, F., et al. Trends in herpes simplex virus type 1 and type 2 seroprevalence in the United States. JAMA. 2006; 296: p. 964–973. DOI:10.1001/jama.296.8.964 10.1001.

[13] Horowitz, R., et al. Herpes simplex virus infection in a university health population: clinical manifestations, epidemiology, and implications. J Am Coll Health. 2011; 59: p. 69–74. DOI:10.1080/07448481.2010.483711.

[14] Bernstein, D.I., et al. Epidemiology, clinical presentation, and antibody response to primary infection with herpes simplex virus type 1 and type 2 in young women. Clin Infect Dis. 2013; 56: p. 344–351. DOI:10.1093/cid/cis891.

[15] Samra, Z., E. Scherf, and M. Dan. Herpes simplex virus type 1 is the prevailing cause of genital herpes in the Tel Aviv area, Israel. Sex Transm Dis. 2003; 30: p. 794–796. DOI: 10.1097/01.OLQ.0000079517.04451.79.

[16] Manavi, K., A. McMillan, and M. Ogilvie. Herpes simplex virus type 1 remains the principal cause of initial anogenital herpes in Edinburgh, Scotland. Sex Transm Dis. 2004; 31: p. 322–324.

[17] Kortekangas-Savolainen, O., et al. Epidemiology of genital herpes simplex virus type 1 and 2 infections in southwestern Finland during a 10-year period (2003–2012). Sex Transm Dis. 2014; 41: p. 268–271. DOI:10.1097/OLQ.0000000000000101.

[18] Nieuwenhuis, R.F., et al. Importance of herpes simplex virus type-1 (HSV-1) in primary genital herpes. Act Derm Venereol. 2006; 86: p. 129–134. DOI:10.2340/00015555-0029.

[19] Ryder, N., et al. Increasing role of herpes simplex virus type 1 in first-episode anogenital herpes in heterosexual women and younger men who have sex with men, 1992-2006. Sex Transm Infect. 2009; 85: p. 416–419. DOI:10.1136/sti.2008.033902 10.1136.

[20] Farooq, A.V. and D. Shukla. Herpes simplex epithelial and stromal keratitis: an epidemiologic update. Surv Ophthalmol. 2012; 57: p. 448–462. DOI:10.1016/j.survophthal.2012.01.005.

[21] Kaye, S. and A. Choudhary. Herpes simplex keratitis. Prog Retin Eye Res. 2006; 25: p. 355–380. DOI:10.1016/j.preteyeres.2006.05.001.

[22] Lafferty, W.E., et al. Recurrences after oral and genital herpes simplex virus infection. Influence of site of infection and viral type. N Engl J Med. 1987; 316: p. 1444–1449. DOI: 10.1056/NEJM198706043162304.

[23] Kaneko, H., et al. Evaluation of mixed infection cases with both herpes simplex virus types 1 and 2. J Med Virol. 2008; 80: p. 883–887. DOI:10.1002/jmv.21154.

[24] Obara, Y., et al. Distribution of herpes simplex virus types 1 and 2 genomes in human spinal ganglia studied by PCR and in situ hybridization. J Med Virol. 1997; 52: p. 136–142.

[25] Solomon, L., et al. Epidemiology of recurrent genital herpes simplex virus types 1 and 2. Sex Transm Infect. 2003; 79: p. 456–459.

[26] Janier, M., et al. Virological, serological and epidemiological study of 255 consecutive cases of genital herpes in a sexually transmitted disease clinic of Paris (France): a prospective study. Int J STD AIDS. 2006; 17: p. 44–49. DOI: 10.1258/095646206775220531.

[27] Benedetti, J., L. Corey, and R. Ashley. Recurrence rates in genital herpes after symptomatic first-episode infection. Ann Intern Med. 1994; 121: p. 847–854.

[28] Krummenacher, C., et al. Comparative usage of herpesvirus entry mediator A and nectin-1 by laboratory strains and clinical isolates of herpes simplex virus. Virology. 2004; 322: p. 286–299. DOI:10.1016/j.virol.2004.02.005.

[29] Grinde, B. Herpesviruses: latency and reactivation—viral strategies and host response. J Oral Microbiol. 2013; 5:22766. DOI:10.3402/jom.v5i0.22766.

[30] Mogensen, T.H. Pathogen recognition and inflammatory signaling in innate immune defenses. Clin Microbiol Rev. 2009; 22: p. 240–273. DOI: 10.1128/CMR.00046-08.

[31] Tang, D., et al. PAMPs and DAMPs: signal 0s that spur autophagy and immunity. Immunol Rev. 2012; 249: p. 158–175. DOI:10.1111/j.1600-065X.2012.01146.x.

[32] Johnson, K.E., L. Chikoti, and B. Chandran. Herpes simplex virus 1 infection induces activation and subsequent inhibition of the IFI16 and NLRP3 inflammasomes. J Virol. 2013; 87: p. 5005–5018. DOI:10.1128/JVI.00082-13.

[33] Mogensen, T.H. and S.R. Paludan. Molecular pathways in virus-induced cytokine production. Microbiol Mol Biol Rev. 2001; 65: p. 131–150. DOI: 10.1128/MMBR.65.1.131-150.2001.

[34] Owen, D.J., C.M. Crump, and S.C. Graham. Tegument assembly and secondary envelopment of alphaherpesviruses. Viruses. 2015; 7: p. 5084–5114. DOI:10.3390/v7092861.

[35] Dohner, K., et al. Function of dynein and dynactin in herpes simplex virus capsid transport. Mol Biol Cell. 2002; 13: p. 2795–2809. DOI:10.1091/mbc.01-07-0348.

[36] Triantafilou, K., D. Eryilmazlar, and M. Triantafilou. Herpes simplex virus 2-induced activation in vaginal cells involves Toll-like receptors 2 and 9 and DNA sensors DAI and IFI16. Am J Obstet Gynecol. 2014; 210: p. 122 e1–e10. DOI:10.1016/j.ajog.2013.09.034.

[37] Dawson, M.J. and J.A. Trapani. The interferon-inducible autoantigen, IFI 16: localization to the nucleolus and identification of a DNA-binding domain. Biochem Biophys Res Commun. 1995; 214: p. 152–162. DOI:10.1006/bbrc.1995.2269.

[38] Conrady, C.D., et al. Resistance to HSV-1 infection in the epithelium resides with the novel innate sensor, IFI-16. Mucosal Immunol. 2012; 5: p. 173–183. DOI:10.1038/mi.2011.63.

[39] Orzalli, M.H., et al. cGAS-mediated stabilization of IFI16 promotes innate signaling during herpes simplex virus infection. Proc Natl Acad Sci U S A. 2015; 112: p. E1773–E1781. DOI: 10.1073/pnas.1424637112.

[40] Li, X.D., et al. Pivotal roles of cGAS-cGAMP signaling in antiviral defense and immune adjuvant effects. Science. 2013; 341: p. 1390–1394. DOI:10.1126/science.1244040.

[41] Wu, J.J., et al. Inhibition of cGAS DNA Sensing by a herpesvirus virion protein. Cell Host Microbe. 2015; 18: p. 333–344. DOI:10.1016/j.chom.2015.07.015.

[42] Unterholzner, L., et al. IFI16 is an innate immune sensor for intracellular DNA. Nat Immunol. 2010; 11: p. 997–1004. DOI:10.1038/ni.1932.

[43] Johnson, K.E., et al. IFI16 restricts HSV-1 replication by accumulating on the HSV-1 genome, repressing HSV-1 gene expression, and directly or indirectly modulating histone modifications. PLoS Pathog. 2014; 10: p. e1004503. DOI:10.1371/journal.ppat.1004503.

[44] Reikine, S., J.B. Nguyen, and Y. Modis. Pattern recognition and signaling mechanisms of RIG-I and MDA5. Front Immunol. 2014; 5: p. 342. DOI: 10.3389/fimmu.2014.00342.

[45] Yao, X.D. and K.L. Rosenthal. Herpes simplex virus type 2 virion host shutoff protein suppresses innate dsRNA antiviral pathways in human vaginal epithelial cells. J Gen Virol. 2011; 92: p. 1981–1993. DOI:10.1099/vir.0.030296-0.

[46] Lund, J., et al. Toll-like receptor 9-mediated recognition of Herpes simplex virus-2 by plasmacytoid dendritic cells. J Exp Med. 2003; 198: p. 513–520. DOI:10.1084/jem.20030162.

[47] Krug, A., et al. Herpes simplex virus type 1 activates murine natural interferon-producing cells through toll-like receptor 9. Blood. 2004; 103: p. 1433–1437. DOI: 10.1182/blood-2003-08-2674.

[48] Boivin, N., et al. Modulation of TLR9 response in a mouse model of herpes simplex virus encephalitis. Antiviral Res. 2012; 96: p. 414–421. DOI:10.1016/j.antiviral.2012.09.022.

[49] Ashkar, A.A., et al. Local delivery of CpG oligodeoxynucleotides induces rapid changes in the genital mucosa and inhibits replication, but not entry, of herpes simplex virus type 2. J Virol. 2003; 77: p. 8948–8956.

[50] Shen, H. and A. Iwasaki. A crucial role for plasmacytoid dendritic cells in antiviral protection by CpG ODN-based vaginal microbicide. J Clin Invest. 2006; 116: p. 2237–2243. DOI:10.1172/JCI28681.

[51] Harandi, A.M., K. Eriksson, and J. Holmgren. A protective role of locally administered immunostimulatory CpG oligodeoxynucleotide in a mouse model of genital herpes infection. J Virol. 2003; 77: p. 953–962.

[52] Pyles, R.B., et al. Use of immunostimulatory sequence-containing oligonucleotides as topical therapy for genital herpes simplex virus type 2 infection. J Virol. 2002; 76: p. 11387–11396.

[53] Kang, R. and D. Tang. PKR-dependent inflammatory signals. Sci Signal. 2012; 5: p. pe47. DOI: 10.1126/scisignal.2003511.

[54] Carr, D.J.J., et al. RNA-dependent protein kinase is required for alpha-1 interferon transgene-induced resistance to genital herpes simplex virus type 2. J Virol. 2005; 79: p. 9341–9345. DOI:10.1128/JVI.79.14.9341.

[55] Leib, D.A., et al. Specific phenotypic restoration of an attenuated virus by knockout of a host resistance gene. Proc Natl Acad Sci U S A. 2000; 97: p. 6097–6101. DOI: 10.1073/pnas.100415697.

[56] He, B., M. Gross, and B. Roizman. The gamma(1)34.5 protein of herpes simplex virus 1 complexes with protein phosphatase 1alpha to dephosphorylate the alpha subunit of the eukaryotic translation initiation factor 2 and preclude the shutoff of protein synthesis by double-stranded RNA-activated protein kinase. Proc Natl Acad Sci U S A. 1997; 94: p. 843–848.

[57] Poppers, J., et al. Inhibition of PKR activation by the proline-rich RNA binding domain of the herpes simplex virus type 1 Us11 protein. J Virol. 2000; 74: p. 11215–11221.

[58] Miller, R.L., et al. Treatment of primary herpes simplex virus infection in guinea pigs by imiquimod. Antiviral Res. 1999; 44: p. 31–42.

[59] Hirokawa, D., et al. Treatment of recalcitrant herpes simplex virus with topical imiquimod. Cutis. 2011; 88: p. 276–277.

[60] Kan, Y., et al. Imiquimod suppresses propagation of herpes simplex virus 1 by upregulation of cystatin A via the adenosine receptor A1 pathway. J Virol. 2012; 86: p. 10338–10346. DOI:10.1128/JVI.01196-12.

[61] Lascaux, A.S., et al. Successful treatment of aciclovir and foscarnet resistant herpes simplex virus lesions with topical imiquimod in patients infected with human immunodeficiency virus type 1. J Med Virol. 2012; 84: p. 194–197. DOI:10.1002/jmv.23188.

[62] Deza, G., et al. Successful treatment of hypertrophic herpes simplex genitalis in HIV-infected patient with topical imiquimod. J Dermatol. 2015; 42: p. 1176–1178. DOI: 10.1111/1346-8138.12969.

[63] Alexopoulou, L., et al. Recognition of double-stranded RNA and activation of NF-kappaB by Toll-like receptor 3. Nature. 2001; 413: p. 732–738. DOI: 10.1038/35099560.

[64] Reinert, L.S., et al. TLR3 deficiency renders astrocytes permissive to herpes simplex virus infection and facilitates establishment of CNS infection in mice. J Clin Invest. 2012; 122: p. 1368–1376. DOI:10.1172/JCI60893.

[65] Liu, Z., et al. HSV-1 activates NF-kappaB in mouse astrocytes and increases TNF-alpha and IL-6 expression via Toll-like receptor 3. Neurol Res. 2013; 35: p. 755–762. DOI: 10.1179/016164113X13703372991516.

[66] Casrouge, A., et al. Herpes simplex virus encephalitis in human UNC-93B deficiency. Science. 2006; 314: p. 308–312. DOI:10.1126/science.1128346.

[67] Zhang, S.Y., et al. TLR3 deficiency in patients with herpes simplex encephalitis. Science. 2007; 317: p. 1522–1527. DOI:10.1126/science.1139522.

[68] Guo, Y., et al. Herpes simplex virus encephalitis in a patient with complete TLR3 deficiency: TLR3 is otherwise redundant in protective immunity. J Exp Med. 2011; 208: p. 2083–2098. DOI:10.1084/jem.20101568.

[69] Mork, N., et al. Mutations in the TLR3 signaling pathway and beyond in adult patients with herpes simplex encephalitis. Genes Immun. 2015; 16: p. 552–566. DOI:10.1038/gene.2015.46.

[70] Lafaille, F.G., et al. Impaired intrinsic immunity to HSV-1 in human iPSC-derived TLR3-deficient CNS cells. Nature. 2012; 491: p. 769–773. DOI:10.1038/nature11583.

[71] Lim, H.K., et al. TLR3 deficiency in herpes simplex encephalitis: high allelic heterogeneity and recurrence risk. Neurology. 2014; 83: p. 1888–1897. DOI:10.1212/WNL.0000000000000999.

[72] Andersen, L.L., et al. Functional IRF3 deficiency in a patient with herpes simplex encephalitis. J Exp Med. 2015; 212: p. 1371–1379. DOI:10.1084/jem.20142274.

[73] Ashkar, A.A., et al. Toll-like receptor (TLR)-3, but not TLR4, agonist protects against genital herpes infection in the absence of inflammation seen with CpG DNA. J Infect Dis.. 2004; 190: p. 1841–1849. DOI:10.1086/425079.

[74] Gianni, T. and G. Campadelli-Fiume. AlphaVbeta3-integrin relocalizes nectin1 and routes herpes simplex virus to lipid rafts. J Virol. 2012; 86: p. 2850–2855. DOI:10.1128/JVI.06689-11.

[75] Gianni, T., V. Leoni, and G. Campadelli-Fiume. Type I interferon and NF-kappaB activation elicited by herpes simplex virus gH/gL via alphavbeta3 integrin in epithelial and neuronal cell lines. J Virol. 2013; 87: p. 13911–1396. DOI: 10.1128/JVI.01894-13.

[76] Gianni, T., et al. Alphavbeta3-integrin is a major sensor and activator of innate immunity to herpes simplex virus-1. Proc Natl Acad Sci U S A. 2012; 109: p. 19792–19797. DOI:10.1073/pnas.1212597109.

[77] Ariza, M.E., R. Glaser, and M.V. Williams. Human herpesviruses-encoded dUTPases: a family of proteins that modulate dendritic cell function and innate immunity. Front Microbiol. 2014; 5: p. 504. DOI:10.3389/fmicb.2014.00504.

[78] Sato, A., M.M. Linehan, and A. Iwasaki. Dual recognition of herpes simplex viruses by TLR2 and TLR9 in dendritic cells. Proc Natl Acad Sci U S A. 2006; 103: p. 17343–17348. DOI:10.1073/pnas.0605102103.

[79] Kurt-Jones, E.A., et al. Herpes simplex virus 1 interaction with Toll-like receptor 2 contributes to lethal encephalitis. Proc Natl Acad Sci U S A. 2004; 101: p. 1315–1320. DOI:10.1073/pnas.0308057100.

[80] Schachtele, S.J., et al. Herpes simplex virus induces neural oxidative damage via microglial cell Toll-like receptor-2. J Neuroinflammation. 2010; 7: p. 35. DOI: 10.1186/1742-2094-7-35.

[81] Shu, M., et al. Selective degradation of mRNAs by the HSV host shutoff RNase is regulated by the UL47 tegument protein. Proc Natl Acad Sci U S A. 2013; 110: p. E1669–E1675. DOI:10.1073/pnas.1305475110.

[82] Taddeo, B., W. Zhang, and B. Roizman. The herpes simplex virus host shutoff RNase degrades cellular and viral mRNAs made before infection but not viral mRNA made after infection. J Virol. 2013; 87: p. 4516–4522. DOI:10.1128/JVI.00005-13.

[83] Finnen, R.L., et al. The herpes simplex virus 2 virion-associated ribonuclease vhs interferes with stress granule formation. J Virol. 2014; 88: p. 12727–12739. DOI: 10.1128/JVI.01554-14.

[84] Schoggins, J.W. Interferon-stimulated genes: roles in viral pathogenesis. Curr Opin Virol. 2014; 6: p. 40–46. DOI:10.1016/j.coviro.2014.03.006.

[85] Theofilopoulos, A.N., et al. Type I interferons (alpha/beta) in immunity and autoimmunity. Annu Rev Immunol. 2005; 23: p. 307–336. DOI:10.1146/annurev.immunol.23.021704.115843.

[86] Al-khatib, K., et al. Distinctive roles for 2′,5′-oligoadenylate synthetases and double-stranded RNA-dependent protein kinase R in the in vivo antiviral effect of an adenoviral vector expressing murine IFN-beta. J Immunol. 2004; 172: p. 5638–5647.

[87] Diebold, S.S., et al. Innate antiviral responses by means of TLR7-mediated recognition of single-stranded RNA. Science. 2004; 303: p. 1529–1531. DOI: 10.1126/science.1093616.

[88] Hemmi, H., et al. Small anti-viral compounds activate immune cells via the TLR7 MyD88-dependent signaling pathway. Nat Immunol. 2002; 3: p. 196–200. DOI:10.1038/ni758.

[89] Donnelly, R.P. and S.V. Kotenko. Interferon-lambda: a new addition to an old family. J Interferon Cytokine Res. 2010; 30: p. 555–564. DOI:10.1089/jir.2010.0078.

[90] Peng, T., et al. Evasion of the mucosal innate immune system by herpes simplex virus type 2. J Virol. 2009; 83: p. 12559–12568. DOI:10.1128/JVI.00939-09.

[91] Lin, R., et al. The herpes simplex virus ICP0 RING finger domain inhibits IRF3- and IRF7-mediated activation of interferon-stimulated genes. J Virol. 2004; 78: p. 1675–1684.

[92] Wang, S., et al. Herpes simplex virus 1 serine/threonine kinase US3 hyperphosphorylates IRF3 and inhibits beta interferon production. J Virol. 2013; 87: p. 12814–12827. DOI: 10.1128/JVI.02355-13.

[93] Xing, J., et al. Herpes simplex virus 1-encoded tegument protein VP16 abrogates the production of beta interferon (IFN) by inhibiting NF-kappaB activation and blocking IFN regulatory factor 3 to recruit its coactivator CBP. J Virol. 2013; 87: p. 9788–9801. DOI:10.1128/JVI.01440-13.

[94] Wang, S., et al. Herpes simplex virus 1 ubiquitin-specific protease UL36 inhibits beta interferon production by deubiquitinating TRAF3. J Virol. 2013; 87: p. 11851–11860. DOI:10.1128/JVI.01211-13.

[95] Milligan, G.N. and D.I. Bernstein. Interferon-gamma enhances resolution of herpes simplex virus type 2 infection of the murine genital tract. Virology. 1997; 229: p. 259–268. DOI:10.1006/viro.1997.8441.

[96] Johnson, K.E., B. Song, and D.M. Knipe. Role for herpes simplex virus 1 ICP27 in the inhibition of type I interferon signaling. Virology. 2008; 374: p. 487–494. DOI:10.1016/j.virol.2008.01.001.

[97] Chee, A.V. and B. Roizman. Herpes simplex virus 1 gene products occlude the interferon signaling pathway at multiple sites. J Virol. 2004; 78: p. 4185–4196.

[98] Johnson, K.E. and D.M. Knipe. Herpes simplex virus-1 infection causes the secretion of a type I interferon-antagonizing protein and inhibits signaling at or before Jak-1 activation. Virology. 2010; 396: p. 21–29. DOI:10.1016/j.virol.2009.09.021.

[99] Fung, K.Y., et al. Interferon-epsilon protects the female reproductive tract from viral and bacterial infection. Science. 2013; 339: p. 1088–1092. DOI: 10.1126/science.1233321.

[100] Hermant, P., et al. IFN-epsilon is constitutively expressed by cells of the reproductive tract and is inefficiently secreted by fibroblasts and cell lines. PLoS One. 2013; 8: p. e71320. DOI:10.1371/journal.pone.0071320.

[101] Mangan, N., et al. A role for interferon epsilon in the innate immune response in the female reproductive tract. Cytokine. 2014; 70: p. 58.

[102] Shupack, J., et al. Topical alpha-interferon ointment with dimethyl sulfoxide in the treatment of recurrent genital herpes simplex. Dermatology. 1992; 184: p. 40–44.

[103] Luker, G.D., et al. Bioluminescence imaging reveals systemic dissemination of herpes simplex virus type 1 in the absence of interferon receptors. J Virol. 2003; 77: p. 11082–11093. DOI: 10.1128/JVI.77.20.11082-11093.2003

[104] Zhang, S.Q., et al. Interleukin 29 enhances expression of Toll receptor 3 and mediates antiviral signals in human keratinocytes. Inflamm Res. 2011; 60: p. 1031–1037. DOI: 10.1007/s00011-011-0364-z.

[105] Zhou, L., et al. IL-29/IL-28A suppress HSV-1 infection of human NT2-N neurons. J Neurovirol. 2011; 17: p. 212–219. DOI:10.1007/s13365-011-0031-8.

[106] Iversen, M.B., et al. Expression of type III interferon (IFN) in the vaginal mucosa is mediated primarily by dendritic cells and displays stronger dependence on NF-kappaB than type I IFNs. J Virol. 2010; 84: p. 4579–4586. DOI: 10.1128/JVI.02591-09.

[107] Green, D.R. and F. Llambi. Cell death signaling. Cold Spring Harb Perspect Biol. 2015; 7:a006080. DOI:10.1101/cshperspect.a006080.

[108] Aubert, M., E.M. Krantz, and K.R. Jerome. Herpes simplex virus genes Us3, Us5, and Us12 differentially regulate cytotoxic T lymphocyte-induced cytotoxicity. Viral Immunol. 2006; 19: p. 391–408. DOI:10.1089/vim.2006.19.391.

[109] Wang, X., C. Patenode, and B. Roizman. US3 protein kinase of HSV-1 cycles between the cytoplasm and nucleus and interacts with programmed cell death protein 4 (PDCD4) to block apoptosis. Proc Natl Acad Sci U S A. 2011; 108: p. 14632–14636. DOI: 10.1073/pnas.1111942108.

[110] Yamauchi, Y., et al. Herpes simplex virus UL14 protein blocks apoptosis. Microbiol Immunol. 2003; 47: p. 685–689. DOI: 10.1111/j.1348-0421.2003.tb03432.x

[111] Golembewski, E.K., et al. The HSV-2 protein ICP10PK prevents neuronal apoptosis and loss of function in an in vivo model of neurodegeneration associated with glutamate excitotoxicity. Exp Neurol. 2007; 203: p. 381–393. DOI:10.1016/j.expneurol.2006.08.022.

[112] Sieg, S., et al. Herpes simplex virus type 2 inhibition of Fas ligand expression. J Virol. 1996; 70: p. 8747–8751.

[113] Morton, E.R. and J.A. Blaho. Herpes simplex virus blocks Fas-mediated apoptosis independent of viral activation of NF-kappaB in human epithelial HEp-2 cells. J Interferon Cytokine Res. 2007; 27: p. 365–376. DOI:10.1089/jir.2006.0143.

[114] Rogge, M., et al. Therapeutic use of soluble Fas ligand ameliorates acute and recurrent herpetic stromal keratitis in mice. Invest Ophthalmol Vis Sci. 2015; 56: p. 6377–6386. DOI:10.1167/iovs.15-16588.

[115] Jerome, K.R., et al. HSV and glycoprotein J inhibit caspase activation and apoptosis induced by granzyme B or Fas. J Immunol. 2001; 167: p. 3928–3935.

[116] Zhou, G., et al. Glycoprotein D or J delivered in trans blocks apoptosis in SK-N-SH cells induced by a herpes simplex virus 1 mutant lacking intact genes expressing both

glycoproteins. J Virol. 2000; 74: p. 11782–11791. DOI:10.1128/JVI.74.24.11782-11791.2000.

[117] Guo, H., et al. Herpes simplex virus suppresses necroptosis in human cells. Cell Host Microbe. 2015; 17: p. 243–251. DOI:10.1016/j.chom.2015.01.003.

[118] Bosnjak, L., et al. Herpes simplex virus infection of human dendritic cells induces apoptosis and allows cross-presentation via uninfected dendritic cells. J Immunol. 2005; 174: p. 2220–2227. DOI:10.4049/jimmunol.174.4.2220.

[119] Stefanidou, M., et al. Herpes simplex virus 2 (HSV-2) prevents dendritic cell maturation, induces apoptosis, and triggers release of proinflammatory cytokines: potential links to HSV-HIV synergy. J Virol. 2013; 87: p. 1443–1453. DOI:10.1128/JVI.01302-12.

[120] Kather, A., et al. Herpes simplex virus type 1 (HSV-1)-induced apoptosis in human dendritic cells as a result of downregulation of cellular FLICE-inhibitory protein and reduced expression of HSV-1 antiapoptotic latency-associated transcript sequences. J Virol. 2010; 84: p. 1034–1046. DOI:10.1128/JVI.01409-09.

[121] Iannello, A., et al. Herpes simplex virus type 1-induced FasL expression in human monocytic cells and its implications for cell death, viral replication, and immune evasion. Viral Immunol. 2011; 24: p. 11–26. DOI:10.1089/vim.2010.0083.

[122] Huang, Z., et al. RIP1/RIP3 binding to HSV-1 ICP6 initiates necroptosis to restrict virus propagation in mice. Cell Host Microbe. 2015; 17: p. 229–242. DOI:10.1016/j.chom.2015.01.002.

[123] Wang, X., et al. Direct activation of RIP3/MLKL-dependent necrosis by herpes simplex virus 1 (HSV-1) protein ICP6 triggers host antiviral defense. Proc Natl Acad Sci U S A. 2014; 111: p. 15438–15443. DOI: 10.1073/pnas.1412767111.

[124] Himmelein, S., et al. Latent herpes simplex virus 1 infection does not induce apoptosis in human trigeminal Ganglia. J Virol. 2015; 89: p. 5747–5750. DOI: 10.1128/JVI.03481-14.

[125] Carpenter, D., et al. The herpes simplex virus type 1 (HSV-1) latency-associated transcript (LAT) protects cells against cold-shock-induced apoptosis by maintaining phosphorylation of protein kinase B (AKT). J Neurovirol. 2015; 21: p. 568–575. DOI: 10.1007/s13365-015-0361-z.

[126] Dev, A., et al. NF-kappaB and innate immunity. Curr Top Microbiol Immunol. 2011; 349: p. 115–143. DOI: 10.1007/82_2010_102.

[127] Wang, K., et al. Herpes simplex virus 1 protein kinase US3 hyperphosphorylates p65/RelA and dampens NF-kappaB activation. J Virol. 2014; 88: p. 7941–7951. DOI: 10.1128/JVI.03394-13.

[128] Zhang, J., et al. Herpes simplex virus 1 DNA polymerase processivity factor UL42 inhibits TNF-alpha-induced NF-kappaB activation by interacting with p65/RelA and

p50/NF-kappaB1. Med Microbiol Immunol. 2013; 202: p. 313–325. DOI:10.1007/s00430-013-0295-0.

[129] Zhang, J., et al. Herpes simplex virus 1 E3 ubiquitin ligase ICP0 protein inhibits tumor necrosis factor alpha-induced NF-kappaB activation by interacting with p65/RelA and p50/NF-kappaB1. J Virol. 2013; 87: p. 12935–12948. DOI:10.1128/JVI.01952-13.

[130] Patel, A., et al. Herpes simplex type 1 induction of persistent NF-kappa B nuclear translocation increases the efficiency of virus replication. Virology. 1998; 247: p. 212–222.

[131] Gregory, D., et al. Efficient replication by herpes simplex virus type 1 involves activation of the IkappaB kinase-IkappaB-p65 pathway. J Virol. 2004; 78: p. 13582–13590. DOI: 10.1128/JVI.78.24.13582-13590.2004.

[132] Ferreira, V.H., et al. Proinflammatory cytokines and chemokines—but not interferon-beta—produced in response to HSV-2 in primary human genital epithelial cells are associated with viral replication and the presence of the virion host shutoff protein. Am J Reprod Immunol. 2013; 70: p. 199–212. DOI: 10.1111/aji.12133.

[133] Huang, W., et al. Herpes simplex virus type 2 infection of human epithelial cells induces CXCL9 expression and CD4+ T cell migration via activation of p38-CCAAT/enhancer-binding protein-beta pathway. J Immunol. 2012; 188: p. 6247–6257. DOI:10.4049/jimmunol.1103706.

[134] Thapa, M., et al. CXCL9 and CXCL10 expression are critical for control of genital herpes simplex virus type 2 infection through mobilization of HSV-specific CTL and NK cells to the nervous system. J Immunol. 2008; 180: p. 1098–1106. DOI:10.4049/jimmunol.180.2.1098

[135] Conrady, C.D., et al. IFN-alpha-driven CCL2 production recruits inflammatory monocytes to infection site in mice. Mucosal Immunol. 2013; 6: p. 45–55. DOI: 10.1038/mi.2012.46.

[136] Stock, A.T., J.M. Smith, and F.R. Carbone. Type I IFN suppresses Cxcr2 driven neutrophil recruitment into the sensory ganglia during viral infection. J Exp Med. 2014; 211: p. 751–759. DOI:10.1084/jem.20132183.

[137] Conrady, C.D., et al. Microglia and a functional type I IFN pathway are required to counter HSV-1-driven brain lateral ventricle enlargement and encephalitis. J Immunol. 2013; 190: p. 2807–2817. DOI:10.4049/jimmunol.1203265.

[138] Chucair-Elliott, A.J., et al. Microglia-induced IL-6 protects against neuronal loss following HSV-1 infection of neural progenitor cells. Glia. 2014; 62: p. 1418–1434. DOI: 10.1002/glia.22689.

[139] Aoki, R., et al. Mast cells play a key role in host defense against herpes simplex virus infection through TNF-alpha and IL-6 production. J Invest Dermatol. 2013; 133: p. 2170–2179. DOI: 10.1038/jid.2013.150.

[140] Boivin, N., et al. The combination of valacyclovir with an anti-TNF alpha antibody increases survival rate compared to antiviral therapy alone in a murine model of herpes simplex virus encephalitis. Antiviral Res. 2013; 100: p. 649–653. DOI: 10.1016/j.antiviral.2013.10.007.

[141] Masson, L., et al. Defining genital tract cytokine signatures of sexually transmitted infections and bacterial vaginosis in women at high risk of HIV infection: a cross-sectional study. Sex Transm Infect. 2014; 90: p. 580–587. DOI:10.1136/sextrans-2014-051601.

[142] Wasserheit, J.N. Epidemiological synergy. Interrelationships between human immunodeficiency virus infection and other sexually transmitted diseases. Sex Transm Dis. 1992; 19: p. 61–77.

[143] Barnabas, R.V., et al. Impact of herpes simplex virus type 2 on HIV-1 acquisition and progression in an HIV vaccine trial (the Step study). J Acquir Immune Defic Syndr. 2011; 57: p. 238–244. DOI: 10.1097/QAI.0b013e31821acb5.

[144] Freeman, E.E., et al. Herpes simplex virus 2 infection increases HIV acquisition in men and women: systematic review and meta-analysis of longitudinal studies. Aids. 2006; 20: p. 73–83.

[145] Corey, L., et al. The effects of herpes simplex virus-2 on HIV-1 acquisition and transmission: a review of two overlapping epidemics. J Acquir Immune Defic Syndr. 2004; 35: p. 435–445.

[146] Nixon, B., et al. Genital herpes simplex virus type 2 infection in humanized HIV-transgenic mice triggers HIV shedding and is associated with greater neurological disease. J Infect Dis.. 2014; 209: p. 510–522. DOI:10.1093/infdis/jit472.

[147] Johnson, K.E., et al. Effects of HIV-1 and herpes simplex virus type 2 infection on lymphocyte and dendritic cell density in adult foreskins from Rakai, Uganda. J Infect Dis. 2011; 203: p. 602–609. DOI: 10.1093/infdis/jiq091.

[148] Rebbapragada, A., et al. Negative mucosal synergy between Herpes simplex type 2 and HIV in the female genital tract. Aids. 2007; 21: p. 589–598. DOI:10.1097/QAD.0b013e328012b896.

[149] Goode, D., et al. HSV-2-driven increase in the expression of alpha4beta7 correlates with increased susceptibility to vaginal SHIV(SF162P3) infection. PLoS Pathog. 2014; 10: p. e1004567. DOI:10.1371/journal.ppat.1004567.

[150] Marsden, V., et al. Herpes simplex virus type 2-infected dendritic cells produce TNF-alpha, which enhances CCR5 expression and stimulates HIV production from adjacent infected cells. J Immunol. 2015; 194: p. 4438–4445. DOI:10.4049/jimmunol.1401706.

[151] Sartori, E., et al. Herpes simplex virus type 2 infection increases human immunodeficiency virus type 1 entry into human primary macrophages. Virol J. 2011; 8: p. 166. DOI: 10.1186/1743-422X-8-166.

[152] Martinelli, E., et al. HSV-2 infection of dendritic cells amplifies a highly susceptible HIV-1 cell target. PLoS Pathog. 2011; 7: p. e1002109. DOI:10.1371/journal.ppat.1002109.

[153] de Jong, M.A., et al. Herpes simplex virus type 2 enhances HIV-1 susceptibility by affecting Langerhans cell function. J Immunol. 2010; 185: p. 1633–1641. DOI: 10.4049/jimmunol.0904137.

[154] Svensson, A., et al. Protective immunity to genital herpes simplex [correction of simpex] virus type 2 infection is mediated by T-bet. J Immunol. 2005; 174: p. 6266–6273. DOI: 10.4049/jimmunol.174.10.6266.

[155] Bird, M.D., et al. Early resolution of herpes simplex virus type 2 infection of the murine genital tract involves stimulation of genital parenchymal cells by gamma interferon. J Virol. 2007; 81: p. 423–426. DOI:10.1128/JVI.01455-06.

[156] Khan, A.A., et al. Phenotypic and functional characterization of herpes simplex virus glycoprotein B epitope-specific effector and memory CD8+ T cells from symptomatic and asymptomatic individuals with ocular herpes. J Virol. 2015; 89: p. 3776–3792. DOI: 10.1128/JVI.03419-14.

[157] Sato, A., et al. Vaginal memory T cells induced by intranasal vaccination are critical for protective T cell recruitment and prevention of genital HSV-2 disease. J Virol. 2014; 88: p. 13699–13708. DOI:10.1128/JVI.02279-14.

[158] Johnson, A.J., et al. Herpes simplex virus (HSV)-specific T cells activated in the absence of IFN-gamma express alternative effector functions but are not protective against genital HSV-2 infection. J Reprod Immunol. 2010; 84: p. 8–15. DOI:10.1016/j.jri.2009.09.007.

[159] Tegla, C.A., et al. Membrane attack by complement: the assembly and biology of terminal complement complexes. Immunol Res. 2011; 51: p. 45–60. DOI:10.1007/s12026-011-8239-5.

[160] McNearney, T.A., et al. Herpes simplex virus glycoproteins gC-1 and gC-2 bind to the third component of complement and provide protection against complement-mediated neutralization of viral infectivity. J Exp Med. 1987; 166: p. 1525–1535.

[161] Friedman, H.M., et al. Glycoprotein C of herpes simplex virus 1 acts as a receptor for the C3b complement component on infected cells. Nature. 1984; 309: p. 633–635. DOI: 10.1038/309633a0.

[162] Hook, L.M., et al. Herpes simplex virus type 1 and 2 glycoprotein C prevents complement-mediated neutralization induced by natural immunoglobulin M antibody. J Virol. 2006; 80: p. 4038–4046. DOI:10.1128/JVI.80.8.4038-4046.2006.

[163] Lubinski, J.M., et al. Herpes simplex virus type 1 evades the effects of antibody and complement in vivo. J Virol. 2002; 76: p. 9232–9241. DOI: 10.1128/JVI.76.18.9232-9241.2002

[164] Kim, M., et al. Herpes simplex virus antigens directly activate NK cells via TLR2, thus facilitating their presentation to CD4 T lymphocytes. J Immunol. 2012; 188: p. 4158–4170. DOI:10.4049/jimmunol.1103450.

[165] Frank, G.M., et al. Early responding dendritic cells direct the local NK response to control herpes simplex virus 1 infection within the cornea. J Immunol. 2012; 188: p. 1350–1359. DOI:10.4049/jimmunol.1101968.

[166] Rajasagi, N.K., et al. CD4+ T cells are required for the priming of CD8+ T cells following infection with herpes simplex virus type 1. J Virol. 2009; 83: p. 5256–5268. DOI:10.1128/JVI.01997-08.

[167] Vogel, K., et al. Both plasmacytoid dendritic cells and monocytes stimulate natural killer cells early during human herpes simplex virus type 1 infections. Immunology. 2014; 143: p. 588–600. DOI: 10.1111/imm.12337.

[168] Grauwet, K., et al. Modulation of CD112 by the alphaherpesvirus gD protein suppresses DNAM-1-dependent NK cell-mediated lysis of infected cells. Proc Natl Acad Sci U S A. 2014; 111: p. 16118–16123. DOI:10.1073/pnas.1409485111.

[169] Schepis, D., et al. Herpes simplex virus infection downmodulates NKG2D ligand expression. Scandinavian J Immunol. 2009; 69: p. 429–436. DOI:10.1111/j.1365-3083.2009.02241.x.

[170] Tomazin, R., et al. Stable binding of the herpes simplex virus ICP47 protein to the peptide binding site of TAP. EMBO J. 1996; 15: p. 3256.

[171] Campbell, T.M., et al. Varicella-Zoster Virus and herpes simplex virus 1 differentially modulate NKG2D ligand expression during productive infection. J Virol. 2015; 89: p. 7932–7943. DOI: 10.1128/JVI.00292-15.

[172] Halford, W.P., J.L. Maender, and B.M. Gebhardt. Re-evaluating the role of natural killer cells in innate resistance to herpes simplex virus type 1. Virol J. 2005; 2: p. 56. DOI: 10.1186/1743-422X-2-56.

[173] Nandakumar, S., et al. Natural killer cells as novel helpers in anti-herpes simplex virus immune response. J Virol. 2008; 82: p. 10820–10831. DOI:10.1128/JVI.00365-08.

[174] Godfrey, D.I., et al. Antigen recognition by CD1d-restricted NKT T cell receptors. Seminars Immunol. 2010; 22: p. 61–67. DOI:10.1016/j.smim.2009.10.004.

[175] Rao, P., et al. Herpes simplex virus 1 glycoprotein B and US3 collaborate to inhibit CD1d antigen presentation and NKT cell function. J Virol. 2011; 85: p. 8093–8104. DOI:10.1128/JVI.02689-10.

[176] Yuan, W., A. Dasgupta, and P. Cresswell. Herpes simplex virus evades natural killer T cell recognition by suppressing CD1d recycling. Nat Immunol. 2006; 7: p. 835–842. DOI:10.1038/ni1364.

[177] Xiong, R., et al. Herpes simplex virus 1 US3 phosphorylates cellular KIF3A to down-regulate CD1d expression. J Virol. 2015; 89: p. 6646–6655. DOI: 10.1128/JVI.00214-15.

[178] Iversen, M.B., et al. NKT cell activation by local alpha-galactosylceramide administration decreases susceptibility to HSV-2 infection. Immunobiology. 2015; 220: p. 762–768. DOI:10.1016/j.imbio.2014.12.019.

[179] Raftery, M.J., et al. NKT cells determine titer and subtype profile of virus-specific IgG antibodies during herpes simplex virus Infection. J Immunol. 2014; 192: p. 4294–4302. DOI:10.4049/jimmunol.1300148.

[180] Carreno, L.J., et al. Modulation of the dendritic cell-T-cell synapse to promote pathogen immunity and prevent autoimmunity. Immunotherapy. 2011; 3: p. 6–11. DOI:10.2217/imt.11.38.

[181] Gonzalez, P.A., et al. Respiratory syncytial virus impairs T cell activation by preventing synapse assembly with dendritic cells. Proc Natl Acad Sci U S A. 2008; 105: p. 14999–15004. DOI:10.1073/pnas.0802555105.

[182] Banchereau, J., et al. Immunobiology of dendritic cells. Annu Rev Immunol. 2000; 18: p. 767–811. DOI:10.1146/annurev.immunol.18.1.767.

[183] Gonzalez, P.A., et al. Modulation of immunological synapse by membrane-bound and soluble ligands. Cytokine Growth Factor Rev. 2007; 18: p. 19–31. DOI: 10.1016/j.cytogfr.2007.01.003.

[184] Tobar, J.A., P.A. Gonzalez, and A.M. Kalergis. Salmonella escape from antigen presentation can be overcome by targeting bacteria to Fc gamma receptors on dendritic cells. J Immunol. 2004; 173: p. 4058–4065. DOI: 10.4049/jimmunol.173.6.4058.

[185] Tobar, J.A., et al. Virulent Salmonella enterica serovar typhimurium evades adaptive immunity by preventing dendritic cells from activating T cells. Infect Immun. 2006; 74: p. 6438–6448. DOI:10.1128/IAI.00063-06.

[186] Raftery, M.J., et al. CD1 antigen presentation by human dendritic cells as a target for herpes simplex virus immune evasion. J Immunol. 2006; 177: p. 6207–6214. DOI: 10.4049/jimmunol.177.9.6207.

[187] Majumder, B., et al. Human immunodeficiency virus type 1 Vpr impairs dendritic cell maturation and T-cell activation: implications for viral immune escape. J Virol. 2005; 79: p. 7990–8003. DOI: 10.1128/JVI.79.13.7990-8003.2005.

[188] Morrow, G., et al. Varicella-zoster virus productively infects mature dendritic cells and alters their immune function. J Virol. 2003; 77: p. 4950–4959. DOI: 10.1128/JVI.77.8.4950-4959.2003

[189] Bueno, S.M., et al. The capacity of Salmonella to survive inside dendritic cells and prevent antigen presentation to T cells is host specific. Immunology. 2008; 124: p. 522–533. DOI:10.1111/j.1365-2567.2008.02805.x.

[190] Jones, C.A., et al. Herpes simplex virus type 2 induces rapid cell death and functional impairment of murine dendritic cells in vitro. J Virol. 2003; 77: p. 11139–11149. DOI: 10.1128/JVI.77.20.11139-11149.2003.

[191] Gobeil, P.A. and D.A. Leib. Herpes simplex virus gamma34.5 interferes with autophagosome maturation and antigen presentation in dendritic cells. mBio. 2012; 3: p. e00267–12. DOI:10.1128/mBio.00267-12.

[192] Yordy, B., et al. A neuron-specific role for autophagy in antiviral defense against herpes simplex virus. Cell Host Microbe. 2012; 12: p. 334–345. DOI: 10.1016/j.chom.2012.07.013.

[193] Elboim, M., et al. HSV-2 specifically down regulates HLA-C expression to render HSV-2-infected DCs susceptible to NK cell killing. PLoS Pathog. 2013; 9: p. e1003226. DOI:10.1371/journal.ppat.1003226.

[194] Wu, B., et al. Herpes simplex virus 1 suppresses the function of lung dendritic cells via caveolin-1. Clin Vaccine Immunol. 2015; 22: p. 883–895. DOI:10.1128/CVI.00170-15.

[195] Kim, M., et al. Relay of herpes simplex virus between Langerhans cells and dermal dendritic cells in human skin. PLoS Pathog. 2015; 11: p. e1004812. DOI:10.1371/journal.ppat.1004812.

[196] Mott, K.R. and H. Ghiasi. Role of dendritic cells in enhancement of herpes simplex virus type 1 latency and reactivation in vaccinated mice. Clin Vaccine Immunol. 2008; 15: p. 1859–1867. DOI:10.1128/CVI.00318-08.

[197] Mott, K.R., et al. A role for the JAK-STAT1 pathway in blocking replication of HSV-1 in dendritic cells and macrophages. Virol J. 2009; 6: p. 56. DOI: 10.1186/1743-422X-6-56.

[198] Kassim, S.H., et al. In vivo ablation of CD11c-positive dendritic cells increases susceptibility to herpes simplex virus type 1 infection and diminishes NK and T-cell responses. J Virol. 2006; 80: p. 3985–3993. DOI:10.1128/JVI.80.8.3985-3993.2006.

[199] Cairns, T.M., et al. Dissection of the antibody response against herpes simplex virus glycoproteins in naturally infected humans. J Virol. 2014; 88: p. 12612–12622. DOI: 10.1128/JVI.01930-14.

[200] Bournazos, S. and J.V. Ravetch. Fc gamma receptor pathways during active and passive immunization. Immunological reviews. 2015; 268: p. 88–103. DOI: 10.1111/imr.12343.

[201] Lubinski, J.M., et al. The herpes simplex virus 1 IgG fc receptor blocks antibody-mediated complement activation and antibody-dependent cellular cytotoxicity in vivo. J Virol. 2011; 85: p. 3239–3249. DOI:10.1128/JVI.02509-10.

[202] Para, M.F., L. Goldstein, and P.G. Spear. Similarities and differences in the Fc-binding glycoprotein (gE) of herpes simplex virus types 1 and 2 and tentative mapping of the viral gene for this glycoprotein. J Virol. 1982; 41: p. 137–144.

[203] Armour, K.L., et al. The contrasting IgG-binding interactions of human and herpes simplex virus Fc receptors. Biochem Soc Trans. 2002; 30: p. 495–500. DOI: 10.1042/bst0300495.

[204] Dilillo, D.J., et al. Broadly neutralizing hemagglutinin stalk-specific antibodies require Fc gamma R interactions for protection against influenza virus in vivo. Nat Med. 2014; 20: p. 143–151. DOI:10.1038/nm.3443.

[205] Hill, A., et al. Herpes simplex virus turns off the TAP to evade host immunity. Nature. 1995; 375: p. 411–415. DOI:10.1038/375411a0.

[206] Imai, T., et al. Us3 kinase encoded by herpes simplex virus 1 mediates downregulation of cell surface major histocompatibility complex class I and evasion of CD8+ T cells. PLoS One. 2013; 8: p. e72050. DOI:10.1371/journal.pone.0072050.

[207] La, S., et al. Herpes simplex virus type 1 glycoprotein D inhibits T-cell proliferation. Mole Cells. 2002; 14: p. 398–403.

[208] Sloan, D.D., et al. Inhibition of TCR signaling by herpes simplex virus. J Immunol. 2006; 176: p. 1825–1833. DOI: 10.4049/jimmunol.176.3.1825.

[209] Yang, Y., et al. The Us3 protein of herpes simplex virus 1 inhibits T cell signaling by confining linker for activation of T cells (LAT) activation via TRAF6 protein. J Biol Chem. 2015; 290: p. 15670–15678. DOI:10.1074/jbc.M115.646422.

[210] Aubert, M., et al. The virological synapse facilitates herpes simplex virus entry into T cells. J Virol. 2009; 83: p. 6171–6183. DOI:10.1128/JVI.02163-08.

[211] Vanden Oever, M.J. and J.Y. Han. Caspase 9 is essential for herpes simplex virus type 2-induced apoptosis in T cells. J Virol. 2010; 84: p. 3116–3120. DOI: 10.1128/JVI.01726-09.

[212] Veiga-Parga, T., S. Sehrawat, and B.T. Rouse. Role of regulatory T cells during virus infection. Immunol Rev. 2013; 255: p. 182–196. DOI:10.1111/imr.12085.

[213] Fernandez, M.A., et al. T regulatory cells contribute to the attenuated primary CD8+ and CD4+ T cell responses to herpes simplex virus type 2 in neonatal mice. J Immunol. 2008; 180: p. 1556–1564. DOI: 10.4049/jimmunol.180.3.1556.

[214] Suvas, S., et al. CD4+CD25+ T cells regulate virus-specific primary and memory CD8+ T cell responses. J Exp Med. 2003; 198: p. 889–901. DOI: 10.1084/jem.20030171.

[215] Sloan, D.D. and K.R. Jerome. Herpes simplex virus remodels T-cell receptor signaling, resulting in p38-dependent selective synthesis of interleukin-10. J Virol. 2007; 81: p. 12504–12514. DOI:10.1128/JVI.01111-07.

[216] Sharma, S., et al. Herpes virus entry mediator (HVEM) modulates proliferation and activation of regulatory T cells following HSV-1 infection. Microbes Infect. 2014; 16: p. 648–660. DOI:10.1016/j.micinf.2014.06.005.

[217] Fernandez, M.A., et al. Treg depletion attenuates the severity of skin disease from ganglionic spread after HSV-2 flank infection. Virology. 2013; 447: p. 9–20. DOI: 10.1016/j.virol.2013.08.027.

[218] Iyer, A.V., et al. Single dose of Glycoprotein K (gK)-deleted HSV-1 live-attenuated virus protects mice against lethal vaginal challenge with HSV-1 and HSV-2 and induces lasting T cell memory immune responses. Virol J. 2013; 10: p. 317. DOI: 10.1186/1743-422X-10-317.

[219] Lund, J.M., et al. Coordination of early protective immunity to viral infection by regulatory T cells. Science. 2008; 320: p. 1220–1224. DOI:10.1126/science.1155209.

[220] Mertz, G.J., et al. Double-blind, placebo-controlled trial of a herpes simplex virus type 2 glycoprotein vaccine in persons at high risk for genital herpes infection. J Infect Dis. 1990; 161: p. 653–660. DOI: 10.1093/infdis/161.4.653.

[221] Cheshenko, N., et al. HSV activates Akt to trigger calcium release and promote viral entry: novel candidate target for treatment and suppression. FASEB J. 2013; 27: p. 2584–2599. DOI:10.1096/fj.12-220285.

[222] Kim, M., et al. Immunodominant epitopes in herpes simplex virus type 2 glycoprotein D are recognized by CD4 lymphocytes from both HSV-1 and HSV-2 seropositive subjects. J Immunol. 2008; 181: p. 6604–6615. DOI:10.4049/jimmunol.181.9.6604

[223] Chentoufi, A.A., et al. HLA-A*0201-restricted CD8+ cytotoxic T lymphocyte epitopes identified from herpes simplex virus glycoprotein D. J Immunol. 2008; 180: p. 426–437. DOI: 10.4049/jimmunol.180.1.426.

[224] Nicola, A.V., et al. Structure-function analysis of soluble forms of herpes simplex virus glycoprotein D. J Virol. 1996; 70: p. 3815–3822.

[225] Zhu, X.P., et al. HSV-2 vaccine: current status and insight into factors for developing an efficient vaccine. Viruses. 2014; 6: p. 371–390. DOI:10.3390/v6020371.

[226] Retamal-Díaz, A.R., et al. Immune evasion by herpes simplex viruses. Rev Chilena Infectol. 2015; 32: p. 58–70. DOI:10.4067/S0716-10182015000200013.

[227] Belshe, R.B., et al. Efficacy results of a trial of a herpes simplex vaccine. N Engl J Med. 2012; 366: p. 34–43. DOI:10.1056/NEJMoa1103151.

[228] Bernstein, D.I., et al. Safety and immunogenicity of glycoprotein D-adjuvant genital herpes vaccine. Clin Infect Dis. 2005; 40: p. 1271–1281. DOI:10.1086/429240.

[229] Corey, L., et al. Recombinant glycoprotein vaccine for the prevention of genital HSV-2 infection: two randomized controlled trials. Chiron HSV Vaccine Study Group. JAMA. 1999; 282: p. 331–340. DOI:10.1001/jama.282.4.331

[230] Kohl, S., et al. Limited antibody-dependent cellular cytotoxicity antibody response induced by a herpes simplex virus type 2 subunit vaccine. J Infect Dis. 2000; 181: p. 335–339. DOI:10.1086/315208.

[231] Halford, W.P. Antigenic breadth: a missing ingredient in HSV-2 subunit vaccines? Expert Rev Vaccines. 2014; 13: p. 691–710. DOI: 10.1586/14760584.2014.910121.

[232] Chentoufi, A.A., et al. Towards a rational design of an asymptomatic clinical herpes vaccine: the old, the new, and the unknown. Clin Dev Immunol. 2012; 2012: p. 187585. DOI:10.1155/2012/187585.

[233] Petro, C., et al. Herpes simplex type 2 virus deleted in glycoprotein D protects against vaginal, skin and neural disease. Elife. 2015; 4:e06054. DOI:10.7554/eLife.06054

[234] Halford, W.P., et al. A live-attenuated HSV-2 ICP0 virus elicits 10 to 100 times greater protection against genital herpes than a glycoprotein D subunit vaccine. PLoS One. 2011; 6: p. e17748. DOI:10.1371/journal.pone.0017748.

[235] Halford, W.P., et al. Antibodies are required for complete vaccine-induced protection against herpes simplex virus 2. PLoS One. 2015; 10: p. e0145228. 10.1371/journal.pone. 0145228 10.1371/journal.pone.0145228.

[236] Geltz, J.J., E. Gershburg, and W.P. Halford. Herpes simplex virus 2 (HSV-2) infected cell proteins are among the most dominant antigens of a live-attenuated HSV-2 vaccine. PLoS One. 2015; 10: p. e0116091. DOI:10.1371/journal.pone.0116091.

[237] Da Costa, X., et al. Construction, phenotypic analysis, and immunogenicity of a UL5/ UL29 double deletion mutant of herpes simplex virus 2. J Virol. 2000; 74: p. 7963–7971. DOI:10.1128/JVI.74.17.7963-7971.2000.

[238] Mundle, S.T., et al. High-purity preparation of HSV-2 vaccine candidate ACAM529 is immunogenic and efficacious in vivo. PLoS One. 2013; 8: p. e57224. DOI:10.1371/ journal.pone.0057224.

[239] Diaz, F.M. and D.M. Knipe. Protection from genital herpes disease, seroconversion and latent infection in a non-lethal murine genital infection model by immunization with an HSV-2 replication-defective mutant virus. Virology. 2016; 488: p. 61–67. DOI: 10.1016/j.virol.2015.10.033.

[240] Wang, K., et al. A Herpes simplex virus 2 (HSV-2) gD mutant impaired for neural tropism is superior to an HSV-2 gD subunit vaccine to protect animals from challenge with HSV-2. J Virol. 2015; 90: p. 562–574. DOI:10.1128/JVI.01845-15.

[241] Casanova, G., et al. A double-blind study of the efficacy and safety of the ICP10PK vaccine against recurrent genital HSV-2 infections. Cutis. 2002; 70: p. 235–239. DOI:n/d.

[242] Awasthi, S., et al. Live attenuated herpes simplex virus 2 glycoprotein E deletion mutant as a vaccine candidate defective in neuronal spread. J Virol. 2012; 86: p. 4586–4598. DOI:10.1128/JVI.07203-11.

[243] de Bruyn, G., et al. A randomized controlled trial of a replication defective (gH deletion) herpes simplex virus vaccine for the treatment of recurrent genital herpes among

immunocompetent subjects. Vaccine. 2006; 24: p. 914–920. DOI: 10.1016/j.vaccine. 2005.08.088.

[244] Boukhvalova, M., et al. Efficacy of the herpes simplex virus 2 (HSV-2) glycoprotein D/ AS04 vaccine against genital HSV-2 and HSV-1 infection and disease in the cotton rat sigmodon hispidus model. J Virol. 2015; 89: p. 9825–9840. DOI:10.1128/JVI.01387-15.

[245] Srivastava, R., et al. HLA-A02:01-restricted epitopes identified from the herpes simplex virus tegument protein VP11/12 preferentially recall polyfunctional effector memory CD8+ T cells from seropositive asymptomatic individuals and protect humanized HLA-A*02:01 transgenic mice against ocular herpes. J Immunol. 2015; 194: p. 2232–2248. DOI:10.4049/jimmunol.1402606.

[246] Khan, A.A., et al. Therapeutic immunization with a mixture of herpes simplex virus 1 glycoprotein D-derived "asymptomatic" human CD8+ T-cell epitopes decreases spontaneous ocular shedding in latently infected HLA transgenic rabbits: association with low frequency of local PD-1+ TIM-3+ CD8+ exhausted T cells. J Virol. 2015; 89: p. 6619–6632. DOI:10.1128/JVI.00788-15.

[247] Srivastava, R., et al. A herpes simplex virus type 1 human asymptomatic CD8+ T-cell epitopes-based vaccine protects against ocular herpes in a "humanized" HLA transgenic rabbit model. Invest Ophthalmol Vis Sci. 2015; 56: p. 4013–4028. DOI: 10.1167/ iovs.15-17074.

[248] Cattamanchi, A., et al. Phase I study of a herpes simplex virus type 2 (HSV-2) DNA vaccine administered to healthy, HSV-2-seronegative adults by a needle-free injection system. Clin Vaccine Immunol. 2008; 15: p. 1638–1643. DOI:10.1128/CVI.00167-08.

[249] Dutton, J.L., et al. A novel DNA vaccine technology conveying protection against a lethal herpes simplex viral challenge in mice. PLoS One. 2013; 8: p. e76407. DOI: 10.1371/ journal.pone.0076407.

[250] Kolb, A.W., C. Ane, and C.R. Brandt. Using HSV-1 genome phylogenetics to track past human migrations. PLoS One. 2013; 8: p. e76267. DOI:10.1371/journal.pone.0076267.

Section 4

Novel Attempts to Manage and Prevent Herpesvirus Infections

Chapter 6

Review: Biological and Pharmacological Basis of Cytolytic Viral Activation in EBV-Associated Nasopharyngeal Carcinoma

Natalie Oker, Nikiforos-Ioannis Kapetanakis and Pierre Busson

Additional information is available at the end of the chapter

http://dx.doi.org/10.5772/64738

Abstract

Epstein-Barr virus (EBV) infection contributes to the development of different types of human malignancies, especially nasopharyngeal carcinoma. As a herpesvirus, EBV can establish two major modes of virus-cell interactions: a latent or a lytic infection. Latent infection is prevalent in the vast majority of malignant cells in EBV-related malignancies. Inducing a switch from latent to lytic infection in a substantial fraction of malignant cells has long been considered as a potentially interesting therapeutic approach. Therapeutic benefits are expected from (1) the cytotoxic or cytostatic effects of viral products expressed in the context of the lytic cycle; (2) expression of viral enzymes capable of metabolizing pro-drugs selectively inside these cells and (3) broadening the expression spectrum of antigenic viral proteins. In this chapter, addressing non EBV-specialized readers, we first summarize the main aspects of EBV biology with emphasis on the cellular mechanisms known to control latent and lytic infections. Then, we outline the basic principles and requirements of cytolytic EBV activation performed with a therapeutic intent. Finally, we review the main categories of pharmacological agents reported to be active in the switch from latent to lytic infection, including drugs used for conventional anti-tumour chemotherapy, histone-deacetylase inhibitors and various miscellaneous compounds.

Keywords: nasopharyngeal carcinoma, Epstein-Barr virus, lytic cycle, histone-deacetylase inhibitors, epigenetics, immunotherapy, phenotypic screening, compound library

1. Introduction

Nasopharyngeal carcinomas (NPCs) are consistently associated with the Epstein-Barr virus (EBV) [1] and represent a major public health problem worldwide. In order of frequency, it is the third leading cause of virus-related human malignancies, ranking just behind hepatocellular carcinomas linked to the hepatitis B and C viruses and cervix carcinoma involving human papilloma viruses (HPV) [2]. The incidence of NPC is particularly high in Southern China, especially in the Guangdong province (approximately 25 cases per 100,000 persons per year). In addition, there are areas of intermediate incidence in Southeast Asia and North Africa. Men have been shown to be two to three times more likely to develop NPC than women, the most frequent age of disease occurrence being 50–60 years. Regardless of patient geographical origin, NPCs are constantly associated with EBV (except for a very small number of highly differentiated atypical forms related to tobacco and alcohol and a few cases associated with human papilloma viruses [HPV] mainly observed in Europe and North America) (reviewed in [3]). Like other EBV-associated malignancies, NPC is clearly a multifactorial disease. The non-viral risk factors include germline genetic susceptibility involving alleles of the major histocompatibility complex (MHC) region on chromosome 6 [4]. One example of a susceptibility gene not linked to the MHC region is *MST1R*. It encodes a protein detected in the ciliated epithelial cells in normal nasopharyngeal mucosa, which plays a role in the cilia motility, thus being essential for host defence [5]. The action of diet carcinogens, like salt-preserved fish in South China, probably accounts for multiple acquired cellular genetic and epigenetic alterations detected in malignant cells [4].

Investigations on the mechanisms of NPC oncogenesis and novel therapeutic approaches have long been hampered by a lack of biological resources. It has been proven very difficult to derive tumour lines propagated *in vitro* or even patient-derived xenografts (PDXs), which retain the EBV-genome, using clinical NPC specimens. Currently, there is only one EBV-positive NPC tumour line (C666-1), which is routinely propagated *in vitro*, and a small number of EBV-positive NPC PDXs whose cells are not easily handled *in vitro* [6–9]. There is evidence that malignant NPC cells tend to lose the EBV genome when one attempts their propagation *in vitro*. The resulting EBV-negative cell lines seem to have a phenotype, which does not fit with the NPC cell phenotype *in situ*, especially with regard to immunological characteristics (e.g., HONE1) [10]. They are sometimes artificially reinfected by EBV *in vitro*, but this does not restore a typical NPC cell phenotype.

In addition to the latent EBV-infection, the malignant phenotype of NPC cells is explained by a number of genetic and epigenetic alterations. None of these alterations is constant in all NPC tumours, and few are highly specific of NPCs. In most cases, there are no alterations in the *TP53* gene (it is mutated in less than 10% of the cases; [11]). In contrast, many other tumour suppressor genes (TSGs) are frequently silenced in NPC cells, especially *CDKN2A* (chromosome 9p21.3) and *RASSF1* (chromosome 3p21.3). Their inactivation often results from a combination of hemizygous deletion and promoter hypermethylation on the remaining allele. However, deletions of both alleles and inactivating point mutations have been also reported. Silencing of these TSGs often occurs very early in the carcinogenic process [12]. Many TSGs like the gene encoding the Wnt inhibitory factor 1 (*WIF*, 12q14.3) or E-cadherin (*CDH*, 16q22.1) are consistently inactivated by methylation of both alleles [13, 14]. One has to keep in mind that prolonged latent—or even transient EBV infection—favours genome-wide hypermethylation of gene promoters [15]. In addition to the silencing of multiple TSGs, NPC cells exhibit alterations of multiple oncogenes, which are often affected by copy number gains, especially *CCND1* (encoding cyclin D1 on chromosome 11q13.3) and *PIK3CA* (3q26.1) [12, 16]. There are also frequent copy-number gains of the gene encoding the lymphotoxin-β receptor (*LTβR*) on chromosome 12p13.31 [12]. This is a rare – or even unique – example of a genetic alteration which is highly specific of NPC tumours. Two oncogenic fusion genes—*UBR5-ZNF423* and *FGFR-TACC3*—have been identified by high-throughput sequencing of tumour mRNAs (RNAseq), but they are only detected in a minority of NPC specimens, mainly among late stage tumours [17, 18]. Whole exome sequencing of 128 NPC specimens has revealed mutations in genes encoding proteins involved in chromatin remodelling, especially *ARID1a* (about 10% of the specimens) and in the process of DNA methylation (*TET1*, *TET2* and *TET3*, altogether in about 9% of the specimens) [11].

On average, NPCs are more radio-sensitive and chemo-sensitive than other head and neck tumours. However, they still raise serious therapeutic issues: (1) NPCs are often discovered at a late stage whereas lymph node and distant organ metastases occur early in tumour evolution; (2) despite remarkable advances in 3D radiotherapy, irradiation often leads to severe functional sequels (subcutaneous and muscular sclerosis and xerostomia); (3) although metastatic lesions are initially sensitive to chemotherapy, they often escape from treatment control after a few months [19, 20]. In summary, despite the remarkable progress achieved in the recent years, there is still an urgent need for better therapeutic modalities. In this context, the idea of using EBV as a kind of endogenous oncolytic virus has been in the air for a very long time. The proof of principle that pharmacological agents can disrupt latent infection and push at least a fraction of EBV-infected malignant cells towards the reactivation of the viral lytic cycle was presented almost 40 years ago. Sodium butyrate was reported as a potent activator of the lytic cycle in EBV-infected human B-lymphocytes in 1979 [21]. However, the progress of this concept towards therapeutic applications has been very slow, especially regarding NPC. The aim of this review is to assemble key information for a public of non-EBV-specialists who want to understand the cellular, molecular and pharmacological basis of translational research on cytolytic viral activation in nasopharyngeal carcinomas.

2. Main aspects of EBV biology and regulation of the latent/lytic modes of infection

2.1. General aspects of EBV biology

EBV is one of the eight human Herpesviridae. It belongs to the subfamily of the γ-herpesvirinae and to the genus of lymphocryptoviruses. Like all Herpesviridae, it is an enveloped double-stranded DNA virus, containing about 80 genes. It is the causative agent of infectious mononucleosis, and it has an etiological role in several human malignant diseases mainly of

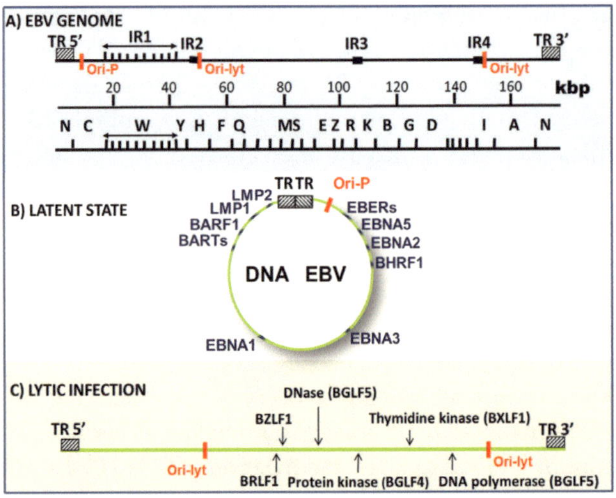

Figure 1. EBV-genome structure and configuration in connection with latent or lytic infection: (A) EBV genome map (linear representation). EBV genome contains about 180 kilobase pairs (kb). Both ends of the viral DNA contain a variable number of repeated non-coding sequences of 500 bp (called TR for terminal repeats). In addition, there are internal repeated sequences called internal repeats (major IR1 and minor IR 2–4). Ori-P is the replication origin of the viral genome used in the latent state of infection. The Ori-lyt are two replication origins used during the lytic infection. The reference restriction map is based on the digestion of the viral DNA by the restriction enzyme BamH1. Restriction fragments are classified from the largest (BamH1A) to the smallest (BamH1Z). Designation of open-reading frames is based on this restriction map. For example, BZLF1 is the first leftward open reading frame in the BamH1 Z fragment (Bam Z leftward open-reading frame 1) (BZLF1 by extension also means the corresponding protein). (B) Configuration of the EBV genome characteristic of the latently infected cells. When the infected cell enters a state of latent infection the viral DNA is circularized probably by recombination of the TRs. This circular form of the genome called episome is contained in the nucleus in combination with cellular chromatin but apart from chromosomes. The episomes are passively replicated by cellular DNA polymerases starting from the Ori-P origin of replication. During latent infection, most viral genes are silent. However, about 10% of them are consistently expressed (in blue). Most of these genes encode final products—viral non-coding RNAs or proteins—with transforming properties. They are called "latent genes" whereas genes expressed only during lytic infection are called "lytic genes". There is no topographical separation between the two categories of genes.(C) Configuration of the EBV-genome characteristic of the lytic infection. As usual in virology, the phase of the lytic cycle which precedes viral DNA replication is called the early phase. As soon as the viral DNA pol starts the autonomous replication of the viral genome, lytically infected cells enter the late phase. Newly synthesized viral genomes are in a linear configuration. Viral proteins expressed at the very beginning of the early phase of the lytic cycle like BZLF1 and BRLF1 are encoded by immediate early genes. Early viral proteins are expressed at a more advanced stage. Many of them are involved in DNA metabolism, for example, the viral thymidine-kinase, DNAse and DNA polymerase. The EBV protein kinase (BGLF4; protein encoded by the Bam G leftward open reading frame 4) can phosphorylate various substrates. It is also one component of the viral particle.

lymphoid and epithelial origin as well as several autoimmune diseases. Examples of EBV-related malignancies are nasopharyngeal carcinomas, several types of lymphomas (endemic Burkitt's Lymphoma (BL), more rarely Hodgkin lymphomas, centro-facial NK-T lymphoma, post-transplant lymphomas and AIDS-associated lymphomas), and approximately 10% of gastric cancers worldwide [22–25]. Examples of autoimmune diseases likely to involve EBV are multiple sclerosis and systemic lupus erythematosus [26, 27]. Like all other herpesviruses, EBV causes lifelong infection following the primo-infection. More than 90% of adult humans are healthy carriers regardless of their geographic origin. Its persistence in healthy carriers is the result of three types of viral characteristics: (1) its capacity to continuously induce bursts of productive infections in various tissues, especially in the upper aerodigestive tract and more specifically in the tonsils, the salivary glands and possibly gingiva; (2) its capacity to achieve latent infection mainly in B-lymphocytes, especially memory B cells in blood, bone marrow and lymphoid organs; (3) its sophisticated strategies of immune evasion [28].

The distinction between two major modes of virus-cell interactions is a key to understanding EBV biology [29]. (1) Latent infections are cellular infection modalities characterized by the absence of viral particle production, a restricted expression of viral genes (often less than 10 out of 80) and a circular configuration of the viral genome (**Figure 1**). (2) Lytic/productive infections are characterized by sequential or concomitant expression of most viral genes, abundant synthesis of linear viral genomes and finally extracellular release of viral particles or virions in a context of mandatory cell death.

2.2. Latent EBV infection in LCL and NPC cells

One major common characteristic of most EBV-related malignancies is the predominance of latent modes of virus-cell interactions. As a rule in EBV-associated tumours, no EBV particles are detected by electron microscopy on tumour sections, whereas the viral DNA can be visualized in the nuclei of malignant cells by *in situ* hybridization. Consistently, very few malignant cells exhibit expression of viral proteins characteristic of the lytic/productive cycle. This minimal expression of lytic viral proteins in EBV-infected malignant cells favours immune evasion. In most latently infected cells, the virus-cell interactions are bidirectional: a few viral genes often modify the phenotype of the host cell, whereas the cellular context contributes to the repression of most viral genes (see subsequent section B3). For laboratory investigations, a model of latent EBV infection is easily obtained *in vitro* by infection of peripheral blood mononuclear cells (PBMCs) from normal donors, which results in the oncogenic transformation of resting B cells. These EBV-transformed B-cell lines are often called lymphoblastoid cell lines (LCLs). LCLs are immortalized and tumorigenic in SCID (severe combined immune-deficiency) mice [30]. They represent a privileged model for *in vitro* investigations of the molecular basis of latent infections.

During latency, the viral genome is conserved under the form of circular copies, called episomes, from one to several tens, which are present in the nuclei apart from the cell chromosomal DNA but also coated with cellular chromatin and replicated by cellular enzymes at each cell division. Most viral genes expressed in EBV-associated malignancies belong to the category of the latent genes, which are expressed in LCLs *in vitro* and contribute to the maintenance of the transformed phenotype. Their oncogenic effects are summarized in **Table 1**. The latent genes encode nuclear proteins like the EBNAs (Epstein-Barr nuclear antigens), membrane proteins like LMP1, LMP-2A and LMP-2B (latent membrane proteins 1, 2A and 2B) and non-coding RNAs. There are two main categories of non-coding viral RNAs: genuine microRNAs and the EBERs (Epstein-Barr virus encoded small RNAs) [31]. Two families of viral microRNAs, called "BHRF1" and "BART" microRNAs, can be transcribed from two distinct regions of the EBV genome, the Bam-H1 H and Bam-H1 A segments, respectively. The BHRF1 (Bam H rightward open reading frame 1) cluster includes at least four microRNAs which are transcribed in LCLs but not detectable in most NPC specimens. They have a key role in the inhibition of apoptosis [32]. In contrast, the microRNAs of the BART (Bam A rightward transcripts) family are abundant in most NPC cells and not detected in LCLs. About 40 BART microRNAs have been identified so far [33, 34]. They target a great variety of mRNAs, for example, those encoding the pro-apoptotic protein Puma (miR-BART5), the tumour suppressor protein PTEN (miR-BART1) or the viral DNA polymerase (miR-BART2) [35–37]. The EBERs are single-stranded RNAs of about 170 nucleotides with a complex secondary structure containing double-stranded segments which can react with various cellular receptors of double-stranded RNAs such as the PKR (protein-kinase RNA-dependent), RIG1 (retinoic acid-inducible gene 1) and TLR3 (Toll-like receptor 3) [38]. These interactions stimulate resistance to interferon and production of growth factors like IGF-1 (insulin-like growth factor 1) [38].

	Type	EBV product	Examples of functions
Latency product	Non-coding latent transcripts	**EBERs 1 and 2** (non-coding RNAs)	Inhibit the RNA dependent protein kinase (PKR) activate the Toll-like receptor 3 (TLR3) [38]
		miR-BART (microRNAs)	Inhibit expression of some viral lytic and cellular pro-apoptotic genes, promote metastases [35, 37, 42]
	Non-membrane protein	**EBNA 1** (nuclear protein)	Episome maintenance, contributes to disruption of PML bodies [43]
		BARF1 (secreted protein)	Ligand of the m-CSF or CSF1 receptor [44]
	Membrane latent protein	**LMP1**	Activator of Bcl3/p50/P50 NF-kB complex [1]
		LMP2A	Activator of PI3 kinase/Akt pathway [1]
		LMP2B	Accelerates the degradation of interferon receptors [1]
Lytic cycle products	Immediate early proteins (IE)	**BZLF1** **BRLF1**	Act as transactivators, enhancing the expression of later lytic genes [45, 46]
	Early proteins (E)	**DNA polymerase**	Lytic replication of the viral genome
		EBV-DNase	Alkaline nuclease with endonuclease and exonuclease activities
		EBV-thymidine kinase (TK)	Phosphokinase with a probable role in the phosphorylation of FIAU [47, 48]
		EBV-protein kinase (PK)	Phosphokinase involved in DNA replication and virion production. Phosphorylates ganciclovir [49, 50]
	Late proteins (L)	**VCA** (viral capsid antigen)	A complex of structural proteins assembled in the viral capsid
		Gp350	Viral envelope glycoprotein binding to the cell membrane receptor CD21 (also known as CR2) [51]

Table 1. Examples of EBV latency and lytic cycle products with clues on their functions.

In comparison to LCLs, latent EBV infection in NPC cells has some specific features. The expression of latent viral proteins is more restricted than in LCLs. Only one latent nuclear protein—EBNA1—is expressed in contrast to six in LCLs. The latent membrane proteins, LMP1 and LMP2, are present in most tumour specimens but often at a low level and with major heterogeneity among tumour cells [39, 40]. Another specific feature of latent EBV-infection in NPCs is the huge abundance of the BART microRNAs which on average account for 20% of total tumour microRNAs [41]).

2.3. The switch from latency to the lytic/productive infection and its regulation

2.3.1. General features of the switch from latent to lytic EBV-infection

Experimental lytic/productive infections by EBV can be achieved in several manners. As explained in the previous section, EBV infection of resting B cells *in vitro* results mostly in transformed cells, which are latently infected. However, EBV-transformed B cells can enter the lytic/productive cycle at a secondary stage triggered by plasmacytic differentiation or treatment with various chemicals (**Table 2**. The experimental systems used for EBV infection of epithelial cells *in vitro* are completely different. First, penetration of viral particles often requires special procedures, as for example, pre-adsorption on B cells [52]. Next, penetration of EBV in epithelial cells often results in direct lytic infection (**Figure 2**) [53, 54]. With most experimental systems, latently infected epithelial cells remain rare, and their isolation usually requires the use of recombinant viruses carrying selectable markers [53]. In some models based on cultured primary epithelial cells, primary lytic infection can be blocked by overexpression of cyclin D1 or inhibition of CDKN2A. So far, most laboratory investigations on EBV lytic/productive infection have been done starting from latently infected cells switching to lytic viral activation (see **Figure 2**). This switch is triggered by external factors and/or modifications of physiological cell conditions, for example, differentiation or senescence. It is the result of a change in the balance of factors either blocking or enhancing the expression of lytic viral genes. As reviewed by Miller et al [29] and more recently by Kenney et al [46] the switch from latent to lytic infection is a sequential process, comprising two main sets of events:

1. Upstream events leading to the expression of the immediate early viral transactivators BZLF1 (also called ZEBRA, Zta or EB-1) and BRLF1 (also called Rta) [29].

2. Downstream events resulting from the interaction of BZLF1 and BRLF1 with a number of viral promoters controlling genes encoding products of the lytic cycle, such as, the EBV DNA-polymerase or EBV-TK (thereafter called lytic promoters) [55].

The genes encoding BZLF1 and BRLF1 are themselves under the control of promoter regions (Zp and Rp), which are regulated by a wide number of cellular factors, either activators or inhibitors. The influence of the inhibitors is predominant in the latently infected cells and vice versa during lytic activation.

Class of drugs	Example
Direct PKC activators	Phorbol-esters [65]
Conventional chemotherapy [30, 60, 74, 88–90]	*cis*-platinum or cisplatin (alkylating agent); paclitaxel (stabilizer of mitotic spindle); 5-fluoro-uracil (pyrimidine analog); gemcitabine (cytidine analog)
Inhibitors of histone deacetylases (HDACi)	Sodium butyrate [21], Trichostatin A [61] Valproic acid [86–88, 104], Panobinostat (LBH-589) [94], Vorinostat (SAHA) [95, 96], Romidepsin [60, 97]
Demethylating agents	5-Azacitidine [100]
Protease inhibitors	Bortezomib [47, 48]
Gamma-secretase inhibitors	Dibenzazepine [101]
Tetrahydrocarbolines and other compounds recently selected by high-throughput assays [103], [102]	
Prodrugs activated by EBV enzymes [59, 80, 105]	Ganciclovir (9-(1,3-dihydroxy-2-propoxyméthyl) guanine or DHPG) FIAU (2′-fluoro-2′-deoxy-β-D-5-iodo-uracil-arabinofuranoside) [47, 48]

Table 2. Summary of the different drugs with reported capacity of lytic EBV activation and prodrugs phosphorylated by EBV-encoded kinases.

BZLF1 and BRLF1 activate one another's promoter and their cooperation is required for optimal activation of many lytic viral promoters [56]. BZLF1 preferentially activates these promoters when they are methylated, whereas BRLF1 is more active on unmethylated promoters [45]. Therefore, they cooperate to induce lytic activation, no matter if the viral genome is methylated or unmethylated. BRLF1 ability to transactivate its target promoters is also dependent on another epigenetic mark, which is the 5-hydroxymethylation of cytosine in promoter CpG islands. Hydroxy-methylation induces an open chromatin conformation, which is critical for optimal action of BRLF1 but not BZLF1 [56].

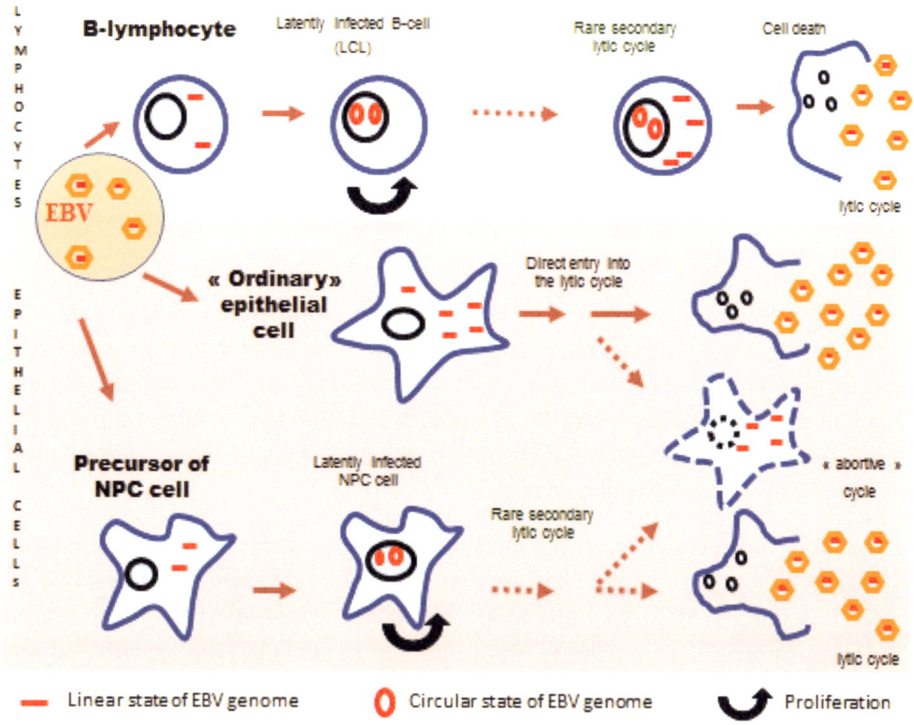

Figure 2. Main modalities of virus-cell interactions in lymphoid and epithelial cells.

– When human resting B-lymphocytes are infected by EBV, a fraction of them enter a state of viral latency requiring the circularization of the EBV genome and the expression of several viral latent genes. Simultaneously, the host cell undergoes an oncogenic transformation driven by the viral latent genes, especially EBNA2, EBNA3A and 3C and LMP1. These transformed B-cells can proliferate indefinitely resulting in LCLs. However, a secondary switch from latency to the lytic cycle can occur in a fraction of them. This fraction is generally very small but it can be increased by some pharmacological agents like HDACi (histone deacetylase inhibitors) or PKC (protein-kinase C) activators.

– EBV infection of epithelial cells *in vitro* requires special experimental systems like co-cultivation with B-cells carrying viral particles . In most of these experiments, penetration of the viral particles results in infections which are directly cytolytic or abortive. There is evidence that the same type of events often occur when epithelial cells are infected *in situ*, for example in the salivary glands or in the tonsil epithelium (normal epithelial cells are depicted by a cell shape named "ordinary epithelial cell") [57, 58].

– However for some reasons, malignant NPC cells undergo a latent infection suggesting a special type of virus-cell interactions at the initial stage of the malignant cell proliferation. There is evidence that the precursor cells have premalignant alterations, especially knock-out of cyclin kinases' inhibitors which make them resistant to virus-induced senescence (cells with pre-malignant lesions are depicted by a cell shape named "precursor of NPC cell"). Obviously, this is not sufficient for the establishment of latency since it is difficult to establish latency in many epithelial cells which are fully transformed and grown *in vitro*. In latently infected NPC cells secondary lytic or abortive cycle can occur spontaneously in a small fraction of the cells. One important aim of cytolytic activation therapy is to dramatically increase the number of the malignant cells undergoing the lytic cycle.

2.3.2. Overview of the cell physiological conditions and transcription factors involved in the switch from latent to lytic EBV infection

The factors controlling the switch from latent to lytic infection are numerous. They are intricate and highly dependent on the cellular context. **Figure 3** is intended to give a concise overview of these factors. As a first approximation, absence of cellular differentiation, cell proliferation, EMT (epithelial to mesenchymal transition) and inflammation tend to favour the maintenance of a latent infection. In contrast, cell differentiation, senescence, DNA damage response and hypoxia favour the entry into the lytic cycle.

Many signalling pathways which favour lytic EBV activation involve protein-kinases C (PKCs). PKCs phosphorylate hydroxyl groups of serine and threonine in multiple protein substrates, including MAP kinases and MARCK proteins. They are involved in multiple and diverse biological processes including transcriptional regulations, cell growth and immune responses. Physiological activation of "conventional" PKCs (α, β, γ) requires stimulation by diacylglycerol and calcium, whereas activation of "novel" PKCs (δ, ε, H, Θ) requires only diacylglycerol. There is evidence for a special contribution of PKCδ to the control of the switch from latent to lytic infection. For example, as explained in sections C1, D2 and D3, PKCδ plays a critical role downstream of various pharmacological agents inducing lytic EBV activation [59–61]. On the contrary, the intracellular form of the cytokine IL-32 has been shown to prevent lytic activation by sequestration of PKCδ [62]. Several PKC isoforms activate cellular immediate early proteins, for example, the FOS and EGR1 (early growth response) transcription

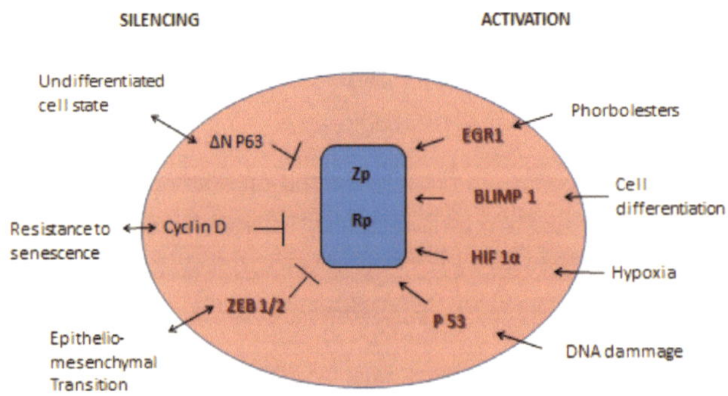

Figure 3. Summary of the physiological cell conditions and transcription factors, which modulate the activity of the *BZLF1* (Zp) and *BRLF1* (Rp) gene promoters in the context of epithelial cells. Both promoters are under the control of inhibitory (left side) and activating (right side) factors. Various physiological cell conditions are enumerated outside the pink circle, whereas the corresponding regulatory proteins are presented inside the pink circle with transcription factors appearing in bold brown letters. Detailed explanations and references are provided in section B3-2.

factors, which have specific binding motifs on the Zp and Rp promoters, respectively [63, 64]. For information, phorbol-esters, which have long been known to induce lytic EBV activation in lymphoid cells, are direct pharmacological agonists of PKCs [65].

The Blimp-1 transcription factor, which is a key player for lymphoid and epithelial cell differentiation, is a strong inducer of lytic EBV activation, especially in epithelial cells; it stimulates the expression of both BZLF1 and BRLF1 [66]. TGF-β has been reported to induce a partial lytic activation in EBV-positive gastric carcinoma cell lines [67]. Various factors, which antagonize senescence, favour the maintenance of EBV latency. As already mentioned, overexpression of cyclin-D1 or loss of CDKN2A, which enhances G0/G1 transition in the cell cycle, prevents lytic activation in some models of EBV latent infection in epithelial cells [53]. Generally speaking, inflammation—for example, inflammation triggered by TNF-α or interferon-γ—is rather seen as a factor which strengthens EBV latency [68]. Activation of NF-κB has been reported to stabilize latency in various γ-herpesviruses [69]. Stat3 is also reported to stabilize latency in EBV-infected cells [63]. However, the influence of inflammatory factors on EBV latency in NPC cells has not been well documented. The ZEB1/ZEB2 transcription factors, which are known to contribute to the EMT in various cell types, have been proven to antagonize EBV lytic activation [46]. Finally, there is evidence that ΔNp63 can contribute to the maintenance of EBV latency. ΔNp63 is a variant of the p63 transcription factor, which is preferentially expressed in undifferentiated basal epithelial cells [46].

The switch of latent to lytic infection is also triggered by various types of cellular stress and adaptive responses. Genotoxic stress and DNA damage response have long been known to favour EBV lytic activation in various cell backgrounds, especially in NPC cells. BRdU treatment was used in one of the oldest reports on lytic EBV activation achieved in an NPC model [70]. Ionizing radiations have been shown to induce lytic activation in LCLs [71]. As explained in details in section D1, many drugs in the arsenal of conventional cancer chemotherapy are inducers of lytic EBV activation in various cellular backgrounds. The ATM (ataxia-telangiectasia mutated) kinase and to a lesser extent TP53 often play a critical role in the sequence of events leading from DNA damage to BZLF1 expression [72, 73]. In addition, there is evidence that ATM is involved in the lytic cascade downstream of BZLF1 [74]. In other words, ATM is apparently involved in the lytic cascade upstream as well as downstream of BZLF1 expression. Endoplasmic reticulum stress, which results from large-scale protein misfolding, has been reported as a condition leading to lytic activation in LCLs [75]. Finally, the cellular stress resulting from hypoxia was reported to favour the switch from latent to lytic infection with a role of the HIF1 transcription factor in the activation of the Zp promoter [46].

2.3.3. *Epigenetic factors control the switch from latent to lytic EBV infection*

This point will be addressed briefly with focus on two epigenetic processes, which are critical for the switch from latent to lytic EBV infection: DNA methylation and transcriptional control by microRNAs. We have previously mentioned that BZLF1 preferentially interacts with methylated lytic promoters, whereas it is the opposite for BRLF1. Therefore, the net impact of the methylation or the demethylation of the viral genome is not easily predicted and is highly dependent on the cell background [56]. Recent work has shed some light on the role of cellular microRNAs in the maintenance of EBV latency. Members of the miR-200 family, like miR-200b, target the transcription factors ZEB1 and ZEB2, thus having the ability to reactivate the EBV lytic gene expression when added to EBV-infected cells [76]. This applies not only to endogenous microRNAs but also to members of the miR-200 family conveyed by extracellular vesicles, which can induce lytic EBV activation in recipient cells [77]. In contrast, other microRNAs of cellular and viral origin have the ability to repress viral reactivation by targeting elements of its machinery [78].

3. Basic principles and requirements of therapies based on viral cytolytic activation in EBV-associated malignancies

Like for all Herpesviridae, production of viral particles is automatically associated with the death of cells infected by EBV. This is the reason why the productive cycle—as opposed to the state of latent infection—is often called the lytic cycle [29]. With this in mind, for a long time —going as far as the end of the seventies—many authors have considered reactivation of the lytic cycle as a possible therapeutic strategy. For a long time, the concept has evolved very slowly. One hurdle was the fact that the state of latent infection is generally very stable. In addition, in most cases it is difficult to go beyond partial reactivation with expression of some proteins of the lytic cycle like the immediate-early BZLF1 transactivator. On the other hand it was recognized that, in many cases, even partial reactivation is sufficient to block cell growth [79]. This intrinsic cytotoxic effect of partial reactivation, the possible induction of the expression of viral enzymes capable to of metabolizing a prodrug and the wish to enlarge the range of viral targets for the immune system are currently the main incentives to investigate the induction of the viral lytic activation as a therapeutic approach [30]. One additional perspective is to use precursors of radio-opaque molecules processed by viral enzymes and selectively retained in the malignant cells for specific medical imaging [73, 48]. Two EBV-encoded enzymes are usually cited as having the potential to metabolize and activate prodrugs: the EBV thymidine kinase (TK) and the EBV protein kinase (PK) encoded by the BXLF1 and BGLF4 genes, respectively. Ganciclovir (GCV) and acyclovir (ACV) are not substrates of EBV-TK. Meng et al. have formally demonstrated that among EBV-encoded kinases, EBV-PK is necessary and sufficient to phosphorylate GCV and ACV [49]. Consistent data had been previously reported by Gustafson et al [80]. The phosphorylated active forms of GCV and ACV inhibits cellular and viral replication. Fialuridine or FIAU (2′-fluoro-2′-deoxy-β-D-5-iodouracil-arabinofuranoside) is also a prodrug activated in EBV-infected cells, presumably by the EBV-TK, but its use is limited by its hepatic and metabolic toxicity [47, 48, 81]. However, it can be used occasionally, at least in animal models, for imaging purpose. Indeed, its phosphorylation by EBV-TK results in its selective retention in malignant cells. Thanks to this property, FIAU can be used for imaging in two ways either as a carrier of iodine atoms, which are opaque to X-ray or when the cold iodine atoms are substituted by radioactive isotopes as a tumour-selective radioactive emitter [47, 48, 73].

Induction of the lytic cycle can also have potentially deleterious effects. Several publications have shown that lytic activation in a small fraction of malignant cells can enhance malignant growth [82]. This is probably due to the increased production of inflammatory cytokines, angiogenic and growth factors in some cells undergoing the lytic cycle [83, 84]. To prevent these deleterious effects, it is important: (a) to ensure that the lytic cycle activation occurs in a large fraction of malignant cells and (b) if possible to combine lytic activation with administration of a cytotoxic prodrug, preferably with a bystander effect (see **Figure 4**).

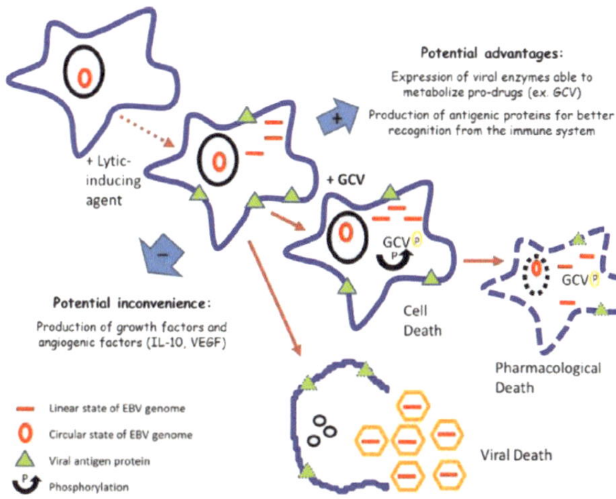

Figure 4. Importance of combining the induction of the lytic cycle with the administration of prodrugs. From a therapeutic point of view, induction of the lytic cycle has both positive and negative consequences. Positive consequences are (1) the expression of viral enzymes, which can activate prodrugs specifically in malignant cells and (2) the broadening of viral antigen expression, which is expected to facilitate specific recognition and destruction of malignant cells by the immune system. One potential drawback is an increase in the production of growth factors and angiogenic factors by malignant cells. Several advantages are expected from the use of a prodrug specifically activated in malignant cells (e.g., ganciclovir or GCV): (1) rapid pharmacological killing of malignant cells including many cells that would not undergo a full lytic cycle and therefore would stay alive for a long time in the absence of the prodrug; (2) reduction in the production of growth and angiogenic factors coming from cells undergoing the lytic cycle; (3) possible bystander killing of cells resistant to lytic cycle induction, for example, by diffusion of phosphorylated GCV through gap junctions.

These experimental approaches will be classified in three categories: (1) one based on drugs used for conventional antitumour chemotherapy; (2) one based on HDAC inhibitors and (3) finally, a miscellaneous category including various agents from PKC activators to demethylating agents.

4. Main categories of pharmacological agents with the potential of cytolytic activation of EBV in the context of NPC cells

4.1. Impact of pharmacological agents used in conventional chemotherapy

A number of drugs used in conventional chemotherapy have the ability to induce the EBV lytic cycle in various lymphoid or epithelial cell backgrounds. The drugs which are the most active in this process—gemcitabine and to a lesser extent doxorubicin, taxol, *cis*-platinum (CDDP), 5-fluoro-uracil (5-FU) and methotrexate, have been empirically identified (*cis*-platinum and 5-FU are only active in epithelial cells; methotrexate probably only in lymphoid cells) [30, 59, 85]. Regarding NPC cells, initial data on this topic have been published by Shannon Kenney's group in 2002. They showed that CDDP, 5-FU and taxol were able to induce —or to enhance—the expression of the lytic proteins BZLF1, BRLF1 and BMRF1 in a gastric carcinoma cell line artificially infected by EBV (AGS-EBV) [59]. Simultaneously in cytotoxicity assays, synergies were found between GCV and *cis*-platinum or 5-FU. Similar results were obtained using the xenografted NPC tumour line, C18. *De novo* expression of BZLF1 and enhancement of BMRF1 expression were observed after treatment with CDDP or 5-FU. In addition, there was a synergy in tumour growth inhibition when GCV was combined with CDDP or 5-FU in intraperitoneal injections to nude mice bearing C18 xenografts. It is noteworthy that the same agents had no impact on lytic EBV-protein expression in two other NPC xenografts, C15 and C17. One specific feature of C18 shared with AGS-EBV is that, even in the absence of drug treatment, it has a low level of constitutive lytic protein expression. This is not the case for the two other NPC xenografts ([7] and P. Busson, unpublished data).

Subsequently, regardless of the cell background, gemcitabine has been confirmed as the most potent inducer of EBV lytic activation among all drugs routinely used in conventional chemotherapy [30, 73, 86]. Its capacity to contribute to lytic activation in NPC cells has been well documented by Wildeman et al. (2012) and to a lesser extent by Hsu et al. (2015) [86, 87]. In both cases, induction of lytic activation in the C666-1 cell line was stronger when gemcitabine (in the range of 3 μM *in vitro*) was combined with valproic acid (in the range of 300 μM *in vitro*). Valproic acid is a short chain fatty acid typically used as an anti-epileptic drug, which behaves, to some extent, as an HDAC inhibitor. Using the gemcitabine/valproic acid combination *in vitro* more than 80% C666-1 cells were positive for BZLF1 by immunofluorescence [86]. Wildeman's publication also provided substantial clinical data. Objective tumour responses were reported for three end-stage NPC patients subjected to a three-drug regimen combining gemcitabine, valproic acid and GCV [86]. Interestingly, 3 years later, partial tumour responses were again reported by the same group for five out of eight NPC patients refractory to conventional treatments and subjected to the almost same regimen except that GCV was replaced by valganciclovir [88]. The median survival was 9 months (95% confidence interval 7–17 months).

In some epithelial cell backgrounds, the combination of gemcitabine with an HDAC inhibitor is not mandatory for induction of the lytic cycle. Using a naturally EBV-infected gastric carcinoma cell-line, SNU-719, Lee et al. have observed induction of BZLF1 expression by gemcitabine alone at low concentrations (in the 10 nM range *in vitro*) [73]. Consistently, they have observed a synergy of gemcitabine with GCV in the treatment of SCID mice xenografted with SNU-719 gastric carcinoma cells. As pointed by the authors, a synergy between GCV and gemcitabine has also been reported in treatment of non-EBV-related malignant cells but much higher concentrations of gemcitabine were required (about 10 μM) [73, 89].

The mechanisms of lytic activation induced by drugs of conventional chemotherapy are complex and probably diverse. In the case of AGS-EBV cells, Kenney's group has highlighted several signalling pathways suspected to link cell response to *cis*-platinum and 5-FU with the expression of immediate-early viral proteins: the MAPK/ERK, p38 MAPK and PKCδ pathways. However, all these data resulted from experiments based on chemical inhibitors. Therefore, they would probably need verifications by other approaches. As previously mentioned, endoplasmic reticulum (ER) stress is one possible cell alteration leading to lytic activation [75]. However, ER stress markers are not modified in gastric carcinoma cells subjected to lytic activation driven by gemcitabine [73]. Signalling pathways involved in the response to genotoxic stress seem to contribute more consistently to viral lytic activation, especially in epithelial cells. In SNU-719 cells, knocking-down expression of ATM and TP53 by RNA-interference antagonizes BZLF1 induction by gemcitabine [73].

4.2. Impact of HDAC inhibitors

Histone deacetylases (HDAC) belong to a class of enzymes that remove acetyl groups from histones, allowing them to wrap the DNA more tightly and therefore to decrease gene expression in the corresponding part of the genome. Therefore, depending on the cell context, HDAC inhibitors (HDACi) lead to transcriptional activation of a fraction of cellular genes, which are epigenetically silenced. Many HDACi have anti-oncogenic properties. They inhibit cell proliferation and favour cell cycle arrest, differentiation or apoptosis. These effects are at least partially related to re-expression of tumour suppressor genes such as *CDKN2A* or *ATM*. Their use for viral lytic induction is based on the assumption that histone acetylation is one epigenetic mechanism contributing to the silencing of most viral genes in latently infected cells. In addition, they can have less direct effects by increasing the expression of cellular proteins involved in the lytic cycle like the ATM kinase.

The first generation of HDACi includes different categories of compounds, for example, trichostatin A (one member of the hydroxamic acid family) or short chain fatty acids such as butyrate and valproic acid. As mentioned in the introduction of this chapter, as early as 1979, sodium butyrate was shown to induce lytic EBV activation in lymphoid cells [21]. At this date, the capacity of butyrate to inhibit histone deacetylases was not known, and the exact mechanism of the lytic induction remained raveled. It is noteworthy that, much later, in the years 2000, arginine butyrate was used in combination with GCV by Faller et al. in the first clinical trial aiming at lytic EBV activation in a group of patients bearing EBV-associated malignancies. Fifteen patients with refractory EBV-associated lymphoid malignancies were included in this phase I/II trial. Significant clinical responses were obtained for 10 of them including some complete clinical and pathological responses, although with important secondary effects [90].

The impact of valproic acid on lytic EBV gene expression has been mentioned in the previous part (D1) of this chapter. In contrast with more recent HDACi, very high concentrations of valproic acid are required for lytic gene induction, often in the range of 300 μM *in vitro*. In addition, valproic acid often has limited effects on lytic gene expression when it is not combined with another drug acting by a distinct mechanism, like gemcitabine. Recent studies published by G. Miller's group have shown that valproic acid has more complex biological effects than other HDACi. In some circumstances, it behaves as an antagonist of other HDACi and as an inhibitor of EBV lytic reactivation [63, 91]. Trichostatin A has been reported to induce

EBV lytic activation in an epithelial cell line artificially infected by EBV through pathways involving activation of the PKCδ and its phosphorylation of the Sp1 transcription factor (specificity protein 1) [61]. It is noteworthy that trichostatin has also been reported to induce activation of chromosomally integrated genomes of human herpesvirus 6 (HHV6), at least *in vitro* [92, 93].

HDACi of the second generation are compounds, which have been specifically designed to inhibit HDAC enzymes. They include the hydroxamic acids like vorinostat (suberoyl anilide hydroxamic acid or SAHA) and panobinostat (LBH589) and benzamides like entinostat (MS275). Most of them have the ability to inhibit HDAC enzymes of the class I (HDAC-1, HDAC-2, HDAC-3 and HDAC-8) and class II (HDAC-4, HDAC-5, HDAC-6, HDAC-7, HDAC-9 and HDAC-10). In 2012, Faller's group has reported an interesting comparative investigation of a series of HDACi mainly of the second generation, with an assessment of their relative strength in the induction of lytic EBV activation in lymphoid cells [94]. The most potent agent was panobinostat. Entinostat and apicidin, although less effective, were active in the nanomolar range. Vorinostat, which is active in epithelial cells as mentioned below, was not active in the panel of lymphoid cells used by the authors. Panobinostat has obtained approval from the European Medicines Agency and the Food and Drug Administration (USA) for the treatment of multiple myeloma.

Information on the impact of HDACi on epithelial cells, especially NPC cells, is available in a series of reports published by A.K.S. Chiang and collaborators from Hong Kong [95, 96]. Hui et al. reported in 2010 that in AGS-EBV cells, expression of BZLF1, BMRF1 and gp350 and even production of infectious viral particles were induced by Vorinostat used at μM concentrations [96]. As in previous studies, it was observed that the AGS-EBV cells had a certain level of spontaneous lytic activation in basal conditions prior to any drug treatment [59]. It was also confirmed that Vorinostat was a poor inducer of lytic EBV activation in lymphoid cells in contrast with data obtained using epithelial cells. In 2012, the same group has reported *in vitro* induction by Vorinostat (5 μM) of BZLF1 and BMRF1 but not gp350 in the NPC cell line C666-1. The induction of BZLF1 in C666-1 cells needed higher concentration of SAHA and a longer incubation time than for the artificial EBV(+) epithelial cell lines like HK1-EBV and HONE1-EBV. Nevertheless, induction of BZLF1 was achieved using Vorinostat *in vivo* by systemic treatment of C666-1 cells xenografted into nude mice (50 mg/kg, 5 days a week) [95]. Finally, in a report of 2016, Hui et al. have used a more selective HDACi, a bacterial product called romidepsin derived from *Chromobacterium violaceum* [60]. Romidepsin has selective inhibitory action against class I HDAC enzymes (mainly HDAC-1, HDAC-2 and HDAC-3). Romidepsin was shown to induce BZLF1, BRLF1 and BMRF1 in artificially EBV-infected epithelial cells using concentrations ranging from 0.5 to 5 nM. In mice xenografted with C666-1 cells, combined systemic administration of romidepsin (0.375 mg/kg, 2 days a week) and GCV (50 mg/kg, 5 days a week) resulted in a substantial tumour growth reduction [60]. The impact of romidepsin on lytic protein expression was abrogated by a chemical inhibitor of PKCδ but not inhibitors of PI3K, MEK, p38 MAPK, JNK. Interestingly lytic activation was not impaired by an ATM kinase inhibitor in contrast with observations made on SNU-719 gastric carcinoma cells treated with gemcitabine (see part D1 of this chapter and Lee et al.) [73]. Romidepsin is approved by the FDA (Food and Drug Administration) but not the EMA (European Medicines Agency) for the treatment of cutaneous T-cell lymphomas. Adverse effects are nausea, vomiting, thrombocytopenia and leucopenia [97]. For future research, data on romidepsin underline the potential of novel more selective HDACi whose design is based on now-solved HDAC structures (third generation HDACi, for more information see Stahl et al. [98]).

4.3. Impact of miscellaneous pharmacological agents

In this section, we will briefly introduce other agents that have been used for lytic EBV activation but less consistently than HDAC inhibitors or conventional anti-cancer agents like gemcitabine. Phorbol-esters (like 12-*O*-tetradecanoylphorbol-13-acetate) are compounds, which activate proteins of the PKC family. In the history of EBV research, they have been among the first pharmacological agents along with sodium butyrate and BRdU used for induction of EBV lytic activation. However, to our knowledge, phorbol-esters have not been used in experiments involving NPC cells [65]. Nevertheless, as previously mentioned, one protein of the PKC family, PKCδ was reported to contribute to lytic EBV activation induced in epithelial cells by *cis*-platinum and 5-FU on the one hand and by romidepsin, an inhibitor of class I HDAC enzymes, on the other hand (see sections D1 and D2, respectively) [60, 59].

Bortezomib requires a special mention because it has been selected by a systematic screening of an FDA library of hundreds of chemical compounds to identify novel inducers of the lytic cycle (not published data but quoted by [48]). In Burkit lymphoma cells, the effect of Bortezomib on lytic activation has been reported to be dependent on the b-ZIP transcription factor C-EBP β (CCAAT/enhancer-binding protein β [99]). Bortezomib has proven to induce BZLF1 and EBV-TK expression in EBV-positive Burkitt lymphoma or gastric carcinoma cells xenografted on SCID mice [47, 48]. This process has been exploited for selective accumulation of FIAU in tumour cells expressing EBV-TK. Either for imaging purpose using this iodinated compound labelled with [^{125}I] or with therapeutic intent after labelling FIAU with [^{131}I]. To our knowledge, this approach has not been extended to NPC models. As explained in section C of this chapter, the use of FIAU in patients is compromised by the risk of acute metabolic or hepatic toxicity [81]. In more recent publication, the same group was involved in a new systematic screening of another compound library (John Hopkins Drug Library), which has identified gemcitabine as the best candidate for combination treatment with GCV [73].

Demethylating agents, especially 5-azacytidine, have been considered as potential inducers of EBV lytic activation in NPC cells. As reported by Chan et al., eight NPC patients were treated with 5-aza for one to six cycles: only mild lytic activation was recorded by RT-PCR and immunohistochemistry of lytic EBV products [100]. This relative weakness of 5-azacytidine might be explained by some distinct characteristics of BZLF1 and BRLF1 transactivation, which have been observed in the context of epithelial cells. BZLF1 transactivation of lytic gene promoters is enhanced by DNA methylation whereas it is the opposite for BRLF1 [45]. This is bad news for the impact of demethylating agents since cooperation of BZLF1 and BRLF1 is crucial for the optimal progression of lytic EBV activation.

A Notch2 inhibitor—dibenzazepine—has been shown to induce lytic EBV activation in Burkit and LCL cells by Giunco et al [101]. According to the authors, this effect depends on the downregulation of the BATF transcription factor, which modulates BZLF1 expression. To our knowledge, lytic induction based on Notch2 inhibitors has not been investigated in NPC cells.

Finally, two groups have recently selected novel inducers of the lytic activation by high-throughput phenotypic screening from large chemical libraries containing several ten thousands of compounds [102, 103]. Tikhmyanova et al. have reported five structurally related tetrahydrocarboline derivatives, which are active in the range of 150–170 nM in various EBV-positive cell-lines including the C666-1 NPC cell line [103]. Choi et al. have published data on five novel compounds, which are distinct from PKC agonists and HDACi, one of which activates the MAPK pathways and bears structural resemblance to iron chelators [102].

5. Conclusions

The idea of inducing EBV lytic activation in malignant NPC cells with a therapeutic intent has been in the air for more than 30 years [21]. However, this therapeutic approach is still facing major obstacles. First, there is evidence that EBV latency is heavily locked in NPC cells, and several locking mechanisms are probably intimately connected with the oncogenic alterations at the levels of genome, epigenome and cell phenotype. For example, there is evidence that the wild-type ATM kinase plays a critical role at several steps of lytic EBV activation (although not under treatment by romidepsin) [60, 72, 74]. In fact, ATM is frequently down-regulated in NPC cells [106]. There is also evidence that Stat3 activation prevents EBV lytic activation. Again, constitutive Stat3 activation is a common feature of malignant NPC cells. Hydroxy-methylation marks often disappear from the DNA of NPC cells [107, 108]. In a fraction of tumours, this alteration is a consequence of inactivating mutations in the *TET1*, *TET2* or *TET3* genes [11]. Regardless of its mechanism, the loss of DNA hydroxyl-methylation promotes malignant transformation and simultaneously makes the lytic promoters less sensitive to the action of BRLF1 [56].

Another difficulty is the absence of biomarkers for early identification of NPC tumours that will be responsive to various agents expected to induce the lytic cycle. We suggest that, in general, the most sensitive tumours will be those where there is a spontaneous expression of lytic genes prior to any treatment, a point that would deserve a specific investigation. In spite of all these difficulties, significant progress has been accomplished. Several objective tumour responses have been obtained in NPC patients treated with a combination of gemcitabine, valproic acid and GCV [86, 88]. Since HDACi more effective than valproic acid are now available, there is room for progress using similar patterns of treatment. At a time when the success of immunotherapies based on checkpoint inhibitors has a dramatic impact on our approach of cancer biology and therapy, several authors rightly emphasize the importance of EBV lytic activation as a mean to increase the antigenicity of malignant cells [109]. This trend is even stronger since major changes are taking place at the confluence of epigenetics, virology and tumour immunology: recent publications have shown that demethylating agents can increase tumour cell antigenicity by removing the inhibition of endogenous retroviruses [110].

However, combining the inducers of EBV lytic activation with prodrugs specifically activated by viral enzymes remains a valuable goal. It is striking that while remarkable progress is being made concerning lytic inducers, almost nothing seems to happen regarding the prodrug candidates. So far, most investigators rely on GCV (ganciclovir), which was not designed for EBV-infected cells but is used by default. Nevertheless, a change seems to be in the air in this field too. A recent systematic proteomic analysis of EBV-PK substrates has identified hundreds of cellular proteins involved in DNA damage response, mitosis and cell cycle. More importantly, in terms of pharmacology, the analysis of the phosphosites of these substrates reveals a proline-rich motif signature, which will probably be helpful for the design of artificial substrates [50].

Competing interests

The authors declare no financial or non-financial competing interests.

Acknowledgements

Natalie Oker was the recipient of a fellowship from the "Union des Blessés de la Face et de la Tête—Les Gueules Cassées" (2014).

Author details

Natalie Oker[1,2], Nikiforos-Ioannis Kapetanakis[1] and Pierre Busson[1*]

*Address all correspondence to: pbusson@igr.fr

1 CNRS UMR 8126, Gustave Roussy and University of Paris-Sud/Paris-Saclay, Villejuif, France

2 Department of Otorhinolaryngology, Cervicofacial, Maxillofacial and Plastic Surgery, Lariboisière Hospital (Assistance Publique Hôpitaux de Paris) and University of Denis Diderot, Paris, France

References

[1] Busson P, editor. Nasopharyngeal Carcinoma. Keys for Translational Medicine and Biology. New York/Austin: Landes/Springer; 2012. 205 p.

[2] Busson P, Keryer C, Ooka T, Corbex M. EBV-associated nasopharyngeal carcinomas: from epidemiology to virus-targeting strategies. Trends Microbiol. 2004;12:356–60.

[3] Chua ML, Wee JT, Hui EP, Chan AT. Nasopharyngeal carcinoma. Lancet. 2016 Mar 5;387(10022):1012–24. DOI: 10.1016/S0140-6736(15)00055-0. pii: S0140-6736(15)00055-0.

[4] Feng BJ. Descriptive, environmental and genetic epidemiology of nasopharyngeal carcinoma. In: Bussson P, editor. Nasopharyngeal Carcinoma: Keys for Translational Medicine and Biology. Austin/New York: Landes/Springer; 2013. p. 23–41.

[5] Dai W, Zheng H, Cheung AK, Tang CS, Ko JM, Wong BW, et al. Whole-exome sequencing identifies MST1R as a genetic susceptibility gene in nasopharyngeal carcinoma. Proc Natl Acad Sci USA. 2016;113:3317–22. DOI: 10.1073/pnas.1523436113.

[6] Cheung ST, Huang DP, Hui AB, Lo KW, Ko CW, Tsang YS, et al. Nasopharyngeal carcinoma cell line (C666-1) consistently harbouring Epstein-Barr virus. Int J Cancer. 1999;83:121–6.

[7] Busson P, Ganem G, Flores P, Mugneret F, Clausse B, Caillou B, et al. Establishment and characterization of three transplantable EBV-containing nasopharyngeal carcinomas. Int J Cancer. 1988;42:599–606.

[8] Gressette M, Verillaud B, Jimenez-Pailhes AS, Lelievre H, Lo KW, Ferrand FR, et al. Treatment of nasopharyngeal carcinoma cells with the histone-deacetylase inhibitor abexinostat: cooperative effects with *cis*-platin and radiotherapy on patient-derived xenografts. PLoS One. 2014;9:e91325. DOI: 10.1371/journal.pone.0091325.

[9] Hoe SL, Tan LP, Jamal J, Peh SC, Ng CC, Zhang WC, et al. Evaluation of stem-like side population cells in a recurrent nasopharyngeal carcinoma cell line. Cancer Cell Int. 2014;14:101. DOI: 10.1186/s12935-014-0101-0.

[10] Glaser R, Zhang HY, Yao KT, Zhu HC, Wang FX, Li GY, et al. Two epithelial tumor cell lines (HNE-1 and HONE-1) latently infected with Epstein-Barr virus that were derived from nasopharyngeal carcinomas. Proc Natl Acad Sci USA. 1989;86:9524–8.

[11] Lin DC, Meng X, Hazawa M, Nagata Y, Varela AM, Xu L, et al. The genomic landscape of nasopharyngeal carcinoma. Nat Genet. 2014;46:866–71. DOI: 10.1038/ng.3006.

[12] Lo K, Chung GT, To KF. Acquired genetic and epigenetic alterations in nasophryngeal carcinomas. In: Busson P, editor. Nasopharyngeal Carcinoma—Keys for Translational Medicine and Biology. Austin/New York: Landes/Springer; 2013. p. 61–81.

[13] Ayadi W, Karray-Hakim H, Khabir A, Feki L, Charfi S, Boudawara T, et al. Aberrant methylation of p16, DLEC1, BLU and E-cadherin gene promoters in nasopharyngeal carcinoma biopsies from Tunisian patients. Anticancer Res. 2008;28:2161–7.

[14] Chan SL, Cui Y, van Hasselt A, Li H, Srivastava G, Jin H, et al. The tumor suppressor Wnt inhibitory factor 1 is frequently methylated in nasopharyngeal and esophageal carcinomas. Lab Invest. 2007;87:644–50. DOI: 10.1038/labinvest.3700547.

[15] Birdwell CE, Queen KJ, Kilgore PC, Rollyson P, Trutschl M, Cvek U, et al. Genome-wide DNA methylation as an epigenetic consequence of Epstein-Barr virus infection of immortalized keratinocytes. J Virol. 2014;88:11442–58. DOI: 10.1128/JVI.00972-14.

[16] Hui AB, Or YY, Takano H, Tsang RK, To KF, Guan XY, et al. Array-based comparative genomic hybridization analysis identified cyclin D1 as a target oncogene at 11q13.3 in nasopharyngeal carcinoma. Cancer Res. 2005;65:8125–33.

[17] Chung GT, Lung RW, Hui AB, Yip KY, Woo JK, Chow C, et al. Identification of a recurrent transforming UBR5-ZNF423 fusion gene in EBV-associated nasopharyngeal carcinoma. J Pathol. 2013;231:158–67. DOI: 10.1002/path.4240.

[18] Yuan L, Liu ZH, Lin ZR, Xu LH, Zhong Q, Zeng MS. Recurrent FGFR3-TACC3 fusion gene in nasopharyngeal carcinoma. Cancer Biol Ther. 2014;15:1613–21. DOI: 10.4161/15384047.2014.961874.

[19] Guigay J. Advances in nasopharyngeal carcinoma. Curr Opin Oncol. 2008;20:264–9.

[20] Lee AW, Ma BB, Ng WT, Chan AT. Management of nasopharyngeal carcinoma: current practice and future perspective. J Clin Oncol. 2015 Oct 10;33(29):3356–64.. DOI: 10.1200/JCO.2015.60.9347.

[21] Luka J, Kallin B, Klein G. Induction of the Epstein-Barr virus (EBV) cycle in latently infected cells by *n*-butyrate. Virology. 1979;94:228–31.

[22] Tse E, Kwong YL. How I treat NK/T-cell lymphomas. Blood. 2013;121:4997–5005. DOI: 10.1182/blood-2013-01-453233.

[23] Flavell KJ, Murray PG. Hodgkin's disease and the Epstein-Barr virus. Mol Pathol. 2000;53:262–9.

[24] Epstein MA, Barr YM. Cultivation in vitro of human lymphoblasts from Burkitt's malignant lymphoma. Lancet. 1964;1:252–3.

[25] Iizasa H, Nanbo A, Nishikawa J, Jinushi M, Yoshiyama H. Epstein-Barr virus (EBV)-associated gastric carcinoma. Viruses. 2012;4:3420–39.

[26] Ascherio A, Munger KL, Lunemann JD. The initiation and prevention of multiple sclerosis. Nat Rev Neurol. 2012;8:602–12. DOI: 10.1038/nrneurol.2012.198.

[27] Draborg AH, Duus K, Houen G. Epstein-Barr virus in systemic autoimmune diseases. Clin Dev Immunol. 2013;2013:535738. DOI: 10.1155/2013/535738.

[28] Hu Z, Usherwood EJ. Immune escape of gamma-herpesviruses from adaptive immunity. Rev Med Virol. 2014 Nov;24(6):365–78. DOI: 10.1002/rmv.1791.

[29] Miller G, El-Guindy A, Countryman J, Ye J, Gradoville L. Lytic cycle switches of oncogenic human gammaherpesviruses. Adv Cancer Res. 2007;97:81–109. DOI: 10.1016/S0065-230X(06)97004-3.

[30] Feng WH, Hong G, Delecluse HJ, Kenney SC. Lytic induction therapy for Epstein-Barr virus-positive B-cell lymphomas. J Virol. 2004;78:1893–902.

[31] Skalsky RL, Cullen BR. EBV noncoding RNAs. Curr Top Microbiol Immunol. 2015;391:181–217. DOI: 10.1007/978-3-319-22834-1_6.

[32] Klinke O, Feederle R, Delecluse HJ. Genetics of Epstein-Barr virus microRNAs. Semin Cancer Biol. (Review). 2014;26:52–9. DOI: 10.1016/j.semcancer.2014.02.002.

[33] Amoroso R, Fitzsimmons L, Thomas WA, Kelly GL, Rowe M, Bell AI. Quantitative studies of Epstein-Barr virus-encoded microRNAs provide novel insights into their regulation. J Virol. 2011;85:996–1010. DOI: 10.1128/JVI.01528-10.

[34] Cosmopoulos K, Pegtel M, Hawkins J, Moffett H, Novina C, Middeldorp J, et al. Comprehensive profiling of Epstein-Barr virus microRNAs in nasopharyngeal carcinoma. J Virol. 2009;83:2357–67.

[35] Choy EY, Siu KL, Kok KH, Lung RW, Tsang CM, To KF, et al. An Epstein-Barr virus-encoded microRNA targets PUMA to promote host cell survival. J Exp Med. 2008;205:2551–60.

[36] Barth S, Pfuhl T, Mamiani A, Ehses C, Roemer K, Kremmer E, et al. Epstein-Barr virus-encoded microRNA miR-BART2 down-regulates the viral DNA polymerase BALF5. Nucleic Acids Res. 2008;36:666–75. DOI: 10.1093/nar/gkm1080.

[37] Cai L, Ye Y, Jiang Q, Chen Y, Lyu X, Li J, et al. Epstein-Barr virus-encoded microRNA BART1 induces tumour metastasis by regulating PTEN-dependent pathways in nasopharyngeal carcinoma. Nat Commun. 2015;6:7353. DOI: 10.1038/ncomms8353.

[38] Iwakiri D, Takada K. Role of EBERs in the pathogenesis of EBV infection. Adv Cancer Res. (Review). 2010;107:119–36. DOI: 10.1016/S0065-230X(10)07004-1.

[39] Khabir A, Karray H, Rodriguez S, Rose M, Daoud J, Frikha M, et al. EBV latent membrane protein 1 abundance correlates with patient age but not with metastatic behavior in north African nasopharyngeal carcinomas. Virol J. 2005;2:39.

[40] Heussinger N, Buttner M, Ott G, Brachtel E, Pilch BZ, Kremmer E, et al. Expression of the Epstein-Barr virus (EBV)-encoded latent membrane protein 2A (LMP2A) in EBV-associated nasopharyngeal carcinoma. J Pathol. 2004;203:696–9.

[41] Barth S, Meister G, Grasser FA. EBV-encoded miRNAs. Biochim Biophys Acta. [Research Support, Non-U.S. Gov't]. 2011;1809:631–40. DOI: 10.1016/j.bbagrm.2011.05.010.

[42] Jung YJ, Choi H, Kim H, Lee SK. MicroRNA miR-BART20-5p stabilizes Epstein-Barr virus latency by directly targeting BZLF1 and BRLF1. J Virol. 2014;88:9027–37. DOI: 10.1128/JVI.00721-14.

[43] Frappier L. Role of EBNA1 in NPC tumourigenesis. Semin Cancer Biol. 2012;22:154–61. DOI: 10.1016/j.semcancer.2011.12.002. pii: S1044-579X(11)00103-9.

[44] Strockbine LD, Cohen JI, Farrah T, Lyman SD, Wagener F, DuBose RF, et al. The Epstein-Barr virus BARF1 gene encodes a novel, soluble colony-stimulating factor-1 receptor. J Virol. 1998;72:4015–21.

[45] Wille CK, Nawandar DM, Panfil AR, Ko MM, Hagemeier SR, Kenney SC. Viral genome methylation differentially affects the ability of BZLF1 versus BRLF1 to activate Epstein-Barr virus lytic gene expression and viral replication. J Virol. 2013;87:935–50. DOI: 10.1128/JVI.01790-12.

[46] Kenney SC, Mertz JE. Regulation of the latent-lytic switch in Epstein-Barr virus. Semin Cancer Biol. 2014;26:60–8. DOI: 10.1016/j.semcancer.2014.01.002.

[47] Fu DX, Tanhehco Y, Chen J, Foss CA, Fox JJ, Chong JM, et al. Bortezomib-induced enzyme-targeted radiation therapy in herpesvirus-associated tumors. Nat Med. 2008;14:1118–22. DOI: 10.1038/nm.1864.

[48] Fu DX, Tanhehco YC, Chen J, Foss CA, Fox JJ, Lemas V, et al. Virus-associated tumor imaging by induction of viral gene expression. Clin Cancer Res. 2007;13:1453–8. DOI: 10.1158/1078-0432.CCR-06-2295.

[49] Meng Q, Hagemeier SR, Fingeroth JD, Gershburg E, Pagano JS, Kenney SC. The Epstein-Barr virus (EBV)-encoded protein kinase, EBV-PK, but not the thymidine kinase (EBV-TK), is required for ganciclovir and acyclovir inhibition of lytic viral production. J Virol. 2010;84:4534–42. DOI: 10.1128/JVI.02487-09.

[50] Li R, Liao G, Nirujogi RS, Pinto SM, Shaw PG, Huang TC, et al. Phosphoproteomic profiling reveals Epstein-Barr virus protein kinase integration of DNA damage response and mitotic signaling. PLoS Pathog. 2015;11:e1005346. DOI: 10.1371/journal.ppat.1005346. pii: PPATHOGENS-D-15-01981.

[51] Coghill AE, Bu W, Nguyen H, Hsu WL, Yu KJ, Lou PJ, et al. High levels of antibody that neutralize B-cell infection of Epstein-Barr virus and that bind EBV gp350 are associated with a lower risk of nasopharyngeal carcinoma. Clin Cancer Res. 2016 Jul 15;22(14):3451–7. DOI: 10.1158/1078-0432.CCR-15-2299. pii: clincanres.2299.2015.

[52] Shannon-Lowe CD, Neuhierl B, Baldwin G, Rickinson AB, Delecluse HJ. Resting B cells as a transfer vehicle for Epstein-Barr virus infection of epithelial cells. Proc Natl Acad Sci USA. 2006 May 2;103(18):7065–70.

[53] Tsang CM, Yip YL, Lo KW, Deng W, To KF, Hau PM, et al. Cyclin D1 overexpression supports stable EBV infection in nasopharyngeal epithelial cells. Proc Natl Acad Sci USA. 2012;109:E3473–82. DOI: 10.1073/pnas.1202637109.

[54] Feederle R, Neuhierl B, Bannert H, Geletneky K, Shannon-Lowe C, Delecluse HJ. Epstein-Barr virus B95.8 produced in 293 cells shows marked tropism for differentiat-

ed primary epithelial cells and reveals interindividual variation in susceptibility to viral infection. Int J Cancer. 2007;121:588–94. DOI: 10.1002/ijc.22727.

[55] Quinlivan EB, Holley-Guthrie EA, Norris M, Gutsch D, Bachenheimer SL, Kenney SC. Direct BRLF1 binding is required for cooperative BZLF1/BRLF1 activation of the Epstein-Barr virus early promoter, BMRF1. Nucleic Acids Res. 1993;21:1999–2007.

[56] Wille CK, Nawandar DM, Henning AN, Ma S, Oetting KM, Lee D, et al. 5-Hydroxymethylation of the EBV genome regulates the latent to lytic switch. Proc Natl Acad Sci USA. 2015;112:E7257–65. DOI: 10.1073/pnas.1513432112.

[57] Temple RM, Zhu J, Budgeon L, Christensen ND, Meyers C, Sample CE. Efficient replication of Epstein-Barr virus in stratified epithelium in vitro. Proc Natl Acad Sci USA. 2014;111:16544–9. DOI: 10.1073/pnas.1400818111.

[58] Hadinoto V, Shapiro M, Sun CC, Thorley-Lawson DA. The dynamics of EBV shedding implicate a central role for epithelial cells in amplifying viral output. PLoS Pathog. 2009;5:e1000496. DOI: 10.1371/journal.ppat.1000496.

[59] Feng WH, Israel B, Raab-Traub N, Busson P, Kenney SC. Chemotherapy induces lytic EBV replication and confers ganciclovir susceptibility to EBV-positive epithelial cell tumors. Cancer Res. 2002;62:1920–6.

[60] Hui KF, Cheung AK, Choi CK, Yeung PL, Middeldorp JM, Lung ML, et al. Inhibition of class I histone deacetylases by romidepsin potently induces Epstein-Barr virus lytic cycle and mediates enhanced cell death with ganciclovir. Int J Cancer. 2016;138:125–36. DOI: 10.1002/ijc.29698.

[61] Tsai PF, Lin SJ, Weng PL, Tsai SC, Lin JH, Chou YC, et al. Interplay between PKCdelta and Sp1 on histone deacetylase inhibitor-mediated Epstein-Barr virus reactivation. J Virol. 2011;85:2373–85. DOI: 10.1128/JVI.01602-10.

[62] Lai KY, Chou YC, Lin JH, Liu Y, Lin KM, Doong SL, et al. Maintenance of Epstein-Barr Virus latent status by a novel mechanism, latent membrane protein 1-induced interleukin-32, via the protein kinase c-delta pathway. J Virol. 2015;89:5968–80. DOI: 10.1128/JVI.00168-15.

[63] Gorres KL, Daigle D, Mohanram S, McInerney GE, Lyons DE, Miller G. Valpromide inhibits lytic cycle reactivation of Epstein-Barr virus. MBio. 2016 Mar 1;7(2):e00113;7. DOI: 10.1128/mBio.00113-16 e00113-16.

[64] Ye J, Gradoville L, Miller G. Cellular immediate-early gene expression occurs kinetically upstream of Epstein-Barr virus bzlf1 and brlf1 following cross-linking of the B cell antigen receptor in the Akata Burkitt lymphoma cell line. J Virol. 2010;84:12405–18. DOI: 10.1128/JVI.01415-10.

[65] Nutter LM, Grill SP, Li JS, Tan RS, Cheng YC. Induction of virus enzymes by phorbol esters and *n*-butyrate in Epstein-Barr virus genome-carrying Raji cells. Cancer Res. 1987;47:4407–12.

[66] Vrzalikova K, Vockerodt M, Leonard S, Bell A, Wei W, Schrader A, et al. Down-regulation of BLIMP1alpha by the EBV oncogene, LMP-1, disrupts the plasma cell differentiation program and prevents viral replication in B cells: implications for the pathogenesis of EBV-associated B-cell lymphomas. Blood. 2011;117:5907–17. DOI: 10.1182/blood-2010-09-307710.

[67] Fukuda M, Ikuta K, Yanagihara K, Tajima M, Kuratsune H, Kurata T, et al. Effect of transforming growth factor-beta1 on the cell growth and Epstein-Barr virus reactivation in EBV-infected epithelial cell lines. Virology. 2001;288:109–18. DOI: 10.1006/viro.2001.1071. pii: S0042-6822(01)91071-2.

[68] Li Y, Long X, Huang L, Yang M, Yuan Y, Wang Y, et al. Epstein-Barr Virus BZLF1-mediated downregulation of proinflammatory factors is essential for optimal lytic viral replication. J Virol. 2015;90:887–903. DOI: 10.1128/JVI.01921-15.

[69] Brown HJ, Song MJ, Deng H, Wu TT, Cheng G, Sun R. NF-kappaB inhibits gamma-herpesvirus lytic replication. J Virol. 2003;77:8532–40.

[70] Trumper PA, Epstein MA, Giovanella BC. Activation in vitro by BUdR of a productive EB virus infection in the epithelial cells of nasopharyngeal carcinoma. Int J Cancer. 1976;17:578–87.

[71] Westphal EM, Blackstock W, Feng W, Israel B, Kenney SC. Activation of lytic Epstein-Barr virus (EBV) infection by radiation and sodium butyrate in vitro and in vivo: a potential method for treating EBV-positive malignancies. Cancer Res. 2000;60:5781–8.

[72] Hagemeier SR, Barlow EA, Meng Q, Kenney SC. The cellular ataxia telangiectasia-mutated kinase promotes Epstein-Barr virus lytic reactivation in response to multiple different types of lytic reactivation-inducing stimuli. J Virol. 2012;86:13360–70. DOI: 10.1128/JVI.01850-12.

[73] Lee HG, Kim H, Kim EJ, Park PG, Dong SM, Choi TH, et al. Targeted therapy for Epstein-Barr virus-associated gastric carcinoma using low-dose gemcitabine-induced lytic activation. Oncotarget. 2015;6:31018–29. DOI: 10.18632/oncotarget.5041.

[74] Hau PM, Deng W, Jia L, Yang J, Tsurumi T, Chiang AK, et al. Role of ATM in the formation of the replication compartment during lytic replication of Epstein-Barr virus in nasopharyngeal epithelial cells. J Virol. 2015;89:652–68. DOI: 10.1128/JVI.01437-14.

[75] Taylor GM, Raghuwanshi SK, Rowe DT, Wadowsky RM, Rosendorff A. Endoplasmic reticulum stress causes EBV lytic replication. Blood. 2011;118:5528–39. DOI: 10.1182/blood-2011-04-347112.

[76] Lin Z, Flemington EK. miRNAs in the pathogenesis of oncogenic human viruses. Cancer Lett. 2011;305:186–99. DOI: 10.1016/j.canlet.2010.08.018.

[77] Lin Z, Swan K, Zhang X, Cao S, Brett Z, Drury S, et al. Secreted oral epithelial cell membrane vesicles induce Epstein-Barr virus reactivation in latently infected B cells. J Virol. 2016;90:3469–79. DOI: 10.1128/JVI.02830-15.

[78] Forte E, Luftig MA. The role of microRNAs in Epstein-Barr virus latency and lytic reactivation. Microbes Infect/Institut Pasteur. 2011;13:1156–67. DOI: 10.1016/j.micinf.2011.07.007.

[79] Cayrol C, Flemington EK. The Epstein-Barr virus bZIP transcription factor Zta causes G0/G1 cell cycle arrest through induction of cyclin-dependent kinase inhibitors. EMBO J. 1996;15:2748–59.

[80] Gustafson EA, Chillemi AC, Sage DR, Fingeroth JD. The Epstein-Barr virus thymidine kinase does not phosphorylate ganciclovir or acyclovir and demonstrates a narrow substrate specificity compared to the herpes simplex virus type 1 thymidine kinase. Antimicrob Agents Chemother. 1998;42:2923–31.

[81] McKenzie R, Fried MW, Sallie R, Conjeevaram H, Di Bisceglie AM, Park Y, et al. Hepatic failure and lactic acidosis due to fialuridine (FIAU), an investigational nucleoside analogue for chronic hepatitis B. N Engl J Med. 1995;333:1099–105. DOI: 10.1056/NEJM199510263331702.

[82] Hong GK, Gulley ML, Feng WH, Delecluse HJ, Holley-Guthrie E, Kenney SC. Epstein-Barr virus lytic infection contributes to lymphoproliferative disease in a SCID mouse model. J Virol. 2005;79:13993–4003.

[83] Hsu M, Wu SY, Chang SS, Su IJ, Tsai CH, Lai SJ, et al. Epstein-Barr virus lytic transactivator Zta enhances chemotactic activity through induction of interleukin-8 in nasopharyngeal carcinoma cells. J Virol. 2008;82:3679–88. DOI: 10.1128/JVI.02301-07.

[84] Lee CH, Yeh TH, Lai HC, Wu SY, Su IJ, Takada K, et al. Epstein-Barr virus Zta-induced immunomodulators from nasopharyngeal carcinoma cells upregulate interleukin-10 production from monocytes. J Virol. 2011;85:7333–42. DOI: 10.1128/JVI.00182-11.

[85] Feng WH, Cohen JI, Fischer S, Li L, Sneller M, Goldbach-Mansky R, et al. Reactivation of latent Epstein-Barr virus by methotrexate: a potential contributor to methotrexate-associated lymphomas. J Natl Cancer Inst. 2004;96:1691–702. DOI: 10.1093/jnci/djh313.

[86] Wildeman MA, Novalic Z, Verkuijlen SA, Juwana H, Huitema AD, Tan IB, et al. Cytolytic virus activation therapy for Epstein-Barr virus-driven tumors. Clin Cancer Res. 2012;18:5061–70. DOI: 10.1158/1078-0432.CCR-12-0574.

[87] Hsu CL, Kuo YC, Huang Y, Huang YC, Lui KW, Chang KP, et al. Application of a patient-derived xenograft model in cytolytic viral activation therapy for nasopharyngeal carcinoma. Oncotarget. 2015;6:31323–34. DOI: 10.18632/oncotarget.5544.

[88] Stoker SD, Novalic Z, Wildeman MA, Huitema AD, Verkuijlen SA, Juwana H, et al. Epstein-Barr virus-targeted therapy in nasopharyngeal carcinoma. J Cancer Res Clin Oncol. 2015;141:1845–57. DOI: 10.1007/s00432-015-1969-3.

[89] Boucher PD, Shewach DS. In vitro and in vivo enhancement of ganciclovir-mediated bystander cytotoxicity with gemcitabine. Mol Ther. 2005;12:1064–71. DOI: 10.1016/j.ymthe.2005.07.643. pii: S1525-0016(05)01254-2.

[90] Perrine SP, Hermine O, Small T, Suarez F, O'Reilly R, Boulad F, et al. A phase 1/2 trial of arginine butyrate and ganciclovir in patients with Epstein-Barr virus-associated lymphoid malignancies. Blood. 2007;109:2571–8. DOI: 10.1182/blood-2006-01-024703.

[91] Daigle D, Gradoville L, Tuck D, Schulz V, Wang'ondu R, Ye J, et al. Valproic acid antagonizes the capacity of other histone deacetylase inhibitors to activate the Epstein-barr virus lytic cycle. J Virol. 2011;85:5628–43. DOI: 10.1128/JVI.02659-10.

[92] Arbuckle JH, Medveczky MM, Luka J, Hadley SH, Luegmayr A, Ablashi D, et al. The latent human herpesvirus-6A genome specifically integrates in telomeres of human chromosomes in vivo and in vitro. Proc Natl Acad Sci USA. 2010;107:5563–8. DOI: 10.1073/pnas.0913586107.

[93] Pellett PE, Ablashi DV, Ambros PF, Agut H, Caserta MT, Descamps V, et al. Chromosomally integrated human herpesvirus 6: questions and answers. Rev Med Virol. 2012;22:144–55. DOI: 10.1002/rmv.715.

[94] Ghosh SK, Perrine SP, Williams RM, Faller DV. Histone deacetylase inhibitors are potent inducers of gene expression in latent EBV and sensitize lymphoma cells to nucleoside antiviral agents. Blood. 2012;119:1008–17. DOI: 10.1182/blood-2011-06-362434.

[95] Hui KF, Ho DN, Tsang CM, Middeldorp JM, Tsao GS, Chiang AK. Activation of lytic cycle of Epstein-Barr virus by suberoylanilide hydroxamic acid leads to apoptosis and tumor growth suppression of nasopharyngeal carcinoma. Int J Cancer. 2012;131:1930–40. DOI: 10.1002/ijc.27439.

[96] Hui KF, Chiang AK. Suberoylanilide hydroxamic acid induces viral lytic cycle in Epstein-Barr virus-positive epithelial malignancies and mediates enhanced cell death. Int J Cancer. 2010;126:2479–89. DOI: 10.1002/ijc.24945.

[97] Martinez-Escala ME, Kuzel TM, Kaplan JB, Petrich A, Nardone B, Rosen ST, et al. Durable responses with maintenance dose-sparing regimens of romidepsin in cutaneous T-cell lymphoma. JAMA Oncol. 2016 Jun 1;2(6):790–3.. DOI: 10.1001/jamaoncol.2016.0004.

[98] Stahl M, Gore SD, Vey N, Prebet T. Lost in translation? Ten years of development of histone deacetylase inhibitors in acute myeloid leukemia and myelodysplastic syndromes. Expert Opin Investig Drugs. 2016;25:307–17. DOI: 10.1517/13543784.2016.1146251.

[99] Shirley CM, Chen J, Shamay M, Li H, Zahnow CA, Hayward SD, et al. Bortezomib induction of C/EBPbeta mediates Epstein-Barr virus lytic activation in Burkitt lymphoma. Blood. 2011;117:6297–303. DOI: 10.1182/blood-2011-01-332379.

[100] Chan AT, Tao Q, Robertson KD, Flinn IW, Mann RB, Klencke B, et al. Azacitidine induces demethylation of the Epstein-Barr virus genome in tumors. J Clin Oncol. 2004;22:1373–81. DOI: 10.1200/JCO.2004.04.185.

[101] Giunco S, Celeghin A, Gianesin K, Dolcetti R, Indraccolo S, De Rossi A. Cross talk between EBV and telomerase: the role of TERT and NOTCH2 in the switch of latent/lytic cycle of the virus. Cell Death Dis. 2015;6:e1774. DOI: 10.1038/cddis.2015.145.

[102] Choi CK, Ho DN, Hui KF, Kao RY, Chiang AK. Identification of novel small organic compounds with diverse structures for the induction of Epstein-Barr virus (EBV) lytic cycle in EBV-positive epithelial malignancies. PLoS One. 2015;10:e0145994. DOI: 10.1371/journal.pone.0145994. pii: PONE-D-15-43595.

[103] Tikhmyanova N, Schultz DC, Lee T, Salvino JM, Lieberman PM. Identification of a new class of small molecules that efficiently reactivate latent Epstein-Barr Virus. ACS Chem Biol. 2014;9:785–95. DOI: 10.1021/cb4006326.

[104] Stevens SJ, Zwaan CM, Verkuijlen SA, Middeldorp JM. Epstein-Barr virus (EBV) serology for predicting distant metastases in a white juvenile patient with nasopharyngeal carcinoma and no clinical response to EBV lytic induction therapy. Head Neck. (Case Reports) 2006;28:1040–5. DOI: 10.1002/hed.20466.

[105] Chen MR, Chang SJ, Huang H, Chen JY. A protein kinase activity associated with Epstein-Barr virus BGLF4 phosphorylates the viral early antigen EA-D in vitro. J Virol. 2000;74:3093–104.

[106] Bose S, Yap LF, Fung M, Starzcynski J, Saleh A, Morgan S, et al. The ATM tumour suppressor gene is down-regulated in EBV-associated nasopharyngeal carcinoma. J Pathol. 2009;217:345–52.

[107] Ho Y, Tsao SW, Zeng M, Lui VW. STAT3 as a therapeutic target for Epstein-Barr virus (EBV): associated nasopharyngeal carcinoma. Cancer Lett. 2013;330:141–9. DOI: 10.1016/j.canlet.2012.11.052.

[108] Kung CP, Meckes DG, Jr., Raab-Traub N. Epstein-Barr virus LMP1 activates EGFR, STAT3, and ERK through effects on PKCdelta. J Virol. 2011;85:4399–408. DOI: 10.1128/JVI.01703-10.

[109] Hutajulu SH, Kurnianda J, Tan IB, Middeldorp JM. Therapeutic implications of Epstein-Barr virus infection for the treatment of nasopharyngeal carcinoma. Ther Clin Risk Manag. 2014;10:721–36. DOI: 10.2147/TCRM.S47434.

[110] Chiappinelli KB, Strissel PL, Desrichard A, Li H, Henke C, Akman B, et al. Inhibiting DNA methylation causes an interferon response in cancer via dsRNA including endogenous retroviruses. Cell. 2015;162:974–86. DOI: 10.1016/j.cell.2015.07.011. pii: S0092-8674(15)00848-X.

Chapter 7

Herpes Simplex Virus 1 and 2 Vaccine Design: What can we Learn from the Past?

Vladimíra Ďurmanová, Marian Adamkov and
Július Rajčáni

Additional information is available at the end of the chapter

http://dx.doi.org/10.5772/64447

Abstract

This chapter is devoted to the topics of not yet marketed HSV vaccine, which is still in the focus of interest, especially from the point of immunotherapeutic use. To understand the principles of vaccination strategies (prophylactic and/or immunotherapeutic), the pathogenesis of herpes simplex virus 1 (HSV-1) and/or HSV-2 infections in animal models is briefly outlined. Even when both herpesviruses may spread via bloodstream, which is especially true in the immunocompromised host, the main route of their transmission is along peripheral nerves. Both viruses establish latency in ganglion cells, and after reactivation, they spread along axons back to the site of primary infection. Since neither the establishment of latency nor its reactivation can be fully controlled by virus-neutralizing antibodies, the outcome of immune response greatly depends on the activity of cytotoxic CD8+ T lymphocytes. The majority of important antigenic epitopes is located in envelope glycoproteins (such as gB, gD, gE, gC and gG) that are related to virus adsorption and penetration into susceptible cells. The HSV-1 and/or HSV-2 experimental vaccines designed so far were either purified virion products derived from infected cells (subunit vaccines), purified recombinant immunogenic herpes simplex virus HSV-coded proteins (especially gD), and/or attenuated live viruses lacking some of virulence tools (such as gH and/or gE). We bring a comprehensive overview of the efficacy of experimental HSV-1/HSV-2 vaccines and discuss our own data. In conclusion, we believe in the continued demand of HSV-1 and HSV-2 vaccines, at least for their immunotherapeutic use, suggesting unified evaluation criteria for clinical trials to reach consent at their interpretation.

Keywords: herpes simplex virus 1 and herpes simplex virus 2, candidate vaccine, clinical trials, efficacy in animals, humoral and cell-mediated immune response, antigenic epitopes

1. Introduction

This review will be devoted to the topics of not yet marketed HSV vaccine(s), which design is still in the focus of interest, especially from the point of view of immunotherapeutic use. The human herpesvirus 1 (common name herpes simplex virus 1, HSV-1) is one of the first human viruses discovered [1] and belongs among the most intensively investigated viruses. In the span of the last 45 years, the PubMed portal has registered nearly 11,000 papers devoted to various aspects of HSV-1/HSV-2, starting from virus structure, continued by the molecular mechanisms of lytic replication versus latency maintenance, through the virus spread in the body and the eliciting of different forms of immune response, not omitting many clinical and epidemiological studies. In the second half of the last century, two subtypes of herpes simplex virus (HSV) have been described [2] and were designated HSV type 1 and HSV type 2 [3]. While the former (HSV type 1) has been predominantly isolated from the orofacial area and upper respiratory airways, the latter was believed to infect the urogenital tract and occasionally the newborn. According to recent classification, the HSV-2 represents a distinct species of the *Simplexvirus* genus, which along with the *Varicellovirus* genus belongs to subfamily *Herpesvirinae* of the *Herpesviridae* family. Nevertheless, both species are closely related, since they differ only in a few antigenic domains (and/or epitopes) located in the envelope glycoproteins, namely, in an entirely distinct gG and/or in the partially unrelated gC [4].

2. The molecular biology of HSV: virion structure, lytic replication and latency

The HSV virion consists of four elements: (a) a core containing the viral DNA (vDNA), (b) an icosahedral capsid surrounding the core, (c) an unstructured proteinaceous layer called the *tegument* that surrounds the capsid, and (d) an outer lipid bilayer envelope exhibiting spikes on its surface. The core contains the double-stranded (ds) DNA (dsDNA) genome wrapped as a toroid or spool in a liquid crystalline state. A small fraction of the virion DNA may be circular, but the bulk of packaged HSV DNA is linear and double-stranded. The enveloped virion is a spherical particle with an average diameter of 186 nm, which might extend to 225 nm with the spikes included, while the internal capsid has a constant diameter of 110 nm (reviewed at [5]). The HSV virion contains more than 30 proteins that were designated as virion polypeptides (VPs). Out of these approximately known and additional 10 suspected virion proteins (VPs), at least 11 are located within the envelope at the surface of virion (predominantly accessible to antibody), from which at least 10 are glycosylated (reviewed at [6]).

The HSV genes were classified into at least three general kinetic classes: alpha or immediate-early (IE), beta or early (E), and gamma or late (L) genes. The IE mRNAs are transcribed by the help of a transcription-inducing cofactor present in the virion tegument, also called alpha-TIF/VP16. In brief, the tegument protein VP16 is becoming a part of a tripartite complex comprised of octamer-binding protein 1 (Oct-1) and host cell factor 1 (HCF-1). At least two of the IE proteins (ICP0 and ICP4; **Figure 1**) are transactivators needed for initiation of transcription of the E/beta mRNAs (the first checkpoint) and later also for transcription of gamma/L mRNAs. The latter are mainly structural virion proteins in contrast to E transcripts specifying nonstructural polypeptides. The structural proteins are transcribed in two waves, called gamma1/L and gamma2/L. The former occurs more closely related with the E transcription phase (second checkpoint) and requires predominantly ICP4. The expression of beta polypeptides as well as that of group gamma1/L genes requires ICP4 and at low multiplicities of infection also ICP0. The expression of gamma2/L genes, controlled at the third checkpoint, requires ongoing DNA synthesis as well as the presence of ICP4 and ICP0 [7].

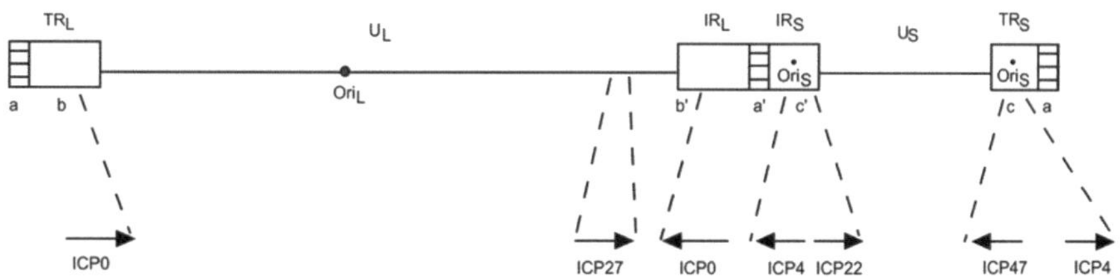

Figure 1. The IE genes and positions of their ORFs in the HSV genome.

The HSV genome consists of two covalently linked sequence components, designated as L (long) and S (short). Each component consists of unique (U) sequences bracketed by inverted repeats (IR) [6].

The entry of HSV into cells involves the interaction of at least five virion surface glycoproteins (gB, gC, gD, gH and gL) with several receptors on the cell surface following fusion of the envelope with a cellular membrane. The HSV glycoproteins along with other proteins important for pathogenicity are listed in **Table 1**. The first step in the process of entry is the binding of virions to glycosaminoglycans (GAGs) on the cell surface. The interaction of virions with GAGs is mediated by two glycoproteins: gC and gB. The next step in virus entry consists of the interaction of gD with its receptors and execution of fusion between the envelope and the cellular membrane by the heterodimer gH/gL and also by gB. The interaction of gD with its receptors has been extensively studied in several laboratories. The consensus is that, for entry, gD interacts with one of three natural receptors (reviewed at [8]). The receptors are nectins, a protein-designated herpesvirus entry mediator (HVEM) and a selected form of 3-O-sulfated heparan sulfate (3-OS HS). Nectins are intracellular adhesion molecules expressed on epithelial and neural cells and are members of the extended immunoglobulin (Ig) family. Earlier studies showed that gD of HSV-1 interacts with the amino-terminal V1 domain of nectin 1. The wild-type HSV-2 can enter susceptible cells via an alternative receptor, namely, nectin 2. HVEM is a member of the extended tumor necrosis factor receptor (TNFR) family, expressed mainly on T lymphocytes but occasionally also on natural killer (NK) cells. Its natural ligand is LIGHT (homologous to lymphotoxins, exhibits inducible expression), which is constitutively expressed on T and natural killer (NK) cells and appears to be a regulator of mucosal immune system. The LIGHT receptor competes with HVEM for the gD (reviewed at [9]). The role of gD with respect to gB and gH/gL is to recruit and position them properly to enable interaction with GAGs and with the lipid bilayers of the cellular membranes [10].

Gene	Protein	Function
RL1	γ34.5	L protein, cofactor for ribosomal translation
RL2	ICP0	IE protein, spliced, three exons, a RING finger motif, acts as a nonspecific transactivator of any beta and gamma gene
UL1	gL	Late glycoprotein, forms the gH/gL complex, *syn* mutation
UL5		E class protein, part of the helicase/primase complex
UL9		E/L class, *ori*-binding protein, cooperates with ICP8 at initiation of vDNA replication
UL10	gM	L class, glycosylated polypeptide, interacts with gN, participates in exocytosis and in cell-to-cell spread
UL18	VP24	L class, capsid component, participates in triplex formation
UL19	VP5	L class protein, the major capsid component (149/150K)
UL21		L class tegument protein weakly capsid-associated, binds to microtubules at axonal transport
UL22	gH	L class, glycosylated protein, essential for penetration to cells, needs complexing with gL
UL23	TK	E class, tegument protein, thymidine kinase, virulence factor
UL26		L class, "scaffolding" capsid protein, the N-terminus required for virion assembly
UL27	gB	L class glycoprotein, essential for adsorption and membrane fusion, syn3 locus
UL29	ICP8	E class, ssDNA binding, required for vDNA synthesis, keeping the DNA fork apart
UL30	DNA pol	E/L class protein, DNA polymerase (elongation enzyme), virulence factor
UL35	VP26	L class virion protein, hexon component, also termed NC7
UL36	VP1/ VP2	L class, large tegument protein, important for egress through cytoplasm and re-envelopment
UL38	VP19C	L class capsid protein, triplet component with VP23 (1:2), connects the hexons and pentons
UL39	RR	E class protein, large subunit of RR, membrane-anchored protein kinase
UL40	RR	E class protein, the small subunit of RR
UL41	*vhs*	L class, tegument protein, interferes with the host cell proteosynthesis, virulence factor
UL44	gC	L class, glycoprotein, reacts with GAG on cell surface, binds C3 and/or C5, virulence factor
UL48	Alpha-TIF /VP16	L class tegument protein, alpha-transinducing factor
UL49.5	gN	L class membrane-associated small glycoprotein, complexes with gM
UL53	gK	L class glycoprotein (40K), localizes to Golgi and ER, involved in egress, syn1 locus
UL54	ICP27/ IE63	IE class protein, blocks cellular mRNA transport to cytoplasm
RS1	ICP4	IE class protein, transactivator for E and L promoters
US1	ICP22	IE class regulatory protein, essential in animal experiments, cellular cyclin A and B degradation

Gene	Protein	Function
US4	gG	L class, glycosylated protein and envelope component, HSV-2 specific
US6	gD	E/L class, glycosylated protein, 56K, adsorption to nectin 1 and HVEM protein receptors, essential for entry to cells, neural uptake
US7	gI	L class glycoprotein, forms heterodimer with gE, the complex facilitates cell-to-cell spread, neural uptake
US8	gE	L class glycoprotein, complexes with gI, essential for neural uptake
US12	ICP47	IE class protein, blocks the transport of viral antigenic epitopes
LAT		Three categories of RNAs (8.5 kb, 2.0, and 1.5 kb), the small LATs terminate antisense to ICP0 ORF. Latency regulator

Abbreviations: vDNA = viral DNA; ICP = infected cell protein; VP = virion protein (structural); IE = immediate-early kinetics (class); E = early kinetics (class); L = late kinetics (class); K = 1,000 kDa (Mr); RR = ribonucleotide reductase; *vhs* = virion host shutoff; LAT = latency-associated transcript(s); RNA molecules without capping, do not interact with ribosomes; UL = unique long (DNA segment); US = unique short; RL = repeat long; RS = repeat short; HVEM = herpes virus entry mediator)
[a]Modified according to Roizman et al. [6].

Table 1. HSV-1 genes and corresponding proteins regarded for importance in virulence[a].

The gB belongs to class III fusion protein that after GAG interaction facilitates fusion of the virion envelope bilayer with the cellular membrane. A recent study showed that gB can also bind to the paired immunoglobulin-like type 2 receptor-α (PILRα) to trigger viral fusion in certain cell types; however, the precise role of this interaction in viral entry remains to be determined [11]. The gH and gL appear to form a tight complex, since neither protein is stable without the other. In contrast to gB, the structural studies of gH/gL showed no homology with fusion domains of other viral glycoproteins. The exact role of gH/gL has not been determined; however, one hypothesis is that the interaction of gD with its receptors changes the conformation of gH/gL, which in turn induces gB to adopt its fusion conformation [12]. Even that gE had been regarded for not essential in cell culture, it has been shown very important at entering nerve endings (neural uptake) and subsequent neural spread [13].

The latency of HSV can be characterized by circularized state of the HSV genome in the absence of IE and/or E transcription, especially lacking the expression of the two most important beta/gamma transcription activators, namely, ICP0 and ICP4 (reviewed at [14]). We pointed at the possibility that the IE block in question might be "leaky" since small amounts of ICP4 mRNA could be found in the non-cultured ganglion explants which would later on yield infectious virus [15]. Overwhelming literature deals with the hypotheses that the small latency-associated transcripts RNA (LATs), RNA molecules expressed during latency contribute to the silencing of ICP0 mRNA transcription as well as to the maintenance of latency [16]. It has been shown that LAT can reduce the expression of viral genes and suppress HSV replication in cultured cells. In addition, LAT probably protects the HSV DNA carrying neuron from apoptosis. The anti-apoptosis activity of LAT has been independently confirmed in tissue culture and in the mouse ocular model [17]. Further data suggest the participation of LAT in reactivation of the latent genome [18, 19].

3. Pathogenesis of HSV-1 and/or HSV-2 infections

The crucial event in HSV pathogenesis is, when the virus, which has reached the pseudounipolar neuron of the regional sensory ganglion via the quick axonal transmission, may but need not undergo productive replication. Thus, latency can be established from the very beginning, that is, in the absence of any transcription provided by the virus-coded alpha-transinducing factor (alpha-TIF). As described by Efstathiou et al. [20], the latent genome resides in the nuclei of neurons in the form of a circularized nonintegrated plasmid-like structure. This structure survives within the carrier neuron. the carrier neuron, so that neural cells harbor the viral DNA for their lifetime. The tegument-bound alpha-transinducing factor (alpha-TIF) might be "lost" during intra-axonal transport [21]. Some axons might be as long as 500 mm (as a rule about 100 mm), while the minimum speed for HSV capsid transmission is about 1–2 mm/h. The quick axonal transport along neurotubules is provided by the dynein molecule, which binds the capsid component UL21. The environment within sensory neurons favors the establishment of latency rather than productive virus replication also because the neuronal transcription cofactors such as Oct-2 and/or Brn-3 repress the IE promoters [22, 23].

During reactivation, the blocked IE checkpoint of virus replication must be overcome especially by overwhelming expression of ICP0 protein in order to achieve productive virus replication and infectious HSV production [24]. The reactivation process can be hampered by two different mechanisms. One depends on viral genome products interacting with cellular cofactors of transcription within neurons. It may not be excluded that due to the existence of at least two activation checkpoints, controlling the expression gamma1 or E/L proteins (glycoproteins) and the gamma2/L proteins (glycoproteins), also incomplete virus particles may be formed. The E and/or E/L proteins may be synthesized in the absence of complete virion formation, or assembly of virions with defective vDNA occurs. However, the presence of virus-coded antigens (even in the absence of infectious virus particles) could induce a potent immune response (including the accumulation of cytotoxic T cells in the vicinity of HSV carrier neurons). It should be also mentioned that the IE protein ICP47 acts by immune evasion. Alternative effects inhibiting the antiviral defense can be exerted by gC [25], which binds complement, and by the gE molecule, which binds the Fc fragment of immunoglobulins.

If reactivated virus reaches the peripheral tissues by retrograde axonal transport (skin squamous epithelium, non-cornified squamous epithelium of mouth mucous membrane, corneal epithelium), then it starts to replicate and causes inapparent virus shedding or blister formation. A nice example for creating favorable conditions of virus replication at peripheral skin was described in the ear model [26, 27]. These investigators found that prostaglandins produced after skin trauma or UV light irradiation would enhance the replication of recurrent HSV-1. As shown by Walz et al. [28], neurectomy of the trigeminal nerve root reactivated the latent HSV harbored within ganglion cells. The round trip of reactivated virus

http://dx.doi.org/10.5772/64447

usually ends with reinfection of additional neurons within the regional sensory ganglion. Less frequently, the retrograde axonal transport may continue in centripetal direction, that is, to brain stem. Furthermore, the central nervous system (CNS) may become infected via bloodstream (in newborn) or along the olfactory route (reviewed at [29]).

The different manifestations of clinical disease reflect the above-described mechanisms of HSV spread in the body. Essentially, HSV-1 can induce the acute primoinfection (gingivostomatitis) and recurrent disease (classical labial herpes). Alternatively, the ocular herpes, often manifested as herpes keratitis, occurs rather as recurrent disease than primoinfection. In newborn as well as in the immunocompromised host and/or in the case of local inflammation in the skin (e.g., due to allergic manifestations such as atopic eczema), the HSV might cause generalized skin disease or even viral sepsis (i.e., the hepatoadrenal necrosis in newborn or severe meningoencephalitis). In newborn, perinatal infection causes an acute dissemination of HSV-2 via bloodstream. Meningitis and meningoencephalitis of neonates, similarly as various forms of genital infection of man and women, are mainly HSV-2-related. In women, the outer but also the inner genital tract (vagina or cervical mucosa covered with non-cornified squamous epithelium) might become infected. In the skin as well as at the mucous membranes covered by squamous epithelium, both HSV-1 and HSV-2 species replicate within the lower and/or medium squamous cell layers causing blister formation [30].

4. Mechanisms of the immune response to HSV-1 or HSV-2

The immune response to HSV-1 and/or HSV-2 is induced in an early and a late phase. During early phase, the nonspecific antiviral mechanisms are activated, while in the late phase, the HSV-specific reaction is mobilized. The specific immune response culminates by recruiting the CD8+ cytotoxic T lymphocytes important for extracellular latency control, in contrast to the intracellular latency control which has been discussed above. The specific cell-mediated immune response may begin in the regional lymph nodes draining the virus inoculation site (both T-lymphocyte lines are engaged) as well as in the trigeminal ganglia which harbor the latent virus (mainly cytotoxic CD8+ T cells take part).

4.1. The innate immune response

The innate antiviral immunity to HSV-1 and/or HSV-2 is provided by alpha/beta type I interferons (IFNs) as well as by activation of natural killer (NK) cells. The role of type I IFNs in anti-HSV defense was demonstrated in knockout mice deficient in type I IFN production [31, 32]. The type I IFN release is induced by virus constituents called pathogen-associated molecular patterns (PAMPs) interacting with the corresponding pattern recognition receptors (PRRs) at the surface of responding cells. The best known examples are the Toll-like receptors (TLR). For example, the envelope glycoprotein D molecule of the HSV-1 interacts with the TLR-2 receptor on the target cell membrane [33], while the TLR-9 receptor binds to non-methylated CpG motifs of the vDNA present in the nuclei of infected cells [34]. It has been also shown that children with TLR-3 defects are more susceptible to herpes encephalitis [35,

36]. Both types I of IFNs act on the receptors in neighboring cells eliciting the synthesis of antiviral substances such as the 2′,5′-oligoadenylate synthase, RNase L, and/or RNA-dependent protein kinase. The type I IFN also inhibits cell proliferation and enhances the activation of NK cells as well as the expression of MHC class I molecules, but downregulates MHC class II expression. The type III IFNs, also designated as IFN-λ1, IFN-λ2 and IFN-λ3 (IL-29, IL-28A, and IL-28B), have been recently characterized; alike to classical type I IFNs, also IFN-λ induces production of antiviral substances in the infected cells [37]. The participation of type III IFNs in inhibition of HSV replication has been confirmed *in vitro* [38, 39].

In addition to type I IFN formation, the activation of NK cells represents another important arm of nonspecific immune response to HSV-1 and HSV-2 infection [40]. The nonspecific killers belong to the group of class I innate lymphoid cells. Morphologically, they belong to large granular lymphocytes (LGLs), which cytoplasm contains azurophilic granules with perforins and granzymes A and B. They exert cytolytic activities helpful at the elimination of infected cells. The perforins create a transmembrane channel piercing the cell membrane, while granzymes activate the apoptosis of target cells. The NK cells also produce IFN-gamma, which promotes their activation along with the activation of macrophages. In association with this, enhanced death rates were noted in NK-deficient mice infected with HSV [41].

The elimination of HSV-1 and/or HSV-2 infected cells at the portal of entry is mediated by additional immune cells such as neutrophils, dendritic cells (DCs), and macrophages. The neutrophils secrete tumor necrosis factor (TNF) which induces apoptosis of infected cells via caspase-8 activation [42]. Blood monocytes when entering the connective and/or other tissues are altered into macrophages able to engulf the extracellular virus particles but also residues of apoptotic cells. The active macrophages belong to the group of antigen-presenting cells (APCs) that present the external immunogenic peptides to T lymphocytes. This process called antigen presentation launches the specific immune response. Activated macrophages also release several pro-inflammatory cytokines like TNF and IL-6 (participates in B-cell activation), type I IFNs, and several chemokines such as RANTES regulated upon activation normal T-cell expressed and secreted. Finally, nitric oxide (NO) and other substances are produced by macrophages. It has been demonstrated in experiments *in vitro* that the replication of HSV-1 in infected cells may be considerably inhibited in the presence of NO released from macrophages [43]. It should be mentioned here that IFN-gamma (belongs to type II IFNs) is in fact a cytokine released from activated NK cells but also produced by the helper CD4+ T lymphocytes as well as by cytotoxic CD8+ T lymphocytes [44]. The IFN-gamma considerably promotes function of activating macrophages and NK cells, in which it induces a production of cytolytic substances. Taken together, both NK cells and macrophages represent an important first-line defense at the early stage of HSV infection, that is, before the onset of specific immune response.

As already mentioned above, important immune cells participating in the initiation of antigen processing are the dendritic cells (DCs). They represent a relatively heterogenous cell population, from which the most active in antiviral defense are the myeloid (conventional) and the plasmacytoid DCs (pDCs), both derived from the myeloid progenitor cells. The myeloid DCs act as antigen-presenting cells (APCs), which carry the processed antigenic peptides into lymph nodes, where the peptides in question are presented to the T lymphocytes. Based on this presentation event, the specific immune response is induced (activation of T and B cells). In DC-depleted mice infected with HSV-1, encephalitis developed with a significantly higher frequency as compared to conventional mice [45]. The plasmacytoid DCs under physiological conditions participate in the development of peripheral immune tolerance. Upon HSV infection, plasmacytoid DCs start to produce high amounts of IFN-alpha, which not only inhibits the virus replication in the otherwise surrounding susceptible cells but also activates lymphocytes and additional DCs. The HSV dsDNA binds to TLR-9 of the plasmacytoid DC which initiates IFN-alpha production [46].

4.2. The acquired immune response

The acquired immune response encounters the activation of both T-lymphocyte lines, namely, those differentiated either in direction of CD4+ or CD8+ T cells. The acquired immune response then is triggered by the activation of T-cell receptors (TCRs), which recognize the HLA I/CD8 and/or the HLA II/CD4 bound antigenic peptides. While the former T cells are involved in the destruction and elimination of HSV-infected cells, the latter acts as helper T cells at inducing the specific antibody production by B cells. At primary infection, the HSV-1 or HSV-2 particles are engulfed by DCs, which move the viral peptides to the regional lymph nodes, where the naïve (unprimed) lymphocytes get first stimulated. The presentation of exogenous viral peptides is achieved by means of the HLA class II molecules, which are recognized by the TCR of the CD4+ T lymphocytes. In contrast, the immunogenic peptides of the newly (de novo) synthesized HSV proteins are presented by HLA class I molecules at the surface of infected cells where they interact with the TCR of cytotoxic CD8+ T lymphocytes [47]. In certain extent, the so-called cross presentation occurs, at which the exogenous viral antigens are binding into the HLA class I molecules that are recognized by the CD8+ T lymphocytes [48]. The activated helper CD4+ T cells release cytokines such as IL-2 (inducing T-lymphocyte proliferation) and IL-4, IL-5 and IL-6 (promoting the differentiation of B cells into plasma cells).

The plasma cells synthesize the specific virus-neutralizing antibodies reacting mainly with the envelope glycoproteins such as gB and gD. The antibodies may also activate complement; on the other hand, the gC molecule of the HSV-1 envelope binds C3b and in less extent also C5b reducing the availability of complement components for virus neutralization. The low-pathogenic HSV-1 gC minus strains may become pathogenic as was confirmed in a C3 knockout murine model [49]. The HSV-1 antibodies belong to IgM as well as IgG class; the HSV-2 antibodies may be also of the secretory IgA class; the latter participates in virus clearance at the genital tract mucosa [50]. Even though the serum antibodies are of importance at the acute phase of infection, they may not fully eliminate the HSV since it invades the nerve endings and spreads to regional sensory ganglia before the development of antibody response. Some studies have shown that passive immunization with immune serum did not prevent latency after genital infection with HSV-2 [51, 52, 53]. Since the latent HSV (episomal vDNA) is frequently harbored in neural tissue for lifelong, the presence of HSV antibodies in the serum of healthy subjects may be interpreted as infectious immunity.

The cytotoxic CD8+ T lymphocytes represent the mainstream of the specific immune response providing clearance of HSV-1- or HSV-2-infected cells from the body. The activation of cytotoxic CD8+ T cells takes place in the regional lymph nodes by means of viral antigenic peptides presented by HLA class I molecules expressed at the surface of DCs. The IL-2 released from helper T cells acts on the precursor cytotoxic T lymphocytes which differentiate into mature cytotoxic CD8+ T cells. These mature CD8+ T cells accumulate at the peripheral virus inoculation site, where they eliminate the HSV-infected cells. The activated cytotoxic T lymphocytes release substances such as perforins, granzyme and granulysin, which destroy the infected target cell and/or induce apoptosis acting on their FAS receptors. They also release cytokines such as IFN-gamma and the tumor necrosis factor (TNF). IFN-gamma has a multiple effect, since it enhances the expression of HLA class I as well as HLA class II molecules [54] and also induces the expression of antiviral substances such as protein kinase R (PKR). This substance causes inhibition of translation of many viral but also cellular proteins. The increased TNF production also enhances the number and activity of HLA class I molecules.

The clearance of HSV-2 from peripheral tissues such as genital mucosa may be also provided by CD4+ T cells. Transgenic mice, which revealed defects in their CD8+ T-lymphocyte activity, have been still well protected against a lethal dose of HSV-2. In contrast, mice with depleted CD4+ T lymphocytes showed slower clearance and less protection against HSV-2 [55–57]. It can be concluded that the clearance of HSV-2 from genital mucosa requires cooperation of both the helper and cytotoxic T lymphocytes. Both T-cell populations can be found in the skin, in the genital and oral mucosa, in the ocular tissue, and also in the trigeminal ganglia surrounding the infected neurons [58–60].

After healing of the acute phase of HSV infection, about 0.1–1% of memory T cells, which may remain within the circulation, are still able to recognize the HSV antigenic epitopes. These epitopes being recognized by CD4+ and/or CD8+ lymphocytes were not all exactly mapped yet, but until now, 22 of them were defined. The HSV-specific epitopes can be found mainly among VPs (structural envelope glycoproteins, tegument proteins and capsid polypeptides), but are also present on the ICPs, that is, on nonstructural enzymes and regulatory proteins. The CD4+ T lymphocytes generated against the HSV-2-specified structural proteins recognize the epitopes of the RR1/UL39 polypeptide, the epitopes of UL46 tegument protein, and several ones on glycoproteins gD and gB [61].

The CD8+ T lymphocytes, surrounding the neurons of the regional sensory ganglia of mice, rabbits, and humans in which viral latency had been established [62–64], are believed to control reactivation [65]. It was demonstrated, for example, that the ICP4/145K IE protein can be digested by granzyme B, which would prevent virus reactivation [66]. The accumulated CD8+ T cells produce IFN-gamma as well, inhibiting the expression of ICP0/110K IE protein [67].

The most intriguing still unexplained question is why do the CD8+ T lymphocytes accumulated in the neighborhood of latent HSV-harboring neurons, since the expression of IE and E polypeptides is widely hampered in them. Interestingly enough, the great majority of CD8+ T lymphocytes in the trigeminal ganglion of mice in which latency had been established possess a TCR which reacts with gB epitope at aa 498–505, while a smaller proportion of them may be stimulated with RR1 epitope aa 822–829. The reactivity of the other T cells was not identified

[68, 69]. In human trigeminal ganglia, both the CD4+ and CD8+ T cells were described that react with many antigenic epitopes present in the IE polypeptides ICP0 and ICP4, in the E polypeptides such as thymidine kinase (TK) and RRl, as well as with antigenic domains from structural proteins such as the tegument proteins VP11/12 and VP13/14 and envelope glycoproteins gB, gK, and gL, even though an exact identification of all antigenic epitopes in the HSV proteins was not done yet [70, 71].

The phenotype of CD8+ T lymphocytes which can accumulate within the ganglia was not characterized. The permanently present cytotoxic T lymphocytes might belong to the population of so-called tissue-resident memory T lymphocytes (TRM) or to the population referred as T-effector memory cells (TEM cells). Additional markers such as CD44, CD69, CD62L, and CCR7 were described at their surface, but their full definition is still the matter of investigation [72].

5. Survey of experimental HSV-1 and HSV-2 vaccines and their design

Though the first vaccines against HSV-1 and/or HSV-2 were prepared in the sixties of last century [73], no accepted and fully efficient HSV vaccine is available till now. The main problem is the incomplete understanding of the role of cytotoxic CD8+ T cells in the maintenance and/or of elimination neurons carrying the silenced HSV DNA. Another serious problem is the production of immune evasion polypeptides (reviewed at [74]). The optimal HSV vaccine should overcome the ICP47-mediated interference with TAP, which transports the viral peptides inside ER to bind with HLA molecules. Finally, the last but not negligible problem is that at least some of over 20 immunogenic epitopes, which are distributed within about 80 HSV proteins (both structural and nonstructural), should participate in the vaccine but in an optimal composition. An effective HSV vaccine might differ depending of its purpose, which could be either preventive or immunotherapeutic. An ideal vaccine should not allow the acute disease to develop, and it should be able to prevent the establishment of latency. These goals, especially the latter, are difficult to achieve. The minimum effect provided by an immunotherapeutic vaccine would be to minimize the extent of recurrent lesion originating from the reactivation of the latent viral genome. As described above, the cytotoxic T lymphocytes accumulating in vicinity of HSV DNA carrier cells in the regional sensory ganglion seem of great importance when keeping a state of equilibrium probably inhibiting the transcription of IE genes by an unknown mechanism. One could estimate that in the case of the inefficiency and/or complete failure of the function of cytotoxic T-cell virus, reactivation and subsequent retrograde axonal transport of virions occur. In this section, we describe the various HSV vaccines which have been used under experimental conditions, while the next paragraph will describe their efficacy in human volunteers.

5.1. Inactivated virion and subunit vaccines

The inactivated HSV-1 and/or HSV-2 vaccines consist of infected cell extracts, which have been introduced in the 1980s of last century, partially purified and inactivated either by UV light, by thermal treatment, or with formalin [75–77]. The efficacy of these first vaccines was tested mainly in mice, but some of them were used also in human trials (see Section 6). Especially in animal models, a good protective effect against acute virus challenge has been found not to prevent the establishment of latency. However, when testing the effect of a virion-free HSV vaccine prepared by extraction of infected LEP cells with Nonidet P-40 [78] in the rabbit corneal model, Rajčáni et al. [79] concluded that even though vaccination prior to infection did not fully prevent latency, it considerably reduced the number of regional sensory (trigeminal) ganglion cells (neurons), which became the HSV genome carriers. Recently, a formalin-inactivated HSV-2 (FI-HSV2) vaccine mixed with $Al(OH)_3$ adjuvant was tested in combination with monophosphoryl lipid A (MPL) [80]. The latter authors showed that the vaccine protected mice against local vaginal challenge with HSV-2 as well as reduced the extent of latency established in the sensory ganglia of lumbosacral nerve roots.

The subunit vaccines were mainly glycoprotein mixes purified on lectins (e.g., lentil lectin) showing high affinity to the HSV virion envelope antigens. The dominant protective antigens among the 11 HSV glycoproteins are gB and gD, which possess important immunogenic epitopes. The abovementioned glycoproteins elicit virus-neutralizing antibodies, antibodies participating in the antibody-dependent cellular cytotoxic (ADCC) response, and they also activate the T lymphocytes. Several reports described the efficacy of the subunit vaccines of various purity based on either HSV-1 and/or HSV-2 envelope glycoproteins [81–84]. For example, the subunit HSV-1 vaccine (strain HSZP Immuno) had been prepared from chick embryo cells infected with the low-virulent HSZP strain [85]. Tested in cooperation with the Research and Development Department of the former Immuno AG Company in Vienna, the infected cell extract in question was purified on lentil lectin to obtain a glycoprotein mix containing at least four envelope glycoproteins (gB, gC, gD and gG). This subunit vaccine was immunogenic and protective in mice as well as rabbits and showed at least partial cross protection in the HSV-2-challenged guinea pigs infected by the vaginal route.

5.2. Recombinant HSV-1 and HSV-2 vaccines

The next step of HSV vaccine development proceeded from purified (nearly cell DNA-free) subunit vaccines to those composed of recombinant HSV-1/HSV-2 polypeptides [86–90]. Great majority of the recombinant vaccines contained the gB and/or gD polypeptides, and their efficacy was done in mice. The first purified glycoprotein vaccines (gB1 and gD1) were prepared on immunoaffinity columns (with specific-bound MoAbs); such vaccines were found to protect mice against intracerebral challenge with HSV-1 [91–93]. Manservigi et al. [94] expressed the gB ectodomain in mammalian cells. After immunization with the purified gB fragment, the mice developed virus-neutralizing antibodies not only against HSV-1 but also cross-reacting antibodies to HSV-2. In addition, the authors also showed that the animals were resistant to the challenge with a lethal HSV dose. Later on, the recombinant proteins were prepared by transfection of plasmids (carrying the gD and/or gB ORFs) into competent *Escherichia coli* cells, which expressed the corresponding not glycosylated polypeptides [90, 95–100]. Recombinant glycoproteins (including gC) were also prepared in insect and/or mammalian cells, in which the recombinant products could be glycosylated [101].

Immunization with the recombinant gD1 or gD2 alone, or in combination with the gB protected mice against infectious virus challenge given by intraperitoneal or subcutaneous routes and in the case of gD1 vaccination cross protection to HSV-2 was observed as well. Immunization with gD alone was more effective than that with gB alone [87], while immunity provided by gC alone was negligible [95]. In contrast, very high effect was achieved following immunization with the mix of gB1, gD1, and gE1 glycoproteins in combination with the $Al(OH)_3$ adjuvant including the cross protection of guinea pigs challenged with HSV-2 at genital route [99]. A trivalent vaccine containing gD2, gC2 and gE2 prepared in the baculovirus expression system was more immunogenic for mice than the subunit vaccine containing gC2 and gD2 [102]. Furthermore, Awasthi et al. [103] immunized the guinea pigs with recombinant proteins gC2 and gD2 prepared in a baculovirus system (which activated antibody production), with the adenovirus vector carrying the VP5 capsid protein and with the tegument proteins VP13 and VP14 (which activated the T-cell-mediated response). However, no significant difference was detected, which confirmed that the glycoprotein mix gD2/gB2 was sufficient enough.

The alum adjuvant in combination with the recombinant gD polypeptide activates the Th2-type humoral response and therefore may be less suitable for immunotherapeutic use, for which the Th1-type response is essential. To stimulate the Th1 response predominantly, cytokines as adjuvants were tested, such as IL-2 with good results after corneal challenge with the virulent HSV-1 CHR3 strain [104]. The so-called immune-stimulating lipid complexes (ISCOM) combined with HSV-2 immunogenic polypeptides induced both Th1- and Th2-type responses when showing a highly neutralizing antibody response along with the production of IL-2, IFN-gamma, and TNF [105]. Similar strong potentiating effect was observed at immunization with gD2 polypeptide adjuvanted with modified lipid A (AS04) [98]. Furthermore, when using the gD2 fusion polypeptide along with MF59 (squalene) as adjuvant, the local mucosa immune response could neither be stimulated properly, nor the latency reactivation prevented [106]. There is worth mentioning that the so-called autoimmune/inflammatory syndrome induced by adjuvants (ASIA) is an inflammatory syndrome associated with certain adjuvants (such as MF59/squalene); the latter potentiates pathological autoimmune reactions, which may be evident in the case of prophylactic mass immunization campaigns [107].

In contrast to T-lymphocyte stimulation, the local IgA secretion can be enhanced by mistletoe lectins such as ML-1, ML-2, and/or ML-3, the application of which in combination with the gD2 polypeptide elicited a good secretory IgA response at intranasal challenge in mice [108]. The authors also used non-ionized liposome like particles carrying the gB ectodomain and additional polylysine-rich polypeptides. Intranasal application of the product in question provided protection against lethal challenge with HSV-2 and induced a strong Th1-type immune response [109]. Skoberne et al. [110] prepared an experimental vaccine named GEN-003/MM-2, which contained gD2 and the IE protein ICP4/175K expressed in a baculovirus system. In combination with MM2 adjuvants (also called matrix M2 composed of cholesterol, phospholipids, and saponin), the vaccine showed immunotherapeutic effect in guinea pigs when it reduced the frequency of recurrent genital lesions upon HSV-2 challenge.

5.3. Viral vectored and DNA vaccines

The recent idea of DNA vaccines represents a progressive approach for immunization (reviewed at [111]). The advantage of DNA vaccines is that the immune response resembles to that following the administration of live-attenuated virus vaccines, but without the risk of reversion to viral phenotype. The viral DNA vaccines fall into two categories: viral DNA carriers and the recombinant plasmid vaccines (classical DNA vaccines). The viral DNA carriers are in fact nonpathogenic attenuated viruses that genome contains the inserted ORF fragments encoding the desired antigen. The best examples are either the recombinant adenovirus or vaccinia virus, which carry the HSV gD or gB genes. The latter glycoproteins become expressed in the immunized animal, that is, in the mice, which are then protected against HSV challenge [112–115]. The recombinant vesicular stomatitis virus (VSV) was prepared from a plasmid containing the cDNA of the VSV RNA genome and the gD2 ORF US6. This recombinant virus induced a good cell-mediated immune response as well as anti-gD antibody formation. Immunized mice were protected against acute HSV-2 challenge, and the establishment of latency was also reduced [116]. Chiuppesi et al. [117] described the effect of immunization with feline lentiviral vector-based, herpes simplex virus 1 (HSV-1) glycoprotein B vaccine. This lentivirus construct induced HSV-1 antibody formation and also provided cross protection against lethal HSV-2 infection.

Many classical plasmid DNA vaccines were prepared with the inserted HSV DNA fragment. The majority of them encoded HSV-1 and/or HSV-2 glycoproteins such as gB, gD, gC, and gE; their efficacy was tested in mice, guinea pigs, and rabbits [90, 118–124]. The results were obtained after immunization with plasmids encoding the glycoproteins gD and/or gB of either HSV-1 or HSV-2 alone or in combination. Especially the immunization of mice and/or guinea pigs with the gD-expressing plasmid protected against challenge with a lethal dose of HSV-2 [124–128], but without clear-cut reduction of the latency rate. Better results were obtained with plasmids encoding both gB and gD [119, 129, 130]. The efficiency of DNA vaccines could be higher when adding cytokines such as IL-12 which induced the Th type 1 immune response [131, 132] similarly as the presence of IL-18 and/or RANTES [133, 134]. In contrast, the Th2-type response could be better achieved if the gD and IL-4-coding plasmid was used for immunization [133, 135]. The Th type 2 immune response is important for virus clearance from peripheral tissues including the infection of the eye, while the Th1-type response was involved in preventing the latency establishment [135]. The DNA vaccine-encoding gB when combined with DNA plasmid coding for cytokines IL-12 and IL-18 as adjuvant was efficient in prevention of the vaginal infection in mice: gB1/IL-12 and/or gB1/IL-18 elicited a local resistance of genital mucosa and protected mice against lethal HSV-2 challenge. The best results were observed with IL-12, while additional adjuvants did not enhance protection [136]. Another adjuvant tested with the DNA vaccines was the lipid adjuvant Vaxfectin®. In guinea pigs immunized with plasmid-expressing gD2 and VP11/VP12 as well as VP13/14 polypeptides along with a lipid adjuvant, a great prophylactic effect and the reduced HSV-2 replication in the genital tract of experimental animals was observed. The vaccine also showed immunotherapeutic properties when reducing the extent of latency (vDNA contents) in the dorsal root ganglia [137, 138]. Immunization with the recombinant plasmid encoding the fusion protein consisting of the gB and the CCL19 chemokine ORF induced both the Th type 1 and the Th type 2 responses including an increased local secretory IgA antibody production protecting mice against HSV-2 challenge [139]. The enhanced efficiency of DNA vaccines could be achieved by combining genes encoding the envelope glycoproteins with certain nonstructural HSV genes. The recombinant plasmid consisting of gD2, gB2, and ICP27 ORFs elicited a higher cellular as well as humoral response than the plasmid construct encoding the glycoproteins only. The construct in question also provided a higher protection against vaginal challenge with HSV-2 [140].

5.4. Live-attenuated HSV-1 and HSV-2 vaccines

Attenuated HSV vaccines are live HSV-1 and/or HSV-2 viruses derived from the wild-type strains by modifications of their virulence but keep the immunogenic properties. The best known deletion for HSV-1 was the removal of the UL22 ORF-encoding gH glycoprotein [141, 142] and/or the removal of the IR1 sequence encoding the protein γ34.5 gamma, a neurovirulence factor [143]. Furthermore, the deletion of the gE encoding by US8 gene, which is not needed for virus replication in cell culture but is inevitable for neural uptake [144, 145] along with the deletion of the UL41 gene, encoding the virion host shutoff (vhs) protein [146] might be an excellent solution. In this respect, the non-virulent HSZP strain with natural mutations altering the vhs protein, if deleted in the gE gene, would be of special advantage [147]. Another attempts to prepare a live-attenuated HSV strain were made by deleting nonstructural genes, such as the ORF UL54 (encodes the ICP27 IE polypeptide), the ORF RS1 (encodes the transactivation protein ICP4) [146, 148], and/or the ORF RL2 (encoding the ICP0 transactivation protein) as described by Halford et al. [149]. All the above-mentioned attenuated viruses was protective against HSV challenge in various animal models. The HSV-2 deleted in the gH gene designated as disabled infectious single cycle (DISC) and tested as therapeutic vaccine, but no convincing protection was found [150].

Several other attenuated HSV strains were prepared by deleting the nonstructural genes important for virulence. Deleted ORFs for such purpose were the following: (1) the UL23 ORF encoding the thymidine kinase (TK) as described by Morrison and Knipe [151], (2) the UL39 ORF encoding the large RR1 subunit [152], (3) the UL29 ORF encoding the ssDNA-binding ICP8 polypeptide [153], (4) the UL5 ORF encoding a protein of the primase/helicase complex [154, 155], and finally (5) the UL9 ORF encoding the ori-binding protein [156]. The TK minus recombinant R7017 was prepared from the w.t. strain F, which genome was, in addition, deleted in the IR1 ORF sequence encoding the γ34.5 and furthermore manipulated by inserting the gD2, gI2, and gG2 sequences along with a portion of the gE ORF (US4–US8). The TK-reversed recombinant virus was further modified by reinserting the TK gene (R7020 TK plus). Both recombinant viruses protected mice as well as guinea pigs against HSV-2 challenge [148]. The next UL39-/RR1-deleted virus was tested not only in animals but also in man [152, 157]. The phase I and phase II clinical trials showed partial protection against recurrences (in 37.5% of immunized individuals as compared with the placebo group) [157]. The attenuated strain deleted in the genes UL29 and UL5 (called dl29-5) protected mice against ocular infection with HSV-1 and guinea pigs against genital challenge with HSV-2 [158, 159]. Stanfield et al. [160]

prepared an attenuated strain of HSV-2 called VC2, which had mutations in the gK gene and in the UL20 ORF (which is membrane protein inhibiting the neural uptake). This vaccine prevented genital infection upon vaginal challenge with HSV-2 and also inhibited latent infection in the lumbosacral dorsal root ganglia. Finally, the defective HSV-2 designated CJ9-gD2 was used to immunize mice. This virus had mutation in the UL9 ORF which encodes a vDNA replication protein and was deleted in the gD2 ORF (US9). The attenuated vaccine induced a higher antibody response in comparison with the gD2-alum/MPL subunit vaccine (used in a human trial) and protected mice against lethal challenge with HSV-2 [161].

6. Human vaccination trials: prophylactic and therapeutic HSV vaccines

Some of the vaccines mentioned above were tested not only in animal models but also in man at clinical trials. They were designed either as prophylactic vaccines, or they were destined for immunotherapeutic use, having been suggested for prevention or modulation of genital infection predominantly caused by HSV-2. The aim of prophylactic vaccine against HSV-2 infection is not only to prevent a clinical disease at primoinfection but also to interfere with the subsequent establishment of latency. The latter is a hard task, since the majority of vaccines just reduce the number of neurons which are getting HSV DNA carriers but does not fully prevent latent infection. Therefore, it is more reasonable to design a vaccine for immunotherapeutic use aimed to reduce the extent and the frequency of recurrent lesions.

The prophylactic vaccine should induce a satisfactory humoral as well as cell-mediated immune response. For such purpose, subunit, recombinant and DNA vaccines were tested. The first subunit vaccine tested was an HSV-2 glycoprotein mix (gB, gC, gG, gD, and gE) purified from infected chick embryo cells (this product is essentially similar to the subunit HSZP vaccine immuno mentioned above). As shown in 22 seronegative volunteers, this particular vaccine induced both the humoral and the cell-mediated specific response [162]. Alternatively, a similar vaccine (containing gB2 and gG2) was used to immunize 161 seronegative individuals with a less encouraging effect at phase II clinical trial [163]. The company Chiron Corporation sponsored the testing of a recombinant gB2/gG2 vaccine mixed with the MF59 adjuvant used for immunization of 137 persons. The efficiency of this vaccine was reported 9% only [53, 164]. Another study by GlaxoSmithKline uses a recombinant gD2 in combination with alum adjuvant and/or ASO_4; in the latter trial, 7460 volunteers were selected as seronegative before the onset of the phase II trial. Immunization with the vaccine in question induced higher antibody titers than natural infection and also conferred partial protection against natural infection that had a milder course as compared to non-immunized controls [165]. At phase III trial, 847 seronegative individuals (no antibodies to HSV-1 as well as to HSV-2) and 1867 women showing antibodies to HSV-1 but not to HSV-2 were immunized with the same vaccine [166]. The results showed that 73–74% immunized women which were seronegative against both antigens have been protected against HSV-2 primoinfection (as detected by natural seroconversion), but the vaccine was not effective in man and in HSV-1 seropositive women. The GlaxoSmithKline company provided another trial, during which together 8323 seronegative women (for HSV-1 as well as HSV-2) were immunized. This follow-up was less encouraging when showing only 20% efficiency when measured by the seroconversion rate against natural genital HSV-2 infection and about 58% protection against HSV-1 genital infection [167]. In a multicenter study from 2013, the possible role of the abovementioned gD2-ASO_4 vaccine in the etiology of stillbirth was evaluated. Together 19,727 pregnant women were immunized, from which 13.3% really had stillbirth in comparison with 11.00% of pregnant women in the control group that shows a clearly not significant effect [168].

The HSV DNA vaccine was also tested for prophylactic use. In the phase I trial, 62 seronegative women were immunized with the gD2 recombinant plasmid GENEVAX. T-cell-mediated response was found in one out of four volunteers [169]. Another prophylactic candidate vaccine tested was the HSV-2/HSV529-attenuated virus (deleted in genes UL5 and and UL29, also called dl5-29). This vaccine when tested in guinea pigs elicited a satisfactory humoral as well as T-cell response, conferred protection to HSV-2 challenge, and reduced the extent of latency in the regional lumbosacral ganglia [170]. The vaccine efficiency in human will be evaluated by the end of 2016.

As already mentioned, the therapeutic vaccines should decrease the frequency of recurrence episodes as well as their severity. To achieve this, the therapeutic vaccine must induce a potent and specific T-cell-mediated response. Several subunit vaccines were tested with an immunotherapeutic purpose, namely, the semipurified inactivated infected cell extracts, recombinant vaccines, and attenuated viruses. Probably, the first of the purified inactivated HSV-1-infected cell extract tested was the vaccine by Kutinová et al. [171]. A similar vaccine introduced by Skinner et al. [172] was used for immunization of 316 subjects with herpes disease who had recurrent blisters at least six times per year. Though this vaccine induced a detectable increase in the antibody levels and a satisfactory T-cell-mediated response, no difference in the frequency of recurrences was noted during the 1-year observation period. However, the vaccination accelerated the healing of the lesions, which had a less severe course in the immunized persons. Among the recombinant vaccines tested in a therapeutic context, the gD2 vaccine containing alum adjuvant should be mentioned first. This was used for immunization of 98 HSV-2 seropositive persons who had at least four but up to 14 recurrence episodes per year [173]. In this trial, the average of six recurrences per year in the placebo group was siginificantly higher than the average of four recurrences per year in the immunized group ($p = 0.039$). Furthermore, the gB2/gD2 vaccine mixed with the MF59 adjuvant was applied in another trial, in which 202 volunteers were immunized. At the phase II clinical trial, no difference was found in the titers of neutralizing antibodies during the observation period of 8 months, but there was a significant difference in the increased interval between the occurrences of the recurrent lesions following the immunization procedure [174]. Further trials were made using peptide vaccines. An overview of defined T-cell-based epitopes from HSV proteins was reported by Laing et al. ([175], **Table 2**).

Not all known T-cell based epitopes can induce protective immunity. Mapping of T cells in seropositive population found out that CD4+ T cells were mainly stimulated by tegument proteins UL21, UL46, UL47, UL49 and envelope glycoproteins gB and gD. It was observed that gB stimulates both CD4+ and CD8+ T cells, whereas gD induces stronger CD4+ T-cell-dependent immunity [58]. CD8+ T cells were stimulated by gD53–61, gD70–78, and gD278–

286 peptides mainly in HLA-A*02:01-positive HSV-1 and HSV-2 seropositive healthy individuals [190]. Moreover, CD8+ T cells were also induced by tegument protein VP11/VP12 (gene UL46) that would account for another candidate protein to prepare effective HSV vaccine [61].

Protein (gene)	HSV-1 T-cell epitopes		HSV-2 T-cell epitopes		B-cell epitopes	Reference
	CD4	CD8	CD4	CD8		
ICP0 (RL2)		Human	Human	Human		[61]
VP5 (UL19)			Human	Human		[176]
gH I (UL22)		Mice				[69]
TK (UL23)		Human				[177]
VP26 (UL25)		Human, mice		Human		[176, 178]
VP21 (UL26)		Human		Human		[61]
gB (UL27)	Human	Human, mice	Human	Human	Mice	[60, 61, 179–181]
ICP8 (UL29)		Human, mice		Human		[61, 176]
ICP10 (UL39)		Human, mice	Human	Human		[61, 69, 176]
Vhs (UL41)		Human, mice				[61, 69]
gC (UL44)		Human, mice			Mice	[69, 180]
VP11/VP12 (UL46)		Human	Human, mice	Human, mice		[61, 176, 182]
VP13/VP14 (UL47)		Human	Mice	Human, mice		[61, 176, 178]
VP16 (UL48)		Human	Human			[61, 183, 184]
VP22 (UL49)		Human	Human, mice	Human, mice		[61, 182, 183]
gK (UL53)	Mice	Human, mice				[61, 185, 186]
ICP27 (UL54)		Human		Human, mice		[61, 187]
ICP22 (US1)		Human				[61]
gG (US4)		Mice			Mice	[69, 180]
gD (US6)	Rabbit, human	Rabbit, human, mice	Human, mice	Human, mice	Mice	[161, 180, 188–191]
gE (US8)				Human	Mice	[178, 180]
ICP4 (RS1)		Human	Human	Human		[61, 192, 193]

[a]Modified according to Laing et al. [175].

Table 2. Overview of T- and B-cell HSV-1/HSV-2–specific epitopes as tested in human, mice, and rabbits[a].

Vaccine design also requires involvement of epitopes suitable for HLA binding by most people. In most ethnic groups, HLA-A*02:01 and HLA-B*07:02 belong to the most abundant HLA alleles [194]. HLA-A*02:01-restricted epitopes have been found in glycoprotein B (UL27 442–451), tegument protein VP13/VP14 (UL47 551–559), and tegument protein coded for UL25 (UL25 372–380) of HSV-2, and they stimulated CD8+ T-cell response [176, 195]. HLA-B*07:02-restricted epitopes have been reported for tegument protein VP22 (gene UL49) (HSV-2 UL49 49–57, HSV-2 UL49 82–90, HSV-2 UL49 99–108, HSV-2 UL49 131–140, and HSV-1 UL49 291–290) and stimulated CD8+ T-cell response [176]. Samandary et al. [196] found association with high prevalence of herpes infection and disease with the frequency of HLA-A*24, HLA-B*27, and HLA-B*58 alleles. In contrast, low prevalence of herpes infection and disease appeared associated with the high frequency of HLA-B*44 allele.

The effectivity of immune response is also depending on adjuvant type. Cooper et al. [189] found out that vaccine design and adjuvant type can have a significant effect on T-cell epitope utilization. Four epitopes within the gD2 molecule gD2 49–63, gD2 105–119, gD2 245–259 and gD2 333–347 were administered to mice with alum or IL-12. CD4+ T-cell response was induced in mice immunized with gD HSV-2 epitope gD2 245–259 and adjuvant alum. Mice immunized with IL-12 stimulate CD4+ T-cell response to HSV-2 epitope gD2 245–259 as well as to gD2 333–347 [189].

"Epitope" (peptide) vaccines that selectively stimulate T and B cells belong to other herpes simplex vaccine candidates. Wang et al. [180] prepared multi-epitope peptide vaccine that contained six B-cell epitopes from different glycoproteins of HSV-2 (gB2 466–473, gC2 216–223, gD2 6–18, gE2 483–491, gG2 572–579 and gI2 286–295), four CD4+ T-cell-based epitopes (gD2 21–28, gD2 205–224, gD2 245–259 and gB2 162–177) and two CD8+ T-cell-based epitopes (gD2 10–20 and gD2 268–276). All above-described epitopes were inserted into the extracellular fragment (1–290) of HSV-2 glycoprotein D to construct multi-epitope assembly peptides (MEAPs) by replacing some non-epitope amino acid sequences. The genes of the selected peptides were inserted into recombinant plasmid and expressed in *E. coli* strain BL21. The multi-epitope vaccine elicited in mice production of virus-neutralizing antibodies induced Th1 and Th2 immune response and protected mice against intravaginally induced lethal challenge of HSV-2 [180].

Many studies have focused on mapping of protective epitopes that stimulate immunity in asymptomatic individuals, that is, individuals without clinical findings of herpes infection. Analysis of IFN-γ-producing CD4+ T cells in HSV-1 seropositive individuals revealed that gB peptide epitopes (aa 166–180 and aa 666–680) were strongly recognized by CD4+ T cells from asymptomatic individuals, but not from symptomatic individuals. Inversely, CD4+ T cells from symptomatic individuals preferentially recognized gB (aa 661–675) [179]. Another study identified asymptomatic CD8+ T-cell epitopes from glycoprotein D (gD53–61, gD70–78 and gD278–286) [191]. It can be hypothesized that repertoire of T-cell-based epitopes determines either the development of HSV-1 (-2) clinical symptoms or asymptomatic viral shedding.

Finally, some investigators preferred the genetically attenuated virus vaccines, because they induce an immune response essentially similar to that following natural infection. For example, Casanova et al. [157] immunized the volunteers (32 persons having at least five recurrent lesions per year) with an attenuated HSV-2 virus deleted in the UL39 gene (the RR1 protein ORF). The phase I and phase II clinical trials showed the reduction of recurrent clinical manifestations by 37.5% as compared with the placebo-immunized group. Another clinical trial, which was performed in 2006, took the advantage of HSV-2-attenuated virus deleted in the gH gene (the so-called disabled infectious single cycle [DISC] virus). Unfortunately, no significant difference was found in the number of recurrences between the immunized and control mock-immunized subjects during the 1 year follow-up period [150]. The last phase I and II clinical trial which results will be announced nowadays concerns volunteers who had from two to nine recurrent lesions per year; they were immunized with a DNA vaccine-expressing gD2 in combination with the lipid adjuvant Vaxfectin [197].

7. Future perspectives of HSV-1/HSV-2 vaccination with the emphasis on the T-cell response

As described above, an effective vaccine against HSV-1 and HSV-2 infection that would prevent virus reactivation (therapeutic vaccine) should stimulate both humoral and cellular immunity mediated by CD4+ and CD8+ T cells. This immune response can be induced by live-attenuated virus, but such viruses are not safe because of their possible reversion back to the wild-type virus. Therefore, alternative approaches to develop effective herpes simplex vaccine have been attempted during the last decades. Nowadays, T-cell-inducing herpes simplex vaccines bearing "asymptomatic" immunodominant epitopes derived from HSV proteins were designed and tested [180]. Such vaccines possess many advantages over traditional vaccine like (1) induction of specific T-cell-based immunity, (2) inhibition of pathogenic immune response, and (3) safety.

Only few asymptomatic T-cell epitope-based vaccines were prepared and tested until now. The vaccine used by Wald et al. [198] contained 32 synthetic immunogenic HSV-2 peptides, linked to the heat shock protein Hsp 70 in combination with the QS-21 (contains a saponin) adjuvant. In 32 immunized volunteers, the vaccine elicited no complication, but induced a satisfactory CD4+/CD8+ T-lymphocyte response against a wide range of immunogenic HSV-2 peptides used in the stimulation tests *in vitro*. Chentoufi et al. [191] prepared CD8+ T-cell epitope-based vaccine containing three separate pairs of CD4–CD8 lipopeptides. Each of the lipopeptide contained one of the three asymptomatic immunodominant human CD8+ T-cell peptide epitopes from HSV-1 glycoprotein D (gD53–61, gD70–78, and gD278–286) that were joined with a human CD4+ T-cell peptide epitope (gD49–82). Humanized HLA-A*02:01 transgenic rabbits were immunized with a mixture of the three CD4–CD8 HSV-1 gD lipopeptides. Immunization induced an increased production of CD4+ and CD8+ T cells and protected rabbits against ocular HSV disease [191]. The same ASYMP vaccine was used for therapeutic vaccination of HLA transgenic rabbits infected by HSV-1. The vaccine induced production of HSV-specific CD8+ T cells that prevent HSV-1 reactivation ex vivo from latently infected explanted trigeminal ganglia. Moreover, the vaccine significantly reduced HSV-1 shedding and boosted the function of HSV-1 gD epitope-specific CD8+ T cells in draining lymph nodes, conjunctiva, and trigeminal ganglion [199].

The lipopeptide vaccines belong to another herpes simplex vaccine candidate. The lipopeptide vaccine can be easily produced and possesses some advantages over traditional vaccine such as safety and tolerance, bearing protective T-cell epitopes derived from HSV antigens, missing of non-immunogenic harmful epitopes, and missing of viral pathogenic proteins such as ICP47, and lipids have functioned as adjuvant. Previous studies observed that lipopeptide vaccine injected intranasally into mice induced mucosal and systemic B and Th1 immune response [191]. Other authors prefer attenuated genetically modified herpes simplex viruses as successfully vaccine candidates (Section 5.4).

8. Conclusions

In conclusion, the development of successfully therapeutical vaccine against HSV infection should respect the following recommendations: (1) the assessment of putative differences in the recognition of T- and/or B-cell epitopes from envelope, tegument, and regulatory HSV proteins in patients with recurrent herpes disease versus asymptomatic individuals; (2) the production of new safer adjuvants avoiding those claimed to cause the ASIA syndrome; (3) the induction of local mucosal immunity mediated by lipopeptides; (4) the use of humanized susceptible HLA transgenic mice as well as rabbits before human trials; and (5) at last but not least, the efficacy of human trials for an immunotherapeutic vaccine that should be made according to internationally accepted unified criteria in at least three groups of subjects (seronegative individuals, seropositive individuals without recurrent herpes disease, and volunteers with such disease). The tests should include the demonstration of elevated antibody titers after vaccination and *in vitro* testing of the T-lymphocyte response in a blastic transformation test as well as production of selected cytokines; 6. Finally, the application of the therapeutic vaccine in future human trials should be intracutaneous rather than by using other administration routes.

Author details

Vladimíra Ďurmanová[1], Marian Adamkov[2] and Július Rajčáni[3*]

*Address all correspondence to: viruraj@savba.sk

1 Institute of Immunology, Faculty of Medicine, Comenius University in Bratislava, Bratislava, Slovakia

2 Department of Histology and Embryology, Jessenius Faculty of Medicine, Comenius University, Martin, Slovakia

3 Institute of Virology, Slovak Academy of Sciences, Bratislava, Slovakia

References

[1] Gruter W. Das Herpesvirus, seine aetiologische und klinische Bedeutung. Munch Med Wsch 1924, 71: 1058.

[2] Schneweis KE. Untersuchungen zur Typendifferenzierung des Herpesvirus hominis. Z Immun-Forsch 1962, 124: 24–28.

[3] Wildy P. Classification and nomenclature of viruses, pp. 33–34, In: Monographs in Virology, Melnick JL (ed), Karger, Basel, 1971.

[4] Lee EK, Coleman RM, Pereira L, Bailey PD, Tatsuno M, Nahmias AJ. Detection of herpes simplex virus type 2 specific antibody with glycoprotein G. J Clin Microbiol 1985, 22: 641–644.

[5] Liu F, Zhou ZH. Comparative virion structures of human herpesviruses, pp. 27–43, In: Arvin A, Campadelli-Fiume G, Mocarski E, Moore PS, Roizman B, Whitley R and Yamanishi K (eds). Human Herpesviruses: Biology, Therapy and Immunoprophylaxis. Cambridge University Press, 2007.

[6] Roizman B, Knipe DM, Whitley RJ. Herpes Simplex Viruses, pp. 1823–1897, In: Knipe DM, Howley PM (eds) Fields Virology, 6th ed., Walters Cluver/Lippincott Williams and Wilkins, Philadelphia, 2013.

[7] Knipe DM, Cliffe AR. Chromatin control of herpes simplex virus lytic and latent infection. Nat Rev Microbiol 2008, 6: 211–221. doi: 10.1038/nrmicro1794.

[8] Campadelli-Fiume G, Menotti L, Avitabile E, Gianni T. Viral and cellular contributions to herpes simplex virus entry into the cell. Curr Opin Virol 2012, 2: 28–36. doi: 10.1016/j.coviro.2011.12.001.

[9] Rajčáni J, Vojvodová A. The role of herpes simplex virus glycoproteins in the virus replication cycle. Acta Virol 1998, 42: 103–118.

[10] Gianni T, Amasio M, Campadelli-Fiume G. Herpes simplex virus gD forms distinct complexes with fusion executors gB and gH/gL in part through the C-terminal profusion domain. J Biol Chem 2009, 284: 17370–17382. doi: 10.1074/jbc.M109.005728.

[11] Satoh T, Arii J, Suenaga T, Wang J, Kogure A, Uehori J, Arase N, Shiratori I, Tanaka S, Kawaguchi Y, Spear PG, Lanier LL, Arase H. PILRα is a herpes simplex virus-1 entry co-receptor that associates with glycoprotein B. Cell 2008, 132: 935–944. doi: 10.1016/j.cell.2008.01.043.

[12] Stampfer SD, Lou H, Cohen GH, Eisenberg RJ, Heldwein EE. Structural basis of local, pH dependent conformational changes in glycoprotein B from herpes simplex virus type 1. J Virol 2010, 84: 12.924–12.933. doi: 10.1128/JVI.01750-10.

[13] Dingwell KS, Brunetti CR, Hendricks RL, Tang Q, Tang M, Rainbow AJ, Johnson DC. Herpes simplex virus glycoprotein E and I facilitate cell to cell spread in vivo and across junctions of cultured cells. J Virol 1994, 68: 834–845.

[14] Rajčáni J, Ďurmanová V. Early expression of herpes simplex virus (HSV) proteins and reactivation of latent infection. Folia Microbiol 2000, 45: 7–28

[15] Režuchová I, Kúdelová M, Ďurmanová V, Vojvodová A, Košovský J, Rajčáni J. Transcription at early stages of herpes simplex virus 1 infection and during reactivation. Intervirology 2003, 46: 25–34.

[16] Stevens JG, Wagner EK, Devi-Rao GB, Cook ML, Feldman LT. RNA complementary to a herpesvirus alpha gene mRNA is prominent in latently infected neurons. Science 1987, 235: 1056–1059.

[17] Ahmed MM, Lock C, Millerm G. Regions of the herpes simplex virus type 1 latency-associated transcript that protect cells from apoptosis in vitro and protect neuronal cells in vivo. J Virol 2002, 76: 717–722.

[18] Perng GC, Jones C, Ciacci-Zanella J, Stone M, Henderson G, Yukht A, Slanina SM, Hofman FM, Ghiasi H, Nesburn AB, Wechsler SL. Virus induced neuronal apoptosis blocked by the herpes simplex virus latency associated transcript (LAT). Science 2000, 287: 1500–1503.

[19] Perng GC, Maguen B, Jin L, Mott KR, Osorio N, Slanina SM, Yukht A, Ghiasi H, Nesburn AB, Inman M, Henderson G, Jones C, Wechsler SL. A gene capable of blocking apoptosis can substitute for herpes simplex virus type 1 latency associated transcript gene and restore wild type reactivation levels. J Virol 2002, 76: 1224–1235

[20] Efstathiou S, Minson AC, Field HJ, Anderson JR, Wildy P. Detection of herpes simplex virus specific DNA sequences in latently infected mice and in humans. J Virol 1986, 32: 446–455.

[21] Kristie TM and Roizman B. Differentiation and DNA contact points to the host proteins binding at the cis site of for virion-mediated induction of herpes simplex virus 1 alpha genes. J Virol 1988, 62: 1145–1157

[22] Lillycrop KA, Budrahan VS, Lakin ND, Terrenghi G, Wood JN, Polak JM, Latchman DS. A novel POU family transcription factor is closely related to Brn-3 but has a distinct expression pattern in neuronal cells. Nucleic Acids Res 1992, 20: 5093–5096.

[23] Lillycrop KA, Estridge JK, Latchman DS. Functional interaction between different isoforms of the Oct-2 transcription factor expressed in neuronal cells. Biochem J 1994, 298: 245–248.

[24] Preston CM, Efstathiou S. Molecular basis of HSV latency and reactivation, pp. 602–615, In: Arvin A, Campadelli-Fiume G, Mocarski E, Moore PS, Roizman B, Whitley R, Yamanishi K. (eds.) Human Herpesviruses, Biology, Therapy and Immunoprophylaxis, Cambridge University Press, 2007.

[25] Fries LF, Friedman HM, Cohen GH, Eisenberg RJ, Hammer CH, Frank MM. Glycoprotein C of herpes simplex virus 1 is an inhibitor of the complement cascade. J Immunol 1986, 137: 1636–1641.

[26] Hill TJ, Field HJ, Blyth WA. Acute and recurrent infection with herpes simplex virus in the mouse: a model for studying latency and recurrent disease. J Gen Virol 1975, 28: 341–353.

[27] Hill TJ, Blyth HJ. An alternative theory of herpes simplex recurrence and a possible role for prostaglandins. Lancet 1976, 1: 397–398.

[28] Walz M, Price R, Notkins A. Latent ganglionic infection with herpes simplex virus types 1 and 2: viral reactivation after neurectomy. Science 1974, 184: 1185–1187.

[29] Kúdelová M, Rajčáni J. Herpes simplex virus and human CNS infection, pp. 169–214, In: Singh SK, Ružek D. (eds), Neuroviral Infection, 1st ed., Taylor and Francis Group CRC, 2013.

[30] Whitley R, Kimberlin D, Prober Ch. HSV 1 and 2: pathogenesis and disease. pp. 569–601, In: Arvin A, Campadelli-Fiume G, Mocarski E, Moore PS, Roizman B, Whitley R, Yamanishi K. (eds.). Human Herpesviruses, Biology, Therapy and Immunoprophylaxis, Cambridge University Press, 2007.

[31] Svensson A, Bellner L, Magnusson M, Eriksson K. Role of IFN-alpha/beta signaling in the prevention of genital herpes virus type 2 infection. J Reprod Immunol 2007, 74: 114–123.

[32] Conrady CD, Halford WP, Carr DJ. Loss of the type I interferon pathway increases vulnerability of mice to genital herpes simplex virus 2 infection. J Virol 2011, 85: 1625–1633. doi: 10.1128/JVI.01715-10.

[33] Kim M, Osborne NR, Zeng W, Donaghy H, McKinnon K, Jackson DC, Cunningham AL. Herpes simplex virus antigens directly activate NK cells via TLR2, thus facilitating their presentation to CD4 T lymphocytes. J Immunol 2012, 188: 4158–4170. doi: 10.4049/jimmunol.1103450.

[34] Lundberg P, Welander P, Han X, Cantin E. Herpes simplex virus type 1 DNA is immunostimulatory *in vitro* and *in vivo*. J Virol 2003, 77: 11158–11169.

[35] Guo Y, Audry M, Ciancanelli M, Alsina L, Azevedo J, Herman M, Anguiano E, Sancho-Shimizu V, Lorenzo L, Pauwels E, Philippe PB, Pérez de Diego R, Cardon A, Vogt G, Picard C, Andrianirina ZZ, Rozenberg F, Lebon P, Plancoulaine S, Tardieu M, Valérie D, Jouanguy E, Chaussabel D, Geissmann F, Abel L, Casanova JL, Zhang SY. Herpes simplex virus encephalitis in a patient with complete TLR3 deficiency: TLR3 is otherwise redundant in protective immunity. J Exp Med 2011, 208: 2083–2098. doi: 10.1084/jem.20101568.

[36] Herman M, Ciancanelli M, Ou YH, Lorenzo L, Klaudel-Dreszler M, Pauwels E, Sancho-Shimizu V, Pérez de Diego R, Abhyankar A, Israelsson E, Guo Y, Cardon A, Rozen-

berg F, Lebon P, Tardieu M, Heropolitanska-Pliszka E, Chaussabel D, White MA, Abel L, Zhang SY, Casanova JL. Heterozygous TBK1 mutations impair TLR3 immunity and underlie herpes simplex encephalitis of childhood. J Exp Med 2012, 209: 1567–1582. doi: 10.1084/jem.20111316.

[37] Ank N, West H, Bartholdy C, Eriksson K, Thomsen AR, Paludan SR. Lambda interferon (IFN-lambda), a type III IFN, is induced by viruses and IFNs and displays potent antiviral activity against select virus infections in vivo. J Virol 2006, 80: 4501–4509.

[38] Li J, Hu S, Zhou L, Ye L, Wang X, Ho J, Ho W. Interferon lambda inhibits herpes simplex virus type I infection of human astrocytes and neurons. Glia 2011, 59: 58–67. doi: 10.1002/glia.21076.

[39] Lopušná K, Režuchová I, Kabát P, Kúdelová M. Interferon lambda induces antiviral response to herpes simplex virus 1 infection. Acta Virol 2014, 58: 325–332.

[40] Grubor-Bauk B, Arthur JL, Mayrhofer G. Importance of NKT cells in resistance to herpes simplex virus, fate of virus-infected neurons, and level of latency in mice. J Virol 2008, 82: 11073–11083. doi: 10.1128/JVI.00205-08.

[41] Adler H, Beland JL, Del-Pan NC, Kobzik L, Sobel RA, Rimm IJ. In the absence of T cells, natural killer cells protect from mortality due to HSV-1 encephalitis. J Neuroimmunol 1999, 93: 208–213.

[42] Milligan GN. Neutrophils aid in protection of the vaginal mucosae of immune mice against challenge with herpes simplex virus type 2. J Virol 1999, 73: 6380–6386.

[43] Kodukula P, Liu T, Rooijen NV, Jager MJ, Hendricks RL. Macrophage control of herpes simplex virus type 1 replication in the peripheral nervous system. J Virol 1999, 162: 2895–2905.

[44] Buc M. Interferon gamma (IFN-gamma), p. 95, In: Basic and Clinical Immunology, Comenius University, Bratislava, 2008.

[45] Kassim SH, Rajasagi NK, Zhao X, Chervenak R, Jennings SR. In vivo ablation of CD11c-positive dendritic cells increases susceptibility to herpes simplex virus type 1 infection and diminishes NK and T-cell responses. J Virol 2006, 80: 3985–3993.

[46] Hochrein H, Schlatter B, O'Keeffe M, Wagner C, Schmitz F, Schiemann M, Bauer S, Suter M, Wagner H. Herpes simplex virus type-1 induces IFN-alpha production via Toll-like receptor 9-dependent and -independent pathways. Proc Natl Acad Sci U S A 2004, 101: 11416–11421.

[47] den Haan JM, Bevan MJ. Antigen presentation to CD8+ T cells: cross-priming in infectious diseases. Curr Opin Immunol 2001, 13: 437–441.

[48] Ramirez MC, Sigal LJ. The multiple routes of MHC-I cross-presentation. Trends Microbiol 2004, 12: 204–207.

[49] Lubinski J, Wang L, Mastellos D, Sahu A, Lambris JD, Friedman HM. In vivo role of complement-interacting domains of herpes simplex virus type 1 glycoprotein gC. J Exp Med 1999, 190: 1637–1646.

[50] McDermott MR, Brais LJ, Evelegh MJ. Mucosal and systemic antiviral antibodies in mice inoculated intravaginally with herpes simplex virus type 2. J Gen Virol 1990, 71: 1497–1504.

[51] Dudley KL, Bourne N, Milligan GN. Immune protection against HSV-2 in B-cell-deficient mice. Virology 2000, 270: 454–463.

[52] Morrison LA, Zhu L, Thebeau LG. Vaccine-induced serum immunoglobin contributes to protection from herpes simplex virus type 2 genital infection in the presence of immune T cells. J Virol 2001, 75: 1195–1204.

[53] Corey L, Langenberg AG, Ashley R, Sekulovich RE, Izu AE, Douglas JM Jr., Handsfield HH, Warren T, Marr L, Tyring S, DiCarlo R, Adimora AA, Leone P, Dekker CL, Burke RL, Leong WP, Straus SE. Recombinant glycoprotein vaccine for the prevention of genital HSV-2 infection: two randomized controlled trials. Chiron HSV Vaccine Study Group. JAMA 1999, 282: 331–340.

[54] Handunnetthi L, Ramagopalan SV, Ebers GC, Knight JC. Regulation of major histocompatibility complex class II gene expression, genetic variation and disease. Genes Immun 2010, 11: 99–112. doi: 10.1038/gene.2009.83.

[55] Milligan GN, Bernstein DI. Interferon-gamma enhances resolution of herpes simplex virus type 2 infection of the murine genital tract. Virology 1997, 229: 259–268.

[56] Milligan GN, Bernstein DI, Bourne N. T lymphocytes are required for protection of the vaginal mucosae and sensory ganglia of immune mice against reinfection with herpes simplex virus type 2. J Immunol 1998, 160: 6093–6100.

[57] Gill N, Ashkar AA. Overexpression of interleukin-15 compromises CD4-dependent adaptive immune responses against herpes simplex virus 2. J Virol 2009, 83: 918–926. doi: 10.1128/JVI.01282-08.

[58] Koelle DM, Schomogyi M, McClurkan C, Reymond SN, Chen HB. CD4 T-cell responses to herpes simplex virus type 2 major capsid protein VP5: comparison with responses to tegument and envelope glycoproteins. J Virol 2000, 74: 11422–11425.

[59] Zhu J, Koelle DM, Cao J, Vazquez J, Huang ML, Hladik F, Wald A, Corey L. Virus-specific CD8+ T cells accumulate near sensory nerve endings in genital skin during subclinical HSV-2 reactivation. J Exp Med 2007, 204: 595–603.

[60] Khanna KM, Bonneau RH, Kinchington PR, Hendricks RL. Herpes simplex virus-specific memory CD8+ T cells are selectively activated and retained in latently infected sensory ganglia. Immunity 2003, 18: 593–603.

[61] Jing L, Haas J, Chong TM, Bruckner JJ, Dann GC, Dong L, Marshak JO, McClurkan CL, Yamamoto TN, Bailer SM, Laing KJ, Wald A, Verjans GM, Koelle DM. Cross-presen-

tation and genome-wide screening reveal candidate T cells antigens for a herpes simplex virus type 1 vaccine. J Clin Invest 2012, 122: 654–763. doi: 10.1172/JCI60556.

[62] Gebhardt BM, Hill JM. Cellular neuroimmunologic responses to ocular herpes simplex virus infection. J Neuroimmunol 1990, 28: 227–236.

[63] Liu T, Tang Q, Hendricks RL Inflammatory infiltration of the trigeminal ganglion after herpes simplex virus type 1 corneal infection. J Virol 1996, 70: 264–271 (1996).

[64] Liu T, Khanna KM, Chen X, Fink DJ, Hendricks RL. CD8(+) T cells can block herpes simplex virus type 1 (HSV-1) reactivation from latency in sensory neurons. J Exp Med 2000, 191: 1459–1466.

[65] Theil D, Derfuss T, Paripovic I, Herberger S, Meinl E, Schueler O, Strupp M, Arbusow V, Brandt T. Latent herpesvirus infection in human trigeminal ganglia causes chronic immune response. Am J Pathol 2003, 163: 2179–2184.

[66] Knickelbein JE, Khanna KM, Yee MB, Baty CJ, Kinchington PR, Hendricks RL. Noncytotoxic lytic granule-mediated CD8+ T cell inhibition of HSV-1 reactivation from neuronal latency. Science 2008, 322: 268–271. doi: 10.1126/science.1164164.

[67] Decman V, Kinchington PR, Harvey SA, Hendricks RL. Gamma interferon can block herpes simplex virus type 1 reactivation from latency, even in the presence of late gene expression. J Virol 2005, 79: 10339–10347.

[68] Mueller SN, Heath W, McLain JD, Carbone FR, Jones CM. Characterization of two TCR transgenic mouse lines specific for herpes simplex virus. Immunol Cell Biol 2002, 80: 156–163.

[69] St Leger AJ, Peters B, Sidney J, Sette A, Hendricks RL. Defining the herpes simplex virus-specific CD8+ T cell repertoire in C57BL/6 mice. J Immunol 2011, 186: 3927–3933. doi: 10.4049/jimmunol.1003735.

[70] Derfuss T, Segerer S, Herberger S, Sinicina I, Hüfner K, Ebelt K, Knaus HG, Steiner I, Meinl E, Dornmair K, Arbusow V, Strupp M, Brandt T, Theil D. Presence of HSV-1 immediate early genes and clonally expanded T-cells with a memory effector phenotype in human trigeminal ganglia. Brain Pathol 2007, 17: 389–398.

[71] van Velzen M, Jing L, Osterhaus AD, Sette A, Koelle DM, Verjans GM. Local CD4 and CD8 T-cell reactivity to HSV-1 antigens documents broad viral protein expression and immune competence in latently infected human trigeminal ganglia. PLoS Pathog 2013, 9: e1003547. doi: 10.1371/journal.ppat.1003547.

[72] Egan KP, Wu S, Wigdahl B, Jennings SR. Immunological control of herpes simplex virus infections. J Neurovirol 2013, 19: 328–345. doi: 10.1007/s13365-013-0189-3.

[73] Kern A, Schiff B. Vaccine therapy in recurrent herpes simplex. Arch Dermatol 1964, 89: 844–845.

[74] Koelle D. HSV 1 and 2 immunobiology and host response, pp. 616–641, In: Arvin A, Campadelli-Fiume G, Mocarski E, Moore PS, Roizman B, Whitley R, Yamanishi K (eds).

Human Herpesviruses: Biology, Therapy and Immunoprophylaxis. Cambridge University Press, 2007.

[75] Skinner GR, Buchan A, Hartley CE, Turner SP, Williams DR. The preparation, efficacy and safety of 'antigenoid' vaccine NFU1 (S-L+) MRC toward prevention of herpes simplex virus infections in human subjects. Med Microbiol Immunol 1980, 169: 39–51.

[76] Dundarov S, Andonov P, Bakalov B, Nechev K, Tomov C. Immunotherapy with inactivated polyvalent herpes vaccines. Dev Biol Stand 1982, 52: 351–358.

[77] Scriba M. Animal studies on the efficacy of vaccination against recurrent herpes. Med Microbiol Immunol 1982, 171: 33–40.

[78] Kutinová V, Vonka V, Řezáčová D. Production and some properties of antigen extracts for neutralizing of herpes simplex virus. Acta Virol 1977, 19: 189–197.

[79] Rajčáni J, Kutinová L, Vonka V. Restriction of latent herpes virus infection of rabbits immunized with subviral herpes simplex virus vaccine. Acta Virol 1980, 24: 183–193.

[80] Morello CS, Kraynyak KA, Levinson MS, Chen Z, Lee KF, Spector DH. Inactivated HSV-2 in MPL/alum adjuvant provides nearly complete protection against genital infection and shedding following long term challenge and rechallenge. Vaccine 2012, 30: 6541–6550. doi: 10.1016/j.vaccine.2012.08.049.

[81] Dundarov S, Andonov P. Seventeen years of application of herpes vaccines in Bulgaria. Acta Virol 1994, 38: 205–208.

[82] Hilfenhaus J, Christ H, Köhler R, Moser H, Kirchner H, Levy HB. Protectivity of herpes simplex virus antigens: studies in mice on the adjuvant effect of PICLC and on the dependence of protection on T cell competence. Med Microbiol Immunol 1981, 169: 225–235.

[83] Thomson TA, Hilfenhaus J, Moser H, Morahan PS. Comparison of effects of adjuvants on efficacy of virion envelope herpes simplex virus vaccine against labial infection of BALB/c mice. Infect Immun 1983, 41: 556–562.

[84] Metcalf JF, Whitley RJ. Protective immunity against herpetic ocular disease in an outbred mouse model. Curr Eye Res 1987, 6: 167–171.

[85] Rajčáni J, Sabó A, Mucha V, Košťál M, Compel P. Herpes simplex virus type 1 envelope subunit vaccine not only protects against lethal virus challenge, but also may restrict latency and virus reactivation. Acta Virol 1995, 39: 37–49.

[86] Myers MG, Bernstein DI, Harrison CJ, Stanberry LR. Herpes simplex virus glycoprotein treatment of recurrent genital herpes reduces cervicovaginal virus shedding in guinea pigs. Antiviral Res 1988, 10: 83–88.

[87] Blacklaws BA, Krishna S, Minson AC, Nash AA. Immunogenicity of herpes simplex virus type 1 glycoproteins expressed in vaccinia virus recombinants. Virology 1990, 177: 727–736.

[88] York LJ, Giorgio DP, Mishkin EM. Immunomodulatory effects of HSV2 glycoprotein D in HSV1 infected mice: implications for immunotherapy of recurrent HSV infection. Vaccine 1995, 13: 1706–1712.

[89] Mosko T, Kosovský J, Rezuchová I, Durmanová V, Kúdelová M, Rajcáni J. Expression of herpes simplex virus 1 glycoprotein D in prokaryotic and eukaryotic cells. Acta Virol 2004, 48: 97–107.

[90] Durmanová V, Mosko T, Sapák M, Kosovský J, Rezuchová I, Buc M, Rajcáni J. Efficacy of recombinant herpes simplex virus 1 glycoprotein D candidate vaccines in mice. Acta Microbiol Immunol Hung 2006, 53: 459–477.

[91] Long D, Madara TJ, Ponce de Leon M, Cohen GH, Montgomery PC, Eisenberg RJ. Glycoprotein D protects mice against lethal challenge with herpes simplex virus types 1 and 2. Infect Immun 1984, 43: 761–764.

[92] Roberts PL, Duncan BE, Raybould TJ, Watson DH. Purification of herpes simplex virus glycoproteins B and C using monoclonal antibodies and their ability to protect mice against lethal challenge. J Gen Virol 1985, 66: 1073–1085.

[93] Kino Y, Eto T, Nishiyama K, Ohtomo N, Mori R. Immunogenicity of purified glycoprotein gB of herpes simplex virus. Arch Virol 1986, 89: 69–80.

[94] Manservigi R, Grossi MP, Gualandri R, Balboni PG, Marchini A, Rotola A, Rimessi P, Di Luca D, Cassai E, Barbanti-Brodano G. Protection from herpes simplex virus type 1 lethal and latent infections by secreted recombinant glycoprotein B constitutively expressed in human cells with a BK virus episomal vector. J Virol 1990, 64: 431–436.

[95] Broker M, Abel KJ, Köhler R, Hilfenhaus J, Amann E. Escherichia coli-derived envelope protein gD but not gC antigens of herpes simplex virus protect mice against a lethal challenge with HSV-1 and HSV-2. Med Microbiol Immunol 1990, 179: 145–159.

[96] Byars NE, Fraser-Smith EB, Pecyk RA, Welch M, Nakano G, Burke RL, Hayward AR, Allison AC. Vaccinating guinea pigs with recombinant glycoprotein D of herpes simplex virus in an efficacious adjuvant formulation elicits protection against vaginal infection. Vaccine 1994, 12: 200–209.

[97] O'Hagan D, Goldbeck C, Ugozzoli M, Ott G, Burke RL. Intranasal immunization with recombinant gD2 reduces disease severity and mortality following genital challenge with herpes simplex virus type 2 in guinea pigs. Vaccine 1999, 17: 2229–2236.

[98] Bourne N, Bravo FJ, Francotte M, Bernstein DI, Myers MG, Slaoui M, Stanberry LR. Herpes simplex virus (HSV) type 2 glycoprotein D subunit vaccines and protection against genital HSV-1 or HSV-2 disease in guinea pigs. J Infect Dis 2003, 187: 542–549.

[99] Manservigi R, Boero A, Argnani R, Caselli E, Zucchini S, Miriagou V, Mavromara P, Cilli M, Grossi MP, Balboni PG, Cassai E. Immunotherapeutic activity of a recombinant combined gB-gD-gE vaccine against recurrent HSV-2 infections in a guinea pig model. Vaccine 2005, 23: 865–872.

[100] Durmanová V, Sapák M, Kosovský J, Rezuchová I, Kúdelová M, Buc M, Rajcáni J. Immune response and cytokine production following immunization with experimental herpes simplex virus 1 (HSV-1) vaccines. Folia Microbiol (Praha) 2008, 53: 73–83. doi: 10.1007/s12223-008-0011-4.

[101] Fotouhi F, Soleimanjahi H, Roostaee MH, Dalimi Asl A. Expression of the herpes simplex virus type 2 glycoprotein D in baculovirus expression system and evaluation of its immunogenicity in guinea pigs. Iran Biomed J 2008, 12: 59–66.

[102] Awasthi S, Balliet JW, Flynn JA, Lubinski JM, Shaw CE, DiStefano DJ, Cai M, Brown M, Smith JF, Kowalski R, Swoyer R, Galli J, Copeland V, Rios S, Davidson RC, Salnikova M, Kingsley S, Bryan J, Casimiro DR, Friedman HM. Protection provided by a herpes simplex virus 2 (HSV-2) glycoprotein C and D subunit antigen vaccine against genital HSV-2 infection in HSV-1-seropositive guinea pigs. J Virol 2014, 88: 2000–2010. doi: 10.1128/JVI.03163-13.

[103] Awasthi S, Mahairas GG, Shaw CE, Huang ML, Koelle DM, Posavad C, Corey L, Friedman HM. A dual-modality herpes simplex virus 2 vaccine for preventing genital herpes by using glycoprotein C and D subunit antigens to induce potent antibody responses and adenovirus vectors containing capsid and tegument proteins as T cell immunogens. J Virol 2015, 89: 8497–8509. doi: 10.1128/JVI.01089-15.

[104] Inoue T, Inoue Y, Nakamura T, Yoshida A, Inoue Y, Tano Y, Shimomura Y, Fujisawa Y, Aono A, Hayashi K. The effect of immunization with herpes simplex virus glycoprotein D fused with interluekin-2 against murine herpetic keratitis. Nihon Ganka Gakkai Zasshi 2001, 105: 223–229.

[105] Mohamedi SA, Heath AW, Jennings R. A comparison of oral and parenteral routes for therapeutic vaccination with HSV-2 ISCOMs in mice; cytokine profiles, antibody responses and protection. Antiviral Res 2001, 49: 83–99.

[106] Burke RL, Goldbeck C, Ng P, Stanberry L, Ott G, Van Nest G. The influence of adjuvant on the therapeutic efficacy of a recombinant genital herpes vaccine. J Infect Dis 1994, 170: 1110–1119.

[107] Shoenfeld Y, Agmont-Levine N. ASIA: autoimmune/inflammatory syndrome induced by adjuvants. J Autoimmun 2011, 36: 4–8. doi: 10.1016/j.jaut.2010.07.003.

[108] Lavelle EC, Grant G, Pusztai A, Pfüller U, Leavy O, McNeela E, Mills KH, O'Hagan DT. Mistletoe lectins enhance immune responses to intranasally co-administered herpes simplex virus glycoprotein D2. Immunology 2002, 107: 268–274.

[109] Cortesi R, Ravani L, Rinaldi F, Marconi P, Drechsler M, Manservigi M, Argnani R, Menegatti E, Esposito E, Manservigi R. Intranasal immunization in mice with non-ionic surfactants vesicles containing HSV immunogens: a preliminary study as possible vaccine against genital herpes. Int J Pharm 2013, 440: 229–237. doi: 10.1016/j.ijpharm.2012.06.042.

[110] Skoberne M, Cardin R, Lee A, Kazimirova A, Zielinski V, Garvie D, Lundberg A, Larson S, Bravo FJ, Bernstein DI, Flechtner JB, Long D. An adjuvanted herpes simplex virus 2 subunit vaccine elicits a T cell response in mice and is an effective therapeutic vaccine in guinea pigs. J Virol 2013, 87: 3930–3942. doi: 10.1128/JVI.02745-12.

[111] Rajčáni J, MoškoT, Režuchová, I. Current developments in viral DNA vaccines: shall they solve the unsolved? Rev Med Microbiol 2005, 15, 1–23.

[112] Cantin EM, Eberle R, Baldick JL, Moss B, Willey DE, Notkins AL, Openshaw H. Expression of herpes simplex virus 1 glycoprotein B by a recombinant vaccinia virus and protection of mice against lethal herpes simplex virus 1 infection. Proc Natl Acad Sci U S A 1987, 84: 5908–5912.

[113] Willey DE, Cantin EM, Hill LR, Moss B, Notkins AL, Openshaw H. Herpes simplex virus type 1-vaccinia virus recombinant expressing glycoprotein B: protection from acute and latent infection. J Infect Dis 1988, 158: 1382–1386.

[114] Wachsman M, Aurelian L, Smith CC, Perkus ME, Paoletti E. Regulation of expression of herpes simplex virus (HSV) glycoprotein D in vaccinia recombinants affects their ability to protect from cutaneous HSV-2 disease. J Infect Dis 1989, 159: 625–634.

[115] Bernstein DI. Effect of route of vaccination with vaccinia virus expressing HSV-2 glycoprotein D on protection from genital HSV-2 infection. Vaccine 2000, 18: 1351–1358.

[116] Natuk RJ, Cooper D, Guo M, Calderon P, Wright KJ, Nasar F, Witko S, Pawlyk D, Lee M, DeStefano J, Tummolo D, Abramovitz AS, Gangolli S, Kalyan N, Clarke DK, Hendry RM, Eldridge JH, Udem SA, Kowalski J. Recombinant vesicular stomatitis virus vectors expressing herpes simplex virus type 2 gD elicit robust CD4+ Th1 immune responses and are protective in mouse and guinea pig models of vaginal challenge. J Virol 2006, 80: 4447–4457.

[117] Chiuppesi F, Vannucci L, De Luca A, Lai M, Matteoli B, Freer G, Manservigi R, Ceccherini-Nelli L, Maggi F, Bendinelli M, Pistello M. A lentiviral vector-based, herpes simplex virus 1 (HSV-1) glycoprotein B vaccine affords cross-protection against HSV-1 and HSV-2 genital infections. J Virol 2012, 86: 6563–6574. doi: 10.1128/JVI.00302-12.

[118] Daheshia M, Kuklin N, Manickan E, Chun S, Rouse BT. Immune induction and modulation by topical ocular administration of plasmid DNA encoding antigens and cytokines. Vaccine 1998, 16: 1103–1110.

[119] Nass PH, Elkins KL, Weir JP. Antibody response and protective capacity of plasmid vaccines expressing three different herpes simplex virus glycoproteins. J Infect Dis 1998, 178: 611–617.

[120] Stanberry LR, Cunningham AL, Mindel A, Scott LL, Spruance SL, Aoki FY, Lacey CJ. Prospects for control of herpes simplex virus disease through immunization. Clin Infect Dis 2000, 30: 549–566.

[121] Baghian A, Chouljenko VN, Dauvergne O, Newmant MJ, Baghian S, Kousoulas KG. Protective immunity against lethal HSV-1 challenge in mice by nucleic acid-based

immunisation with herpes simplex virus type-1 genes specifying glycoproteins gB and gD. J Med Microbiol 2002, 51: 350–357.

[122] Osorio Y, Cohen J, Ghiasi H. Improved protection from primary ocular HSV-1 infection and establishment of latency using multigenic DNA vaccines. Invest Ophthalmol Vis Sci 2004, 45: 506–514

[123] Hoshino Y, Dalai SK, Wang K, Pesnicak L, Lau TY, Knipe DM, Cohen JI, Straus SE. Comparative efficacy and immunogenicity of replication-defective, recombinant glycoprotein, and DNA vaccines for herpes simplex virus 2 infections in mice and guinea pigs. J Virol 2005, 79: 410–418.

[124] Ghaemi A, Soleimanjahi H, Bamdad T, Soudi S, Arefeian E, Hashemi SM, Ebtekar M. Induction of humoral and cellular immunity against latent HSV-1 infections by DNA immunization in BALB/c mice. Comp Immunol Microbiol Infect Dis 2007, 30: 197–210.

[125] Bourne N, Milligan GN, Schleiss MR, Bernstein DI, Stanberry LR. DNA immunization confers protective immunity on mice challenged intravaginally with herpes simplex virus type 2. Vaccine 1996, 14: 1230–1234.

[126] McClements WL, Armstrong ME, Keys RD, Liu MA. The prophylactic effect of immunization with DNA encoding herpes simplex virus glycoproteins on HSV-induced disease in guinea pigs. Vaccine 1997, 15: 857–860.

[127] Strasser JE, Arnold RL, Pachuk C, Higgins TJ, Bernstein DI. Herpes simplex virus DNA vaccine efficacy: effect of glycoprotein D plasmid constructs. J Infect Dis 2000, 182: 1304–1310.

[128] Jazayeri M, Soleimanjahi H, Fotouhi F, Pakravan N. Comparison of intramuscular and footpad subcutaneous immunization with DNA vaccine encoding HSV-gD2 in mice. Comp Immunol Microbiol Infect Dis 2009, 32: 453–461. doi: 10.1016/j.cimid.2008.05.002.

[129] Lee HH, Cha SC, Jang DJ, Lee JK, Choo DW, Kim YS, Uh HS, Kim SY. Immunization with combined HSV-2 glycoproteins B2: D2 gene DNAs: protection against lethal intravaginal challenges in mice. Virus Genes 2002, 25: 179–188.

[130] Domingo C, Gadea I, Pardeiro M, Castilla C, Fernández S, Fernández-Clua MA, De la Cruz Troca JJ, Punzón C, Soriano F, Fresno M, Tabarés E. Immunological properties of a DNA plasmid encoding a chimeric protein of herpes simplex virus type 2 glycoprotein B and glycoprotein D. Vaccine 2003, 21: 3565–3574

[131] Sin JI, Kim JJ, Arnold RL, Shroff KE, McCallus D, Pachuk C, McElhiney SP, Wolf MW, Pompa-de Bruin SJ, Higgins TJ, Ciccarelli RB, Weiner DB. IL-12 gene as a DNA vaccine adjuvant in a herpes mouse model: IL-12 enhances Th1-type CD4+ T cell-mediated protective immunity against herpes simplex virus-2 challenge. J Immun 1999, 162: 2912–2921.

[132] Cooper D, Pride MW, Guo M, Cutler M, Mester JC, Nasar F, She J, Souza V, York L, Mishkin E, Eldridge J, Natuk RJ. Interleukin-12 redirects murine immune responses to

soluble or aluminum phosphate adsorbed HSV-2 glycoprotein D towards Th1 and CD4+ CTL responses. Vaccine 2004, 23: 236–246.

[133] Sin JI, Kim JJ, Boyer JD, Ciccarelli RB, Higgins TJ, Weiner DB. In vivo modulation of vaccine-induced immune responses toward a Th1 phenotype increases potency and vaccine effectiveness in a herpes simplex virus type 2 mouse model. J Virol 1999, 73: 501–509.

[134] Zhu M, Xu X, Liu H, Liu X, Wang S, Dong F, Yang B, Song G. Enhancement of DNA vaccine potency against herpes simplex virus 1 by co-administration of an interleukin-18 expression plasmid as a genetic adjuvant. J Med Microbiol 2003, 52: 223–228.

[135] Osorio Y, Ghiasi H. Comparison of adjuvant efficacy of herpes simplex virus type 1 recombinant viruses expressing TH1 and TH2 cytokine genes. J Virol 2003, 77: 5774–5783.

[136] Lee S, Gierynska M, Eo SK, Kuklin N, Rouse BT. Influence of DNA encoding cytokines on systemic and mucosal immunity following genetic vaccination against herpes simplex virus. Microbes Infect 2003, 5: 571–578.

[137] Veselenak RL, Shlapobersky M, Pyles RB, Wei Q, Sullivan SM, Bourne N. A Vaxfectin-adjuvanted HSV-2 plasmid DNA vaccine is effective for prophylactic and therapeutic use in the guinea pig model of genital herpes. Vaccine 2012, 30: 7046–7051. doi: 10.1016/j.vaccine.2012.09.057.

[138] Shlapobersky M, Marshak JO, Dong L, Huang ML, Wei Q, Chu A, Rolland A, Sullivan S, Koelle DM. Vaxfectin-adjuvanted plasmid DNA vaccine improves protection and immunogenicity in a murine model of genital herpes infection. J Gen Virol 2012, 93: 1305–1315. doi: 10.1099/vir.0.040055-0.

[139] Yan Y, Hu K, Deng X, Guan X, Luo S, Tong L, Du T, Fu M, Zhang M, Liu Y, Hu Q. Immunization with HSV-2 gB-CCL19 Fusion Constructs Protects Mice against Lethal Vaginal Challenge. J Immunol 2015, 195: 329–338. doi: 10.4049/jimmunol.1500198.

[140] Bright H, Perez DL, Christy C, Cockle P, Eyles JE, Hammond D, Khodai T, Lang S, West K, Loudon PT. The efficacy of HSV-2 vaccines based on gD and gB is enhanced by the addition of ICP27. Vaccine 2012, 30: 7529–7535. doi: 10.1016/j.vaccine.2012.10.046.

[141] Forrester A, Farrell H, Wilkinson G, Kaye J, Davis-Poynter N, Minson T. Construction and properties of a mutant of herpes simplex virus type 1 with glycoprotein H coding sequences deleted. J Virol 1992, 66: 341–348.

[142] McLean CS, Erturk M, Jennings R, Challanain DN, Minson AC, Duncan I, Boursnell ME, Inglis SC. Protective vaccination against primary and recurrent disease caused by herpes simplex virus (HSV) type 2 using a genetically disabled HSV-1. J Infect Dis 1994, 170: 1100–1109.

[143] Whitley RJ, Kern ER, Chatterjee S, Chou J, Roizman B. Replication, establishment of latency, and induced reactivation of herpes simplex virus gamma 1 34.5 deletion mutants in rodent models. J Clin Invest 1993, 91: 2837–2843.

[144] Brittle EE, Wang F, Lubinski JM, Bunte RM, Friedman HM. A replication-competent, neuronal spread-defective, live attenuated herpes simplex virus type 1 vaccine. J Virol 2008, 82: 8431–8441. doi: 10.1128/JVI.00551-08.

[145] Awasthi S, Zumbrun EE, Si H, Wang F, Shaw CE, Cai M, Lubinski JM, Barrett SM, Balliet JW, Flynn JA, Casimiro DR, Bryan JT, Friedman HM. Live attenuated herpes simplex virus 2 glycoprotein E deletion mutant as a vaccine candidate defective in neuronal spread. J Virol 2012, 86: 4586–4598. doi: 10.1128/JVI.07203-11.

[146] Keadle TL, Laycock KA, Morris JL, Leib DA, Morrison LA, Pepose JS, Stuart PM. Therapeutic vaccination with vhs(-) herpes simplex virus reduces the severity of recurrent herpetic stromal keratitis in mice. J Gen Virol 2002, 83: 2361–2365.

[147] Rajčáni J, Kúdelová M, Oravcová I, Vojvodová A, Košovský J, Matis J. Characterization of strain HSZP of herpes simplex virus type 1 (HSV1). Folia Microbiol (Praha) 1999, 44: 713–719.

[148] Meignier B. Genetically engineered attenuated herpes simplex viruses. Rev Infect Dis 1991, 13: S895–897.

[149] Halford WP, Püschel R, Gershburg E, Wilber A, Gershburg S, Rakowski B. A live-attenuated HSV-2 ICP0 virus elicits 10 to 100 times greater protection against genital herpes than a glycoprotein D subunit vaccine. PLoS One 2011, 6: e17748. doi: 10.1371/journal.pone.0017748.

[150] de Bruyn G, Vargas-Cortez M, Warren T, Tyring SK, Fife KH, Lalezari J, Brady RC, Shahmanesh M, Kinghorn G, Beutner KR, Patel R, Drehobl MA, Horner P, Kurtz TO, McDermott S, Wald A, Corey L. A randomized controlled trial of a replication defective (gH deletion) herpes simplex virus vaccine for the treatment of recurrent genital herpes among immunocompetent subjects. Vaccine 2006, 24: 914–920.

[151] Morrison LA, Knipe DM. Immunization with replication-defective mutants of herpes simplex virus type 1: sites of immune intervention in pathogenesis of challenge virus infection. J Virol 1994, 68: 689–696.

[152] Wachsman M, Kulka M, Smith CC, Aurelian L. A growth and latency compromised herpes simplex virus type 2 mutant (ICP10DeltaPK) has prophylactic and therapeutic protective activity in guinea pigs. Vaccine 2001, 19: 1879–1890.

[153] Da Costa XJ, Bourne N, Stanberry LR, Knipe DM. Construction and characterization of a replication-defective herpes simplex virus 2 ICP8 mutant strain and its use in immunization studies in a guinea pig model of genital disease. Virology 1997, 232: 1–12.

[154] Da Costa X, Kramer MF, Zhu J, Brockman MA, Knipe DM. Construction, phenotypic analysis, and immunogenicity of a UL5/UL29 double deletion mutant of herpes simplex virus 2. J Virol 2000, 74: 7963–7971.

[155] Delagrave S, Hernandez H, Zhou C, Hamberger JF, Mundle ST, Catalan J, Baloglu S, Anderson SF, DiNapoli JM, Londoño-Hayes P, Parrington M, Almond J, Kleanthous H. Immunogenicity and efficacy of intramuscular replication-defective and subunit vaccines against herpes simplex virus type 2 in the mouse genital model. PLoS One 2012, 7: e46714. doi: 10.1371/journal.pone.0046714.

[156] Brans R, Yao F. Immunization with a dominant-negative recombinant Herpes Simplex Virus (HSV) type 1 protects against HSV-2 genital disease in guinea pigs. BMC Microbiol 2010, 10: 163. doi: 10.1186/1471-2180-10-163.

[157] Casanova G, Cancela R, Alonzo L, Benuto R, Magana Mdel C, Hurley DR, Fishbein E, Lara C, Gonzalez T, Ponce R, Burnett JW, Calton GJ. A double-blind study of the efficacy and safety of the ICP10deltaPK vaccine against recurrent genital HSV-2 infections. Cutis 2002, 70: 235–239.

[158] van Lint AL, Torres-Lopez E, Knipe DM. Immunization with a replication-defective herpes simplex virus 2 mutant reduces herpes simplex virus 1 infection and prevents ocular disease. Virology 2007, 368: 227–231.

[159] Hoshino Y, Pesnicak L, Dowdell KC, Burbelo PD, Knipe DM, Straus SE, Cohen JI. Protection from herpes simplex virus (HSV)-2 infection with replication-defective HSV-2 or glycoprotein D2 vaccines in HSV-1-seropositive and HSV-1-seronegative guinea pigs. J Infect Dis 2009, 200: 1088–1095. doi: 10.1086/605645.

[160] Stanfield BA, Stahl J, Chouljenko VN, Subramanian R, Charles AS, Saied AA, Walker JD, Kousoulas KG. A single intramuscular vaccination of mice with the HSV-1 VC2 virus with mutations in the glycoprotein K and the membrane protein UL20 confers full protection against lethal intravaginal challenge with virulent HSV-1 and HSV-2 strains. PLoS One 2014, 9:e109890. doi: 10.1371/journal.pone.0109890.

[161] Zhang X, Castelli FA, Zhu X, Wu M, Maillère B, BenMohamed L. Gender-dependent HLA-DR-restricted epitopes identified from herpes simplex virus type 1 glycoprotein D. Clin Vaccine Immunol 2008, 15: 1436–1449. doi: 10.1128/CVI.00123-08.

[162] Mertz GJ, Peterman G, Ashley R, Jourden JL, Salter D, Morrison L, McLean A, Corey L. Herpes simplex virus type-2 glycoprotein-subunit vaccine: tolerance and humoral and cellular responses in humans. J Infect Dis 1984, 150: 242–249.

[163] Mertz GJ, Ashley R, Burke RL, Benedetti J, Critchlow C, Jones CC, Corey L. Double-blind, placebo-controlled trial of a herpes simplex virus type 2 glycoprotein vaccine in persons at high risk for genital herpes infection. J Infect Dis 1990, 161: 653–660

[164] Langenberg AG, Burke RL, Adair SF, Sekulovich R, Tigges M, Dekker CL, Corey L. A recombinant glycoprotein vaccine for herpes simplex virus type 2: safety and immunogenicity. Ann Intern Med 1995, 122: 889–898.

[165] Bernstein DI, Aoki FY, Tyring SK, Stanberry LR, St-Pierre C, Shafran SD, Leroux-Roels G, Van Herck K, Bollaerts A, Dubin G; GlaxoSmithKline Herpes Vaccine Study Group. Safety and immunogenicity of glycoprotein D-adjuvant genital herpes vaccine. Clin Infect Dis 2005, 40: 1271–1281.

[166] Stanberry LR, Spruance SL, Cunningham AL, Bernstein DI, Mindel A, Sacks S, Tyring S, Aoki FY, Slaoui M, Denis M, Vandepapeliere P, Dubin G; GlaxoSmithKline Herpes Vaccine Efficacy Study Group. Glycoprotein-D-adjuvant vaccine to prevent genital herpes. N Engl J Med 2002, 347: 1652–1661.

[167] Belshe RB, Leone PA, Bernstein DI, Wald A, Levin MJ, Stapleton JT, Gorfinkel I, Morrow RL, Ewell MG, Stokes-Riner A, Dubin G, Heineman TC, Schulte JM, Deal CD; Herpevac Trial for Women. Efficacy results of a trial of a herpes simplex vaccine. N Engl J Med 2012, 366: 34–43. doi: 10.1056/NEJMoa1103151.

[168] Tavares F, Cheuvart B, Heineman T, Arellano F, Dubin G. Meta-analysis of pregnancy outcomes in pooled randomized trials on a prophylactic adjuvanted glycoprotein D subunit herpes simplex virus vaccine. Vaccine 2013, 31: 1759–1764. doi: 10.1016/j.vaccine.2013.01.002.

[169] Cattamanchi A, Posavad CM, Wald A, Baine Y, Moses J, Higgins TJ, Ginsberg R, Ciccarelli R, Corey L, Koelle DM. Phase I study of a herpes simplex virus type 2 (HSV-2) DNA vaccine administered to healthy, HSV-2-seronegative adults by a needle-free injection system. Clin Vaccine Immunol 2008, 15: 1638–1643. doi: 10.1128/CVI.00167-08.

[170] Bernard MC, Barban V, Pradezynski F, de Montfort A, Ryall R, Caillet C, Londono-Hayes P. Immunogenicity, protective efficacy, and non-replicative status of the HSV-2 vaccine candidate HSV529 in mice and guinea pigs. PLoS One 2015, 10: e0121518. doi: 10.1371/journal.pone.0121518.

[171] Kutinová L, Benda R, Kalos Z, Dbalý V, Votruba T, Kvícalová E, Petrovská P, Doutlík S, Kamínková J, Domorázková E. Placebo-controlled study with subunit herpes simplex virus vaccine in subjects suffering from frequent herpetic recurrences. Vaccine 1988, 6: 223–228.

[172] Skinner GR, Turyk ME, Benson CA, Wilbanks GD, Heseltine P, Galpin J, Kaufman R, Goldberg L, Hartley CE, Buchan A. The efficacy and safety of Skinner herpes simplex vaccine towards modulation of herpes genitalis; report of a prospective double-blind placebo-controlled trial. Med Microbiol Immunol 1997, 186: 31–36.

[173] Straus SE, Corey L, Burke RL, Savarese B, Barnum G, Krause PR, Kost RG, Meier JL, Sekulovich R, Adair SF. Placebo-controlled trial of vaccination with recombinant glycoprotein D of herpes simplex virus type 2 for immunotherapy of genital herpes. Lancet 1994, 343: 1460–1463.

[174] Straus SE, Wald A, Kost RG, McKenzie R, Langenberg AG, Hohman P, Lekstrom J, Cox E, Nakamura M, Sekulovich R, Izu A, Dekker C, Corey L. Immunotherapy of recurrent genital herpes with recombinant herpes simplex virus type 2 glycoproteins D and B: results of a placebo-controlled vaccine trial. J Infect Dis 1997, 176: 1129–1134.

[175] Laing KJ, Dong L, Sidney J, Sette A, Koelle DM. Immunology in the Clinic Review Series; focus on host responses: T cell responses to herpes simplex viruses. Clin Exp Immunol 2012, 167: 47–58. doi: 10.1111/j.1365-2249.2011.04502.x

[176] Laing KJ, Magaret AS, Mueller DE, Zhao L, Johnston C, De Rosa SC, Koelle DM, Wald A, Corey L. Diversity in CD8(+) T cell function and epitope breadth among persons with genital herpes. J Clin Immun 2010, 30: 703–722. doi: 10.1007/s10875-010-9441-2.

[177] Berger C, Flowers ME, Warren EH, Riddell SR. Analysis of transgene-specific immune responses that limit the in vivo persistence of adoptively transferred HSV-TK-modified donor T cells after allogeneic hematopoietic cell transplantation. Blood 2006, 107: 2294–2302.

[178] Koelle DM, Liu Z, McClurkan CL, Cevallos RC, Vieira J, Hosken NA, Meseda CA, Snow DC, Wald A, Corey L. Immunodominance among herpes simplex virus-specific CD8 T cells expressing a tissue-specific homing receptor. Proc Natl Acad Sci U S A 2003, 100: 12899–12904.

[179] Chentoufi AA, Binder NR, Berka N, Durand G, Nguyen A, Bettahi I, Maillère B, BenMohamed L. Asymptomatic human CD4+ cytotoxic T-cell epitopes identified from herpes simplex virus glycoprotein B. J Virol 2008, 82: 11792–11802. doi: 10.1128/JVI.00692-08

[180] Wang X, Xie G, Liao J, Yin D, Guan W, Pan M, Li J, Li Y. Design and evaluation of a multi-epitope assembly peptide (MEAP) against herpes simplex virus type 2 infection in BALB/c mice. Virol J 2011, 8: 232. doi: 10.1186/1743-422X-8-232.

[181] Liu K, Jiang D, Zhang L, Yao Z, Chen Z, Yu S, Wang X. Identification of B- and T-cell epitopes from glycoprotein B of herpes simplex virus 2 and evaluation of their immunogenicity and protection efficacy. Vaccine 2012, 30: 3034–3041. doi: 10.1016/j.vaccine.2011.10.010.

[182] Muller WJ, Dong L, Vilalta A, Byrd B, Wilhelm KM, McClurkan CL, Margalith M, Liu C, Kaslow D, Sidney J, Sette A, Koelle DM. Herpes simplex virus type 2 tegument proteins contain subdominant T-cell epitopes detectable in BALB/c mice after DNA immunization and infection. J Gen Virol 2009, 90: 1153–1163. doi: 10.1099/vir.0.008771-0.

[183] Koelle DM, Frank JM, Johnson ML, Kwok WW. Recognition of herpes simplex virus type 2 tegument proteins by CD4 T cells infiltrating human genital herpes lesions. J Virol 1998, 72: 7476–7483.

[184] Novak EJ, Liu AW, Gebe JA, Falk BA, Nepom GT, Koelle DM, Kwok WW. Tetramer-guided epitope mapping: rapid identification and characterization of immunodominant CD4+ T cell epitopes from complex antigens. J Immunol 2001, 166: 6665–6670.

[185] Osorio Y, Mott KR, Jabbar AM, Moreno A, Foster TP, Kousoulas KG, Ghiasi H. Epitope mapping of HSV-1 glycoprotein K (gK) reveals a T cell epitope located within the signal domain of gK. Virus Res 2007, 128: 71–80.

[186] Mott KR, Chentoufi AA, Carpenter D, BenMohamed L, Wechsler SL, Ghiasi H. The role of a glycoprotein K (gK) CD8+ T-cell epitope of herpes simplex virus on virus replication and pathogenicity. Invest Ophthalmol Vis Sci 2009, 50: 2903–2912. doi: 10.1167/iovs.08-2957.

[187] Haynes JR, Arrington J, Dong L, Braun RP, Payne LG. Potent protective cellular immune responses generated by a DNA vaccine encoding HSV-2 ICP27 and the *E. coli* heat labile enterotoxin. Vaccine 2006, 24: 5016–5026.

[188] BenMohamed L, Bertrand G, McNamara CD, Gras-Masse H, Hammer J, Wechsler SL, Nesburn AB. Identification of novel immunodominant CD4+ Th1-type T-cell peptide epitopes from herpes simplex virus glycoprotein D that confer protective immunity. J Virol 2003, 77: 9463–9473.

[189] Cooper D, Mester JC, Guo M, Nasar F, Souza V, Dispoto S, Sidhu M, Hagen M, Eldridge JH, Natuk RJ, Pride MW. Epitope mapping of full-length glycoprotein D from HSV-2 reveals a novel CD4+ CTL epitope located at the transmembrane-cytoplasmic junction. Cell Immunol 2006, 239: 113–120.

[190] Chentoufi AA, Zhang X, Lamberth K, Dasgupta G, Bettahi I, Nguyen A, Wu M, Zhu X, Mohebbi A, Buus S, Wechsler SL, Nesburn AB, BenMohamed L. HLA-A*02:01-restricted CD8+ cytotoxic T lymphocyte epitopes identified from herpes simplex virus glycoprotein D. J Immunol 2008, 180: 426–437.

[191] Chentoufi AA, Dasgupta G, Christensen ND, Hu J, Choudhury ZS, Azeem A, Jester JV, Nesburn AB, Wechsler SL, BenMohamed L. A novel HLA (HLA-A*02:01) transgenic rabbit model for preclinical evaluation of human CD8+ T cell epitope-based vaccines against ocular herpes. J Immunol 2010, 184: 2561–2571. doi: 10.4049/jimmunol.0902322.

[192] Posavad CM, Remington M, Mueller DE, Zhao L, Magaret AS, Wald A, Corey L. Detailed characterization of T cell responses to herpes simplex virus-2 in immune seronegative persons. J Immunol 2010, 184: 3250–3259. doi: 10.4049/jimmunol.0900722.

[193] Posavad CM, Magaret AS, Zhao L, Mueller DE, Wald A, Corey L. Development of an interferon-gamma ELISPOT assay to detect human T cell responses to HSV-2. Vaccine 2011, 29: 7058–7066. doi: 10.1016/j.vaccine.2011.07.028.

[194] Maiers M, Gragert L, Klitz W. High-resolution HLA alleles and haplotypes in the United States population. Hum Immunol 2007, 68: 779–788.

[195] Koelle DM, Corey L. Herpes simplex: insights on pathogenesis and possible vaccines. Annu Rev Med 2008, 59: 381–395. doi: 10.1146/annurev.med.59.061606.095540.

[196] Samandary S, Kridane-Miledi H, Sandoval JS, Choudhury Z, Langa-Vives F, Spencer D, Chentoufi AA, Lemonnier FA, BenMohamed L. Associations of HLA-A, HLA-B and HLA-C alleles frequency with prevalence of herpes simplex virus infections and diseases across global populations: implication for the development of an universal CD8+ T-cell epitope-based vaccine. Hum Immunol 2014, 75: 715–729. doi: 10.1016/j.humimm.2014.04.016.

[197] Awasthi S, Friedman HM. Status of prophylactic and therapeutic genital herpes vaccines. Curr Opin Virol 2014, 6: 6–12. doi: 10.1016/j.coviro.2014.02.006.

[198] Wald A, Zeh J, Selke S, Warren T, Ryncarz AJ, Ashley R, Krieger JN, Corey L. Reactivation of genital herpes simplex virus type 2 infection in asymptomatic seropositive persons. N Engl J Med 2000, 342: 844–850.

[199] Khan AA, Srivastava R, Spencer D, Garg S, Fremgen D, Vahed H, Lopes PP, Pham TT, Hewett C, Kuang J, Ong N, Huang L, Scarfone VM, Nesburn AB, Wechsler SL, BenMohamed L. Phenotypic and functional characterization of herpes simplex virus glycoprotein B epitope-specific effector and memory CD8+ T cells from symptomatic and asymptomatic individuals with ocular herpes. J Virol 2015, 89: 3776–3792. doi: 10.1128/JVI.03419-14.

Section 5

Bovine Herpesviruses: a Veterinary Problem but a Model for Studies on Human Pathogenesis

Chapter 8

Herpesvirus in Bovines: Importance of Bovine Herpesvirus Type 1

Gurpreet Kaur and Mudit Chandra

Additional information is available at the end of the chapter

http://dx.doi.org/10.5772/63157

Abstract

The chapter aims at providing readers with the overview of the herpesvirus infection in bovines. It includes the detailed etiology of the infection, discussing the virus characteristics, virus structure, genome, viral proteins, types and subtypes of the virus. Then, the chapter discusses the transmission and pathogenesis of the virus, which are very important as they help to control the virus spread, viral latency and clinical signs observed in the affected animals. Later, the chapter discusses the diagnosis of herpesvirus infection in bovines to help the readers to gain knowledge about the techniques used earlier and nowadays for the diagnosis of the infection. Then, the chapter provides information on the procedures to be adopted for the prevention and control of the infection in bovines. Thus, the chapter provides complete information about the herpesvirus infection in bovines.

Keywords: bovines, herpesvirus, etiology, epidemiology, diagnosis, prevention, control

1. Introduction

Viruses have either RNA or DNA as their genome which is one of the criteria for the classification of viruses. Among the DNA virus families is the Herpesviridae family. It is the largest DNA family and derives its name from the Greek word, "herpein", which means "to creep". The viruses belonging to this family affect a number of species of mammals, birds, reptiles, fishes and amphibians. This chapter discusses the herpesvirus infection in bovines.

There are many bovine herpesviruses belonging to different genus viz. Bovine herpesvirus-1 (BHV-1), BHV-2, BHV-4, BHV-5 in the family Herpesviridae. BHV-2 causes skin lesions, BHV-4 often produces subclinical infection and BHV-5 produces meningoencephalitis. This chapter is written with an aim to focus on the most important disease caused by herpesviruses in bovines; infectious bovine rhinotracheitis caused by BHV-1.

BHV-1 is one of the important viruses responsible for great economic loss to the livestock industry. It causes losses in terms of drop in milk yield, abortion and repeat breeding. BHV-1 is associated with different clinical conditions like respiratory infections, conjunctivitis, vulvovaginitis, abortion and balanoposthitis in males. It is also associated with encephalitis and generalized systemic infections [1] too. The virus is readily transmitted and has world-wide distribution. The virus can remain latent in the ganglia of the infected, but clinically normal, animals [2]. The virus is excreted through nasal and ocular secretions, placenta of aborted animals and through semen. The virus transmission via semen is special concern to cattle breeders.

Mayfield et al. [3] identified 3 strains of BHV-1 namely I, II, III depending on the restriction pattern. Studdert [4] reclassified them as BHV-1.1 (respiratory form), BHV-1.2 (genital form) and BHV-1.3 (encephalitic form). BHV-1 consists of 25–33 polypeptides of which 11 are glycosylated [5–7] and associated with virus envelope [5, 6]. The three sets of enveloped glycoproteins gI, gIII and gIV were characterized earlier which are involved in the immune response [7–12]. Babiuk et al. [13] showed that gIV produces the highest serum-neutralizing antibody titres with gI being the least immunogenic. The strains of BHV-1 with different tissue affinities may exist in the field conditions and these different clinical strains can be differentiated by restriction endonuclease strategies [14]. The monoclonal antibodies specific for the major BHV-1 glycoproteins GVP6/11a/16, GVP7, GVP3/9 and GVP11/b are used to determine the glycoproteins and identify the epitopes involved in neutralization and antibody complement lysis [15]. Both humoral and cell-mediated immune responses are generated against BHV-1, but cell-mediated immune response is the major means of defence mechanisms [16]. The disease can be diagnosed by clinical signs and lesions and by a variety of virologic and immunologic techniques [17].

This chapter is written with an aim to provide information on herpesvirus in bovines to the readers.

2. Taxonomy and nomenclature

In 1973, the International Committee for the Taxonomy of Viruses (ICTV) named the virus as bovid herpesvirus type-1 [18] on the basis of the family of virus and the host it infects. The nomenclature system was further discussed in the International Committee for the Taxonomy of Herpesvirus (ICTH) in 1976 [19]. Then, Gibbs and Rweyemamu [1] adopted a system based on sub-family of Bovidae and named the virus to be BHV-1.

According to ICTV, the Herpesviridae family includes three subfamilies. The three subfamilies are Alphaherpesvirinae, Betaherpesvirinae and Gammaherpesvirinae. Alphaherpesviruses replicate and spread in the host, rapidly destroying the host cells. They establish the latent infection in the sensory ganglia of the host. Betaherpesviruses replicate and spread in the host slowly. They cause infected cells to enlarge, hence they are commonly named as cytomegaloviruses. They become latent in secretory glands and lymphoreticular cells of the host. Gammaherpesviruses infect T and B lymphocytes of the host and produce latent infections in these cells. Some of Gammaherpesviruses also replicate in epithelial and fibroblastic cells causing cytolysis. Many of these viruses lead to neoplastic transformation of lymphocytes.

There are nine genera included in the family Herpesviridae. The genera included in the subfamily Alphaherpesvirinae are Simplexvirus (includes BHV-2), Varicellovirus (includes BHV-1 and BHV-5), Mardivirus and Iltovirus. The genera included in the subfamily Betaherpesvirinae are Cytomegalovirus, Muromegalovirus and Roseolovirus. The genera included in the subfamily Gammaherpesvirinae are Lymphocryptovirus and Rhadinovirus (includes BHV-4). There is a 10th genera including Ictalurid herpes-like viruses which includes herpesviruses of fish. BHV-1 is also known as infectious bovine rhinotracheitis virus; BHV-5 is also known as bovine encephalitis virus and BHV-4 is also known as Movar virus. There is a proposal in ICTV to create the BHV-6 in the new genus Macavirus in the subfamily Gammaherpesvirinae.

Herpesviruses of mammals, birds and reptiles share extensive genetic relationship among themselves. Herpesviruses of fish and amphibians are also related to each other but are related only marginally to herpesviruses of mammals, birds and reptiles. No herpesvirus-specific gene is conserved between the classes, but one gene which encodes the putative ATPase subunit of a DNA-packaging terminase is conserved among all herpesviruses.

3. Virus structure and genome

BHV-1 has icosahedral symmetry approximately 150–200 nm in diameter [1, 20]. The structure of the virus consists of four parts viz.

1. The core which includes the genome having linear double-stranded DNA molecule of 139 Kbp [21, 22] in the form of a torus. The G+C content of the genome ranges from 31 to 75% and contains 60 to 120 genes [23]. Herpesvirus genes are not arranged in operons and in most cases have individual promoters. The genome termini are not covalently closed or covalently linked to a protein. All herpesvirus genomes contain lengthy terminal repeats, both direct and inverted.

2. The core is surrounded by the icosahedral capsid made up of 162 capsomeres.

3. The virus consists of an envelope which forms the outer layer of virion. The lipid bilayer envelope is derived from the nuclear membrane of the host by budding [24, 25]. It consists of unique viral glycoproteins which appear as short spikes embedded in the envelope.

4. Between the capsid and the envelope is a proteinaceous layer known as tegument. It consists of the viral enzymes needed to take control of host cell chemical processes for virion production and also to defend itself from the host cell responses.

The glycoproteins are critical to the virus for attachment to [26] and penetration of the susceptible cells [27] and to the host for virus neutralization [28] by the production of neutralizing antibodies. The glycoproteins are the major targets of immune response both at humoral and cellular level [29]. The major BHV-1 proteins that are involved in the immune response are gI, gIII and gIV enveloped glycoproteins [11].

Replication of herpesvirus occurs in the nucleus of the host cell and the envelope is derived from the nuclear membrane of the host cell. The virions are released by exocytosis. Intranuclear inclusion bodies are formed, which are the characteristic of herpesviruses. Herpesvirus genomes replicate by circularization and production of concatemers, followed by cleavage of unit-length genomes during packaging into capsids [30].

For the replication to initiate, the virion attaches to host cell (heparan sulfate moieties of cellular proteoglycans) with the envelope glycoprotein, gC. The viral envelope fuses to the plasma membrane of the host cell so that the nucleocapsid enters the cytoplasm. The glycoproteins involved during this process are gB, gD and gH. The capsid travels along the cytoskeleton to a nuclear pore where the viral DNA is released. The linear genome enters the nucleus and circularizes. Once in the nucleus, the viral DNA is transcribed into mRNA by cellular RNA polymerase II. The viral gene expression is tightly regulated. First, the tegument protein associates with two cellular proteins and the complex transactivates transcription of immediate-early (IE or alpha) genes. The immediate-early genes encode regulatory proteins and initiates transcription of the early (E or beta) genes. These proteins are enzymes needed for viral replication. Then, the late (L or gamma) genes are activated for production of viral structural proteins. After transcription in the nucleus, all mRNA transcripts are translated into protein in the cytoplasm. Subsequently, the proteins can go to the nucleus, stay in the cytoplasm, or become a part of the membrane bilayer. Capsid proteins assemble in the nucleus to form empty capsids. In these capsids, full-length viral DNA is packaged to form nucleocapsids. The nucleocapsids associate with segments of the nuclear membrane where tegument and glycosylated envelope proteins have bound. This association triggers the formation of envelope by budding through the nuclear membrane. Enveloped virions accumulate in the endoplasmic reticulum. Mature virions are released by exocytosis.

4. Physico-chemical and antigenic properties of BHV-1

The virus is sensitive to ether, chloroform, acetone, alcohol and bile salts. It is inactivated within 10 min at 56°C and in 4 min at 65°C. The virus is labile at pH 4.5 to 5.0, but stable between pH 6 to 9. Virus is extremely susceptible to 0.5% sodium hydroxide, 0.01% $HgCl_2$, 1% phenol and 1% quaternary ammonium compounds. Also, 5% formalin can inactivate the virus in 1 min. Thus, the virus is fragile and sensitive to detergents and lipid solvents. It is unstable in the environment, but can survive in the frozen semen indefinitely.

Antigenically, there is only a single serotype of BHV-1 recognized. There are three strains of BHV-1 (I, II, III) described on the basis of endonuclease pattern of viral DNA [3]. Studdert [4] reclassified them as BHV-1.1 (respiratory subtype), BHV-1.2 (genital subtype) and BHV-1.3

http://dx.doi.org/10.5772/63157

(encephalitic subtype). BHV-1.3 has been reclassified as a distinct herpesvirus designated as BHV-5. BHV-1 is antigenically related to equine rhinopneumonitis virus (EHV-1) in complement fixation test [31]. It also shares one-way relationship with Pseudorabies virus and goat herpesvirus [32]. The virus also shares a common antigen with Marek's disease virus [33] and Burkitts lymphoma virus.

5. Epidemiology and pathogenesis

The virus is host-specific. All ages and breeds of cattle are susceptible. Although cattle is the natural host for infectious bovine rhinotracheitis infection, antibodies against BHV-1 have also been demonstrated in sheep, goat, pigs and wild animals [34]. The disease mostly occurs in animals over 6 months of age. Prevalence of BHV-1 increases with age and is less prevalent in cows under 2 years of age. The virus does not discriminate between sex and breed; however, feed lot cattle are more frequently infected than dairy cattle [35].

The virus is readily transmitted and has worldwide distribution. Transmission of the virus occurs by aerosol route. The virus is also secreted through nasal and ocular secretions, genital secretions and placenta of aborted animals and also in milk [1]. The virus is also transmitted through infected semen during artificial insemination and embryo transfer. It is the most common viral pathogen found in bovine semen [36]. The extensive use of artificial insemination in cattle has facilitated the exchange of genetic characteristics. Therefore, contamination of semen and dissemination of bovine pathogens via semen are of primary concern to cattle breeders. It also poses a potential threat to cattle industry as it can cause a variety of genital tract disorders including endometritis, infertility and abortion [37]. Thus, semen should ideally be collected from bulls that are serologically negative for BHV-1 infection. After primary respiratory or genital infections, animals become lifelong carriers of BHV-1, despite the development of neutralizing antibodies. Reactivation of latent BHV-1 in carrier animals occurs periodically and has been due to stress such as intercurrent diseases, transportation, cold, crowding and corticosteroid treatment.

Pathogenesis depends upon the subtype of virus and route of entry of the virus. If the virus (BHV-1.1) enters by aerosol route, it replicates in the mucous membrane of the upper respiratory tract. Thus, the virus is shed in nasal secretions. The virus enters local nerve cell endings and becomes latent in trigeminal ganglion. Secondary bacterial infection leads to systemic infection and death of the animal. Abortion occurs due to fetal infection. Genital infection is caused by subtype BHV-1.2. In this case, the virus replicates in the mucosa of vagina or prepuce and becomes latent in sacral ganglion. Focal necrotic lesions occur on genital mucosa, which later on forms ulcers. Abortion does not occur in the animals affected by BHV-1.2.

6. Clinical signs

Infectious bovine rhinotracheitis initially had several names such as "red nose", "dust pneumonia", "necrotic rhinitis" or "necrotic rhinotracheitis" based on the signs and symptoms manifested by the virus in different parts of the world [38]. The reproductive form of the disease was reported as early as 1938 and was called "epivag", which means causing epididymitis in males. In 1955, at a meeting of US Livestock Sanitary Association it was designated as infectious bovine rhinotracheitis (IBR) [39].

BHV-1 causes various clinical manifestations in cattle and buffaloes. Type of disease caused by the virus depends mostly on the route of the entry of virus. The incubation period of the disease is 2 to 4 days. In case of the respiratory form of infection, the virus multiplies initially in the tissues of respiratory tract and is extended via the lacrimal ducts to the ocular tissues where a secondary site of infection is established. There is sudden onset of anorexia, fever, severe hyperaemia of the nasal mucosa, serous discharge from the eyes and nose, increased salivation and excitation. There is sharp drop in milk yield. Animal has respiratory distress and sudden death occurs within 24 hours after the first signs appear due to obstructive bronchitis. In prolonged cases, the nasal discharge becomes profuse and purulent and death occurs due to secondary bronchopneumonia. There is either bilateral or unilateral conjunctivitis or keratoconjunctivitis with profuse lacrimation. Various workers [40, 41] have isolated IBR virus from the conjunctival and nasal discharge of calves showing symptoms of the disease. The BHV-1 type causing respiratory form of the disease causes abortions usually during 4–8 months of gestation. Abortion occurs due to fetal infection which results in severe visceral damage, gradual cessation of placental circulation and placental degeneration, leading to detachment and abortion.

Kendrick et al. [42] isolated herpesvirus from genital infection of cows which they termed as infectious pustular vulvo-vaginitis (IPV) caused by the genital form (BHV-1.2) of the virus. The initial signs in the genital form of the disease include reddening of the vaginal mucosa and pustule formation, which lead to mucopurulent vaginal discharge. No abortion is seen in this form of the disease. The respiratory and genital forms of the disease are rarely seen at the same time in a herd. Bouters et al. [43] isolated herpesvirus from bulls with infectious pustular balanoposthitis and orchitis. Thus, in males, there is inflammation of preputial lining with pustule formation. Singh et al. [44] isolated IBR/IPV virus from the semen of Jersey bull and from the placenta and cotyledons of Jersey cow.

7. Diagnosis

Any disease control programme has a prerequisite of diagnosis at the earliest. The serological assays for antibodies to BHV-1 have been widely used for the diagnosis of acute infections, epidemiological studies and the detection of latent carriers in relation to control schemes and international trade. Gibbs and Rweyemamu [1] reviewed the diagnostic tests available for BHV-1. These included the conventional clinical diagnosis based on signs and symptoms; but as the virus has numerous clinical manifestations, diagnosis is difficult and requires laboratory confirmation. So, the specific diagnosis of IBR has been traditionally based on the isolation of the causal agent in the cell culture, together with the detection of active antibody response in the host animal. In the cell culture system, the detection of IBR virus is based on the cytopathic effects (CPE) characterized by rounding of individual cells with shrinkage of some with increased granularity, which progresses rapidly to a characteristic "bunch of grapes". The detection of viral antigen in clinical samples like nasal swabs, conjunctival swabs, vaginal discharge, semen, preputial washings, placenta and aborted fetus can be rapid and economical alternative to cell culture. The most widely applied antigen detection technique has been immunofluorescence, either on smears of cells from nasal or ocular epithelium [45] or on cryostat sections of tissues collected at post-mortem. Electron microscopy is another rapid, reliable method of diagnosis of the antigen, but it is difficult to distinguish all herpesviruses [1]. Immunoenzymatic techniques have been described for the labeling of infected cells [46] and for the detection of soluble antigen in diluted nasal mucus [9]. The fluorescent antibody technique (FAT) is frequently used to diagnose respiratory and reproductive forms of BHV-1 infections. Frank et al. [47] described FAT as the test of choice for diagnosis of IBR/IPV virus. The virus can also be identified by neutralization test with mono-specific antiserum or with the use of monoclonal antibodies. Monoclonal antibodies can differentiate between BHV-1 subtypes like BHV-1.1 and BHV-1.2 [20]. Further characterization can be done by DNA restriction enzyme analysis. Enzyme-linked immunosorbent assay (ELISA) to capture antigen can also be done.

The serological investigations are the faster means of detecting the prevalence of antibody in cattle population. The virus neutralization test is highly specific and reliable for the detection of BHV-1 antibodies. The other serological techniques used for the detection of antibodies include passive hemagglutination test, indirect hemagglutination test, agar gel diffusion test (AGID), counter immunoelectrophoresis and complement fixation test (CFT). ELISAs for antibody detection are also being used frequently. Payment et al. [48] compared serum neutralization test (SNT) with ELISA and reported that the antibody titres detected were 100 times higher than those seen in SNT, which showed the increased sensitivity of enzyme immunoassay. The rapid diagnosis of recent infection to BHV-1 was carried out using ELISA by detecting virus-specific IgM by Edwards et al. [49]. Edwards and Gitao [50] reported that antigen detection using avidin-biotin ELISA increased by 50-fold than compared to simple sandwich ELISA. Renukaradhya et al. [51] and Suresh et al. [52] demonstrated the use of avidin-biotin ELISA for the epidemiological studies against IBR antibodies. A gE ELISA is based on the use of two different monoclonal antibodies against gE of BHV-1. Thus, this ELISA detects antibodies against two different epitopes on gE [53]. The gE ELISA can detect antibodies in milk and in bulk milk samples [54]. The milk samples tested by ELISA have advantages over the SNT for mass field surveys [55]. Perrin et al. [56] reported that paired sample of serum and milk indicated that IBR antibody concentration in serum was about 200 times higher than in milk; hence, negative ELISA results in bulk milk samples would not exclude the possibility of infection in up to 25% animals. Since the antibody concentration in the milk is lower than serum, the antibody in the milk should be concentrated by the addition of rennet and ammonium sulfate and the ELISA should be carried out to a solution of the precipitate. To differentiate between the vaccinated and naturally infected animals (DIVA strategy), gE blocking ELISA can be used [54].

Isolation of the IBR virus was done for the first time by Madin et al. [57]. Their earlier attempts to recover the virus in chicken embryo, in weaning and suckling mice and in guinea pigs were unsuccessful. The failure was followed by successful isolation of the virus in tissue cultures of bovine embryonic kidney. Mehrotra et al. [58] isolated the virus in primary calf kidney cell culture and the virus produced intranuclear inclusions and CPE. The virus was also isolated from semen, placenta and cotyledons employing bovine embryonic kidney and bovine turbinate cell lines [44]. Mehrotra et al. [59] isolated BHV-1 in primary cow calf kidney (PCCK) cell culture and used Madin Darby bovine kidney (MDBK) cell line for subsequent passages and characterization of virus isolate. BHV-1 was isolated from the conjunctiva of affected cow after serial passages in MDBK cell line by Mohan Kumar et al. [60].

Nucleic acid detection methods also have widespread application in routine diagnosis nowadays and they have the advantage of being sensitive and quicker than virus isolation. Engelenburg et al. [61] developed polymerase chain reaction (PCR) assay to detect BHV-1 in bovine semen using a purification method to eliminate interfering components. The results of PCR were achieved in a day compared with virus isolation, which takes 7 days and is less laborious. Wiedmann et al. [62] used a nested PCR assay targeting a portion of the glycoprotein IV gene to detect BHV-1 DNA. Kibenge et al. [63] amplified strains of BHV-1 by PCR with primers in the thymidine kinase gene region. Vilcek et al. [64] employed PCR assay on samples like nasal swabs, lung, lymph nodes and tracheal mucosa. Masri et al. [65] used a rapid nested PCR for detection of BHV-1 in semen of infected bulls in which dexamethasone was given for reactivation of BHV-1 from latency. Santurde et al. [66] detected BHV-1 using PCR amplification of a highly conserved DNA fragment within the glycoprotein gI sequence (323 bp between nucleotide 1491 to nucleotide 1814) of the virus. Ashbaugh et al. [67] used nested PCR for simultaneously detecting and discriminating between BHV-1 and BHV-5 using type-common primers derived from gC sequences. Nested PCR is more sensitive than PCR. Rocha et al. [68] detected BHV-1 in the tissues of a naturally aborted bovine fetus by nested PCR assay. Further, real-time PCR can be used for detection and characterization of BHV-1 virus. The real-time PCR reveals the results in the real time during the time the PCR is running. It is a highly sensitive, specific and reliable assay.

The authors developed monoclonal antibodies against BHV-1 [69] using hybridoma technology. The technology is detailed below:

7.1. Propagation of virus in MDBK cell culture

The virus BHV-1 isolate was propagated in MDBK cell line using Dulbecco's minimum essential medium with 10 and 2% FCS for growth and maintenance, respectively, for preparing antigen in bulk quantity.

7.2. Purification of the virus

The cell culture fluid, after three cycles of freezing and thawing, was centrifuged at 7000 rpm for 20 min at 4°C to collect supernatant. The supernatant was subjected to ultracentrifugation at 105 × g for 1 hour to pellet the virus. The pellet was resuspended in 500 µl of phosphate buffered saline and subjected to 20–40% (w/v) sucrose density gradient centrifugation (the sucrose gradient was prepared in 200 mM tris 50 mM NaCl buffer, pH 8.0) at 105 × g for 2 hours and 30 min to collect the virus at the junction of 20–40% sucrose. The presence of virus was confirmed by agar gel precipitation test (AGPT) as per Le Yeune et al. [70] and the protein content was estimated [71].

7.3. Immunization of BALB/C mice

BALB/C mice of 6–7 weeks of age procured from the National Institute of Nutrition, Hyderabad, India, were used for immunization. Four hundred microgram of purified virus was mixed with equal amount of Freund's complete adjuvant to prepare an emulsion and injected into mice *via* intraperitoneal route. Booster was administered after 14 days with 100 µg of purified virus alone *via* intraperitoneal route. Three days after the second injection, all the mice were tail bled to collect serum which was subjected to ELISA to determine the antiviral antibodies. For this, the ELISA plate was coated with purified virus (10µg/ml) and incubated overnight at 4°C. About 100 µl of each dilution (1:20 and 1:40) of the test serum was added in duplicate wells and the normal serum served as negative control. The plates were incubated at 37°C for 2 hours. After washing the plate three times, 100 µl of anti-mouse IgG-horse radish peroxidase conjugate (1:10,000) was added in each well and further incubated the plate at 37°C for 2 hours. After washing, 100 µl of substrate solution was added to each well and incubated the plate at room temperature for 10 min. After stopping the reaction with 50 µl of 1M H2SO4, optical density was read at 450 nm wavelength.

7.4. Myeloma cell line

Non-secretory myeloma cell line SP2/O/Ag-14, procured from the National Centre for Cell Science, Pune, India, was subcultured and maintained in RPMI-1640 medium with 10% fetal calf serum containing 0.2% streptopenicillin (500×) and 1% glutamine. A day prior to fusion, myeloma cells were subcultured in growth medium containing 2% 8-azaguanine. Myeloma cells growing in log phase of growth were used for fusion.

7.5. Preparation of feeder spleen cell layer

Albino mice procured from Punjab Veterinary Vaccine Institute, Punjab Agricultural University, Ludhiana, India, were used for the preparation of feeder layer. One day prior to fusion, splenocyte feeder cell layer was laid down in the 24 well tissue culture plate in HAT medium having 106 cells/ml/well. The plates were incubated in a humid incubator at 37°C with 5% CO_2 tension.

7.6. Preparation of polyethylene glycol (PEG)

PEG (molecular weight 3000–4000) was autoclaved and immediately suspended in RPMI-1640 medium aseptically by keeping the vial at 56°C in water bath.

7.7. Fusion protocol

Myeloma cells in log phase of growth were brought into suspension by tapping and the suspension was transferred into calibrated centrifuge tube and final volume made to 10 ml with serum-free media. The immunized BALB/C mouse was etherized and disinfected by dipping into 70% alcohol. The spleen was removed into a petri plate and washed with 2 ml of serum-free media twice. The splenocytes were released into the medium by flushing with the medium into the spleen and the cells were collected by centrifugation. The splenocytes and myeloma cells were separately centrifuged at 4000 rpm for 10 min. The supernatant was discarded and pellet was brought into suspension by tapping. Equal number (107) of spleen cells and myeloma cells were mixed and co-pelleted by centrifugation at 4000 rpm for 10 min. To the pellet, 1 ml of PEG was added slowly along the side of tube over 1 min, taking care to swirl the tube gently while adding PEG so as to ensure proper mixing of PEG solution. The tube was incubated at room temperature for 1 min to facilitate fusion of myeloma and lymphocyte cells. Later, PEG was diluted by adding 10 ml of growth medium over 10 min and centrifuged at 4000 rpm for 3min. After discarding the medium, the final pellet was dissolved in 48 ml of HAT medium, and the cell suspension was dispensed in a quantity of 1 ml in two 24 well plates, which had already been seeded with normal mice spleen feeder cells a day before. The plates were incubated at 37° C in 5% CO2 tension. The plates were left undisturbed for 3–4 days and examined daily for signs of growth. When the hybrids started showing growth, the supernatants were collected aseptically and screened for anti-BHV-1 antibody secretion by indirect plate ELISA [72].

7.8. Cloning

After identification of single clone (B6.1), the cells were dislodged and ten-fold serial dilutions were made starting from 10^{-1} to 10^{-6} and dispensed in 1 ml quantity into each well which had feeder layer one day before seeding.

7.9. Isotyping of antibodies

Isotyping of monoclonal antibodies in cell culture supernatants was performed with the indirect ELISA-based isotyping kit.

7.10. Immunoblotting

The specificity of the monoclonal antibody for a particular protein of BHV-1 was determined by immunoblot. For this, discontinuous system of polyacrylamide gel electrophoresis (PAGE) [73] was followed. Electrophoresis on 10% resolving gel with 4% stacking gel in tris glycine buffer was carried out at 140 volts for 3 to 4 hours. Following electrophoresis, the protein was blotted to nitrocellulose membrane (NCM) in transfer buffer. Transfer of pro-

http://dx.doi.org/10.5772/63157

tein was carried out in transblot apparatus at 100 volts for 1 hour. A total of 600 ml of infected cell culture fluid was used for purification of virus.

The importance of monoclonal antibodies lies in the fact that they are the antibodies that can be used to detect the single epitope (protein) of the virus. Thus, they can be used in different assays like ELISA, immunofluorescence, virus neutralization test, AGID, CFT for detecting the virus along with differentiating between the different types of the virus. This can be achieved by producing the monoclonal antibodies against the protein of the virus which differentiates between the types of the virus.

8. Prevention and control

Prevention and control of BHV-1 are based on intensive farm management which includes following hygienic measures at the farm, vaccinating the animals at the right time and detection and removal of infected animals. The practice should be made at the farm to keep the newly introduced cattle in quarantine for the period of 4 weeks and the cattle that are BHV-1 sero-negative should be introduced to a herd. The practice of natural mating should be avoided and artificial insemination should be done using semen from BHV-1 negative bulls. Eradication programmes should be followed. These include test and removal programs in which the infected animals should be detected and culled. Carrier cattle should also be identified and removed from the herd.

Vaccines usually prevent the development of clinical signs and markedly reduce the shedding of virus after infection, but do not completely prevent infection. Vaccination campaigns should be a part of eradication programmes. Since BHV-1 is a highly contagious virus, vaccination is recommended as soon as passive immunity in calves disappears, usually around 4–6 months of age. Currently available vaccines for IBR include modified-live-virus vaccines and inactivated vaccines. The timing of vaccination is also as important as the choice of vaccine. Since maximum protection does not generally occur until approximately 3 weeks after vaccination, calves should be vaccinated 2–3 weeks before weaning at which time they start to be at risk of infection. Single vaccination will reduce the severity of disease, but not provide complete protection. Thus, booster vaccination should be done. The use of marker vaccines can help to distinguish between vaccinated and naturally infected animals.

9. Conclusions

The chapter concludes that the BHV type 1 is an important virus of cattle and buffaloes. As the virus can survive for long in frozen semen, it should be of special concern during artificial insemination and also during national and international trade.

Author details

Gurpreet Kaur* and Mudit Chandra

*Address all correspondence to: gurpreet7502@rediffmail.com

Department of Veterinary Microbiology, College of Veterinary Science, Guru Angad Dev Veterinary and Animal Sciences University, Ludhiana, Punjab, India

References

[1] Gibbs EPJ, Rweyemamu M M. Bovine herpesvirus-1. Veterinary Bulletin. 1977; 47: 317–343.

[2] Pastoret P P, Jelleur P, Aguilar-Setien A, Leroy P, Schwers A, Godart M, Schoenaers F. Effect de la dexamethasone sur le titre et la taille des plages du virus de la rhinotracheite infectieuse bovine (Bovid Herpesvirus 1, IBR). Ann Med Vet. 1979; 123: 397–402.

[3] Mayfield J E, Good P J, Van Oort H J, Campbell A R, Reed D E. Cloning and cleavage site mapping of DNA from BHV-1 (Cooper strain). Journal of Virology. 1983; 47: 259–264.

[4] Studdert M Z. Bovine encephalitis herpesvirus. Veterinary Record. 1989; 125: 584.

[5] Misra V, Blumenthal R M, Babiuk L A. Proteins specified by bovine herpesvirus type-1 (infectious bovine rhinotracheitis virus). Journal of Virology. 1981; 40: 367–378.

[6] Bolton D C, Zee Y C, Ardaus A A. Identification of envelope and nucleocapsid proteins of infectious bovine rhinotracheitis virus by SDS-polyacrylamide gel electrophoresis. Veterinary Microbiology. 1983; 8: 57–68.

[7] Gregersen J P, Pauli G, Ludwig H. Bovine herpesvirus-1. Differentiation of IBR and IPV viruses and identification and functional role of their major immunogenic components. Archives of Virology. 1985; 84: 91–103.

[8] Collins J K, Butchner A C, Reigel C A. Neutralising determinants defined by monoclonal antibodies on polypeptides specified by bovine herpesvirus-1. Journal of Virology. 1984; 52: 403–409.

[9] Collins J K, Butchner A C, Reigel C A. Immune response to bovine herpesvirus type-1 infections: virus-specific antibodies in sera from infected animals. Journal of Clinical Microbiology. 1985; 21: 546–552.

[10] Marshall R L, Rodriguez L L, Letchworth G J. Characterisation of envelope proteins of infectious bovine rhinotracheitis virus (bovine herpesvirus-1) by biochemical and immunological methods. Journal of Virology. 1986; 57: 745.

[11] Marshall R L, Israel B A, Letchworth III G J. Monoclonal antibody analysis of bovine herpesvirus-1 glycoprotein antigenic areas relevant to natural infection. Virology. 1988; 165: 338–347.

[12] Van Drunen Little-VanDen Hurk S, Babiuk L A. Polypeptide specificity of the antibody response after primary and recurrent infection with bovine herpesvirus-1. Journal of Clinical Microbiology. 1986; 23: 274-282.

[13] Babiuk L A, L'Italien J, VanDrunen Little-Van den Hurk S, Zamb T, Lawman M J, Hughes G, Gifford G A. Protection of cattle from bovine herpesvirus type-1 (BHV-1) infection by immunization with individual viral glycoproteins. Virology. 1987; 159: 57–66.

[14] Durhams P J K, Hassard L E, Donkersgoed J Van. Serological studies of infectious bovine rhinotracheitis, parinfluenza-3, bovine viral diarrhea and bovine respiratory syncitial virus in calves following entry to a bull test station. Canadian Veterinary Journal 1991; 32: 427–429.

[15] Van Drunen Little-VanDen Hurk S, VanDen Hurk J V, Gilchrist J E, Misra V, Babuik L A. Interactions of monoclonal antibodies and bovine herpesvirus type-1 (BHV-1) glycoproteins: characterization of their biochemical and immunological properties. Virology. 1984; 135: 466–479.

[16] Srinivasulu T, SuriBabu T, Subba Rao M V. Cell mediated immune response to bovine herpesvirus (BHV-1) infection in experimental animals. Indian Journal of Animal Science. 1998; 68(11): 1109-1113.

[17] Kahrs R F. Infectious bovine rhinotracheitis: A review and update. Journal of American Veterinary Medical Association. 1977; 15: 1055-1064.

[18] Roizmann B. Provisional labels for herpesvirus. Report of the Herpesvirus Study Group, International Committee for the Taxonomy of Viruses. Journal of General Virology. 1973; 20: 417-419.

[19] Fenner F. The classification and nomenclature of viruses. Summary of the results of meetings of the International Committee on Taxonomy of Viruses in Madrid, September 1975. Intervirology. 1976; 6: 1-12.

[20] Wyler R, Engels M, Schuyzer M. Infectious bovine rhinotracheitis vulvovaginitis (BHV-1) In: Herpesvirus Diseases of Cattle, Horses and Pigs. 1989; Chapter 1. Wittmann G (ed.) Kluwer Academic Press, Boston.

[21] Russel W C, Crawford L V. Properties of the nucleic acids from some herpes group viruses. Virology. 1964; 22: 286-292.

[22] Gibbs E P J, Johnson R H, Voyle C A. Differential diagnosis of virus infections of the bovine teat skin by electron microscopy. Journal of Comparative Pathology. 1970; 80: 455-463.

[23] Honess R. W. Herpes simplex and 'the herpes complex': diverse observations and a unifying hypothesis. The Eighth Fleming Lecture. Journal of General Virology. 1984; 65:2077–2107.

[24] Jasty V, Chang P W. Envelopment of infectious bovine rhinotracheitis viral particles in bovine kidney cell cultures: an electron microscopic study. American Journal of Veterinary Research. 1971; 32: 1945–1953.

[25] Silva R F, Amborski R L, White M R, Amborski G F. An electron microscopic study of single cycle infection of Madin Darby bovine Kidney cells by infectious bovine rhinotracheitis virus. Journal of Comparative Pathology. 1973; 83: 161–172.

[26] Fuller A D, Spear P G. Specificities of monoclonal and polyclonal antibodies that inhibits adsorption of herpes simplex virus to cells and lack of inhibition by potent neutralizing antibodies. Journal of Virology. 1985; 55: 475–482.

[27] Epstein A L, Jacquemont B, Machuca I. Infection of a restrictive cell line (XC cells) by intratypic recombinants of HSV-1: relationship between penetration of the virus and relative amounts of glycoprotein C. Virology. 1984; 132: 315–324.

[28] Glorioso J, Schroder C H, Kumel G, Szczesiul M, Levine M. Immunogenicity of herpes simplex virus glycoproteins gC and gB and their role in protective immunity. Journal of Virology. 1984; 15: 805–812.

[29] Simmons A, Nash A. Role of antibody in primary and recurrent herpes simplex virus infection. Journal of Virology. 1985; 53: 944–948.

[30] Boehmer P E, Lehman I R. Herpes simplex virus DNA replication. Annual Review of Biochemistry. 1997; 66:347–384.

[31] Plummer G, Goodheart C R, Henson D, Bowling C P. A comparative study of the DNA density and behaviour in tissue cultures of fourteen different herpesviruses. Virology. 1964; 39: 134-137.

[32] Berrios P E, Mckercher D G. Characterization of caprine herpes virus. American Journal of Veterinary Research. 1975; 36: 1755-1762.

[33] Evans R, Alexander P. Mechanisms of immunologically specific killing of tumour cells by macrophages. Nature. 1972; 236: 168-170.

[34] Brako E E, Fulton R W, Nicholoson S S, Amborski F G. Prevalence of BHV-1, bovine viral diarrhoea, PI-3, goat respiratory syncitial, bovine leukemia, blue tongue viral antibodies in sheep. American Journal of Veterinary Research. 1984; 45: 813-816.

[35] Rosner F. Infectious bovine rhinotracheitis: clinical review, immunity and control. Journal of American Veterinary Medical Association. 1968; 153: 1631-1638.

[36] Afshar A, Eglesome M D. Virus associated with bovine semen. Veterinary Bulletin. 1990; 60: 93-109.

[37] Elazhary MASY, Lamothe P, Silim A, Roy R S. Bovine herpesvirus type 1 in the sperm of a bull from a herd with fertility problems. Canadian Veterinary Journal. 1980; 21: 336-339.

[38] Miller N J. Infectious necrotic rhinotracheitis of cattle. Journal of American Veterinary Medical Association. 1955; 126: 463-467.

[39] McKercher D G, Moulton J E, Jasper D E. Virus and virus like cattle disease entities new to California. Proc. US Livestock Sanit Association. 1955; 58: 260-269.

[40] Mehrotra M L, Rajya B S, Kumar S. Infectious bovine rhinotracheitis (IBR), keratoconjunctivitis in calves. Indian Journal of Veterinary Pathology. 1976; 11: 70–72.

[41] Foldi J, Tanyi J, J-Kaszanyitzky E, Ravasz F. Isolation of infectious bovine rhinotracheitis (IBR) virus from calves with keratoconjunctivitis. Mayyar Allatorvosok Lapja. 1992; 47: 202-206 (Veterinary Bulletin 63: 7108).

[42] Kendrick J W, Gillepse J H, McEntee K. Infectious pustular vulvovaginitis of cattle. Cornell Vet. 1958; 48: 458-495.

[43] Bouters R, Vandeplassche M, Florent A, Leunen J, Devos A. The infectious pustular balanoposthitis in bulls. Flemish Veterinarian Journal. 1960; 29: 171-186 (Veterinary Bulletin, pp. 318).

[44] Singh B K, Sreenivasan M A, Tongaonkar S S, Rama Kant, Roychoudhury P N. Isolation of infectious bovine rhinotracheitis from semen and aborted materials of dairy cattle. Indian Journal of Animal Science 1986; 56 (8): 823-826.

[45] Netlleton P F, Herring J A, Herring A J. Evaluation of an immunofluorescent test for the rapid diagnosis of field infections of infectious bovine rhinotracheitis. Veterinary Record. 1983; 113: 298-300.

[46] Edwards S, Chasey D, White H. Experimental infectious bovine rhinotracheitis: comparison of four antigen detection methods. Research in Veterinary Science. 1983; 34: 42-45.

[47] Frank Y P, Magwood S E, Gray D P. Infectious bovine rhinotracheitis in Canada. Bulletin-Office International des Epizooties. 1975; 84: 153-162.

[48] Payment P, Assaf R, Trudel M, Marios P. Enzyme linked immunosorbent assay for serology of infectious bovine rhinotracheitis infections. Journal of Clinical Microbiology. 1979; 10: 633-636.

[49] Edwards S, Woods S B, Westcott D G, Emmerson M, Jones P C, Phillips A J. An evaluation of five serological tests for the detection of antibody to bovine herpes virus-1 in vaccinated and experimentally infected cattle. Research in Veterinary Science. 1986; 41: 378.

[50] Edwards S, Gitao G C. Highly sensitive antigen detection procedures for the diagnosis of infectious bovine rhinotracheitis: amplified ELISA and reverse passive haemagglutination. Veterinary Microbiology. 1987; 13: 135-141.

[51] Renukaradhya G J, Rajasekhar M, Raghavan R. Prevalence of infectious bovine rhinotracheitis in southern India. Revue Scientifique et Technique (International Office of Epizootics). 1996; 15 (3): 1021-1028.

[52] Suresh K B, Sudarshan K J H, Rajasekhar M. Seroprevalence of infectious bovine rhinotracheitis in India. Indian Veterinary Journal. 1999; 76: 5–9.

[53] Van Oirschot J T, Kaashoek M J, Maris Veldhuis M A, Weerdmeester K, Rijsewijk FAM. An enzyme linked immunoassay to detect antibodies against glycoprotein E of bovine herpes virus 1 allows differentiation between infected and vaccinated cattle. Journal of virological methods. 1997; 67: 23-34.

[54] Wellenberg G J, Verstraten ERAM, Mars M H, Van Oirschot J T. Detection of bovine herpesvirus-1 glycoprotein E antibodies in individual milk samples by enzyme linked immunosorbent assays. Journal of Clinical Microbiology. 1998; 36: 409-412.

[55] Bommeli W, Kihm U. The IBR control programme in Switzerland. Proceedings XII World Congress on Diseases of Cattle, The Netherland 1982; Vol. 1, pp. 153-155.

[56] Perrin B, Tixier G, Dannacher G, Soula A, Moussa A, Goyon M, Legardinier J C, Millet A, Protin P. Infectious bovine rhinotracheitis. Use of an ELISA kit to detect antibodies in serum and milk. Recveil de-Medecine Veterinaire. 1984; 160(9): 755-761.

[57] Madin S H, York C J, McKercher D G. Isolation of infectious bovine rhinotracheitis virus. Science. 1956; 124: 721-722.

[58] Mehrotra M L, Kumar S, Rajya B S. Isolation and characterization of infectious bovine rhinotracheitis/infectious pustular vulvovaginitis (IBR/IPV) virus associated with abortion in cow. Indian Journal of Animal Science. 1979; 49: 346-349.

[59] Mehrotra M L, Singh K P, Khanna P N, Shukla D C. Isolation of BHV-1 from an outbreak of abortion in an organised herd. Indian Journal of Animal Science. 1994; 64: 341-354.

[60] MohanKumar K M, Rajasekhar M, Krishnappa G. Isolation of infectious bovine rhinotracheitis virus in Karnataka. Indian Veterinary Journal. 1994; 71: 109-112.

[61] Engelenburg FAC Van, Maes R K, Oirschat J T Van, Rijsewijk FAM, Van Engelenburg FAC, Van Oirschat J T. Development of a rapid and sensitive polymerase chain reaction assay for detection of bovine herpesvirus type 1 in bovine semen. Journal of Clinical Microbiology. 1993; 31: 3129-3135.

[62] Weidmann M, Brandon R, Wagner P, Dubovi E J, Bott C A. Detection of bovine herpes virus-1 in bovine semen by nested PCR. Journal of Virological Methods. 1993; 44: 129-140.

[63] Kibenge F S B, Harris L M, Mckenna P K, Wadowska D, Yason C V. Amplification of strains of bovine herpesvirus-1 by use of polymerase chain reaction with primers in the thymidine kinase region. American Journal of Veterinary Research. 1994; 55: 1206-1212.

[64] Vilcek S, Nettleton P F, Herring A J. Detection of bovine herpesvirus-1 in clinical samples by polymerase chain reaction. DTW. 1995; 102: 249-250.

[65] Masri S A, Olson W, Nguyen P T, Prins S, Deregt D. Rapid detection of bovine herpesvirus-1 in the semen of infected bulls by a nested polymerase chain reaction assay. Canadian Journal of Veterinary Research. 1996; 60: 100-107.

[66] Santurde G, Silva N Da, Villares R, Tabares E, Solana A, Bautista J M, Castro J M, Da-Silva N. Rapid and high sensitivity test for the direct detection of bovine herpesvirus-1 genome in clinical samples. Veterinary Microbiology. 1996; 49: 81-92.

[67] Ashbaugh S E, Thompson K E, Belknap E B, Schultheirs P C, Chowdhury S, Collins J K. Specific detection of shedding and latency of bovine herpesvirus 1 and 5 using a nested polymerase chain reaction. Journal of Veterinary Diagnostic Investigation. 1997; 9: 387-394.

[68] Rocha M A, Barbosa E F, Guedes R M C, Lage A P, Leite R C, Gouveia A M G. Detection of BHV-1 in a naturally infected bovine fetus by a nested PCR assay. Veterinary Research Communications. 1999; 23: 133-141.

[69] Kaur Gurpreet, P N Dwivedi, Ramneek, N K Maiti. Development of monoclonal antibodies against Bovine herpesvirus-1 (BHV-1). Indian Journal of Animal Sciences. 2012; 82(7): 671-675.

[70] Le Yeune J M, Hart L T, Larson A D, Segev C L. Microdiffusion test for detection of antibodies to infectious bovine rhinotracheitis virus in bovine serum. American Journal of Veterinary Research. 1977; 38(4): 459-463.

[71] Lowry O H, Rosebrough N J, Farr A L, Randall R J. Protein measurement with the folin-phenol reagents. Journal of Biological Chemistry. 1951; 193: 265–275.

[72] Florent C, Demarneffe C. Enzyme linked immunosorbent assay used to monitor serum antibodies to bovine respiratory disease viruses. Veterinary Microbiology. 1986; 11: 309–314.

[73] Laemmli U K. Cleavage of structural proteins during the assembly of the head of bacteriophage T 4. Nature. 1970; 227: 680–685.

Chapter 9

Latency of Bovine Herpesvirus 1 (BoHV-1) in Sensory Neurons

Clinton Jones

Additional information is available at the end of the chapter

http://dx.doi.org/10.5772/63750

Abstract

Bovine herpesvirus 1 (BoHV-1) is an important pathogen of cattle and cofactor for bovine respiratory disease, a polymicrobial disease. Acute infection of cattle leads to abundant expression of lytic cycle viral genes, high levels of virus shedding, and clinical symptoms. Following acute infection, lifelong latency is established in sensory neurons. Only the latency-related (LR) gene locus, which encodes at least two micro-RNAs and several proteins, is abundantly expressed in latently infected neurons. Increased corticosteroids, due to external stressors, disrupt the maintenance of latency and increase the incidence of reactivation from latency, which is crucial for virus transmission. For example, calves latently infected with BoHV-1 consistently reactivate from latency following a single intravenous (IV) injection of the synthetic corticosteroid dexamethasone. In contrast to wild-type BoHV-1, an LR-mutant virus that has three in-frame stop codons at the amino terminus of the first open reading frame in the LR gene (ORF2) does not reactivate from latency following dexamethasone treatment. The ability of dexamethasone to initiate BoHV-1 reactivation from latency in calves makes it an attractive model to identify early events that occur during reactivation from latency. Viral and cellular factors that regulate the BoHV-1 latency-reactivation cycle are discussed in this review.

Keywords: bovine herpesvirus 1, latency, sensory neurons, stress-induced reactivation, glucocorticoid receptor, Wnt signaling pathway, pioneer transcription factors

1. Introduction

Bovine herpesvirus 1 (BoHV-1) is a large double-stranded DNA virus that causes significant economical losses to the cattle industry. Acute infection is typically initiated in mucosal epithelium and leads to high levels of virus shedding. Infection of cattle with BoHV-1 can lead to conjunctivitis, pneumonia, genital disorders, abortions, and bovine respiratory disease complex (BRDC), a life-threatening upper respiratory tract infection, reviewed in [1, 2]. In spite of high levels of viral replication, cellular and humoral immune responses eventually clear the virus.

Like other Alphaherpesvirinae subfamily members, BoHV-1 establishes lifelong latency in ganglionic neurons within the peripheral nervous system [3]. The latency-reactivation cycle can be operationally divided into three distinct phases: (1) establishment, (2) maintenance, and (3) reactivation from latency. In contrast to acute infections where all viral genes are abundantly expressed, the latency-related (LR) gene is the only viral transcript abundantly expressed in sensory neurons within trigeminal ganglia (TG) of latently infected calves during the maintenance of latency [4–6]. LR-RNA is antisense with respect to the bICP0 gene [7, 8], which encodes a major viral transcriptional trans-activator. The LR gene encodes at least two micro-RNAs and more than one protein. These proteins and micro-RNAs are detected in a subset of latently infected neurons [9–11] implying that they regulate certain aspects of the latency-reactivation cycle. LR protein expression is necessary for the latency-reactivation cycle [12]. The synthetic corticosteroid dexamethasone (DEX) consistently induces reactivation from latency in calves or rabbits, reviewed in [1, 2]. Reactivation from latency initiated by DEX reduces LR gene products, which correlates with the induction of lytic cycle viral genes. The ability of BoHV-1 to reactivate from latency is crucial for viral transmission and complicates designing effective modified live vaccines.

BoHV-1 is an attractive model to examine the latency-reactivation cycle of Alphaherpesvirinae subfamily members because reactivation from latency can be consistently induced in calves. Consequently, early events during reactivation from latency can be identified and characterized. In contrast to mouse models used to examine events that control the herpes simplex virus 1 (HSV-1) latency-reactivation cycle, the powerful genetic approaches available in mice are lacking in cattle. In this review, the pathogenic properties of BoHV-1 and details of the latency-reactivation cycle are discussed.

2. Pathogenesis of BoHV-1

2.1. Clinical disease caused by BoHV-1

Three BoHV-1 subtypes have been described: BoHV-1.1 (1), BHV-1.2a (2a), and BHV-1.2b (2b) [13]. Subtype 1 strains are frequently found in cattle located in North America, Europe, and South America. Infection with Subtype 1 isolates can result in infectious bovine rhinotracheitis (IBR) and can be detected in the upper respiratory tract. In addition, Subtype 1 isolates are frequently detected in aborted fetuses suggesting that infection caused the abortion. Subtype 2a can also cause IBR and abortions [14] as well as genital infections that can lead to infectious pustular vulvovaginitis (IPV) or balanopostitis (IBP), reviewed in (2). Subtype 2a strains of BoHV-1 are frequently detected in Brazil and Europe prior to the 1970s

(14). Subtype 2b strains, in general, are less pathogenic than Subtype 1 and frequently detected in Australia and Europe [15]. Subtype 2b strains can be detected in cases of respiratory disease and IPV/IPB, but not in aborted fetuses [14, 16].

In breeding cattle, abortions and genital infections are relatively common. Genital infections occur in bulls (IPB) and cows (IPV) within 1–3 days after mating or close contact with infected animals. Initial clinical signs following genital infection of cows are mild vaginal infection and frequent urination [17]. Lesions are routinely observed on the penis and prepuce in bulls. Inflammation of the uterus and transient infertility with purulent vaginal discharge may persist for several weeks if secondary bacterial infections occur. Transmission, in the absence of visible lesions, can occur following artificial insemination with semen from a bull subclinically infected. Abortions can occur at the same time as respiratory disease, but may also occur up to 100 days after infection, which is presumably due to reactivation from latency.

2.2. BoHV-1 is a cofactor of bovine respiratory disease complex

With respect to feedlot cattle, the respiratory form of BoHV-1 is the most common disease observed and is usually caused by Subtype 1 strains. BoHV-1 is an important cofactor of BRDC [18, 19], a polymicrobial disease initiated by stress as well as virus infection. Increased susceptibility to secondary bacterial infections correlates with depressed cell-mediated immunity after BoHV-1 infection [20–23]. Mucosal surfaces of the upper respiratory tract, which promotes the establishment of *Mannheimia haemolytica (MH)* in the lower respiratory tract, are compromised by BoHV-1 infection [24–26]. Productive infection increases neutrophil adhesion and activation [27], which can also amplify the effects of *MH*. *MH* is a gram-negative bacterium [28] that exists as normal flora in the upper respiratory tract of healthy ruminants [29]. This commensal relationship is disrupted following stress or coinfections [30], and then *MH* is the predominant organism that causes bronchopneumonia [24–26, 31]. BoHV-1 also stimulates inflammasome formation [32], which may contribute to BRDC by enhancing inflammation in the lung.

BoHV-1 interferes with immune responses by several mechanisms. For example, CD8+ T-cell recognition of infected cells is impaired by repressing the expression of major histocompatibility complex class I (MHC I) and transporter associated with antigen presentation [33–35]. The gN orthologs encoded by pseudorabies virus (PRV) and BoHV-1 inhibit transporter-associated antigen processing (TAP)-mediated transport of cytosolic peptides into the endoplasmic reticulum, which then interferes with the assembly of peptide-containing ternary MHC-I complexes in vitro in virus-infected cells [36, 37]. gN also targets the TAP complex for proteosomal degradation [36]. CD4+ T-cell function is impaired during acute infection of calves because BoHV-1 infects CD4+ T cells and induces apoptosis [1].

Stimulation of beta-interferon (IFN-β)-dependent transcription is an immediate-early response following virus infection that does not require de novo protein synthesis [38–43]. Activation of existing transcription factors by protein kinases stimulates IFN-β transcription. In contrast to humans or mice, cattle contain three IFN-β genes regulated by distinct promoters [44, 45]. BoHV-1 infection of primary bovine cells inhibits expression of all three bovine IFN-β genes [46]. Blocking viral protein expression by cycloheximide, a protein synthesis inhibitor, prevents BoHV-1 from suppressing IFN-β responses [46]. In contrast to primary bovine cells, BoHV-1 infection of established bovine kidney cells strongly induces IFN-β3 RNA expression [46]. Two viral regulatory proteins, bovine-infected cell protein 0 (bICP0) [47–49] and bICP27 [50], interfere with IFN-β-promoter activation. The bICP0 protein induces the degradation of a transcription factor, interferon-regulatory factor 3 (IRF3), which is necessary for IFN-β-promoter activation [47]. In addition, bICP0 interacts with interferon-regulatory factor 7 (IRF7), another transcription factor that stimulates IFN-β-promoter activity [49]. bICP0 also induces the degradation of the promyelocytic leukemia protein (PML) [51], a crucial component of an intrinsic antiviral complex localized to the nucleus [52–54].

3. Vaccines directed against BoHV-1

Several commercially available BoHV-1 vaccines are available and can be divided into two categories: modified live attenuated virus (MLV) or killed whole virus [55].

Most MLVs were developed more than 30 years ago by serial passage in tissue culture. MLVs generally induce humoral and cellular immune responses as a result of virus replication. The MLVs establish latency and upon reactivation from latency can readily be transmitted to pregnant cows and cause abortions [56]. One study demonstrated that vaccination with a common MLV reduced the number of live births relative to no vaccination [57]. MLVs can also be pathogenic in small calves because their immune system is not fully developed, and most MLVs are immunosuppressive. Recently, there has been an increase in IBR outbreaks in vaccinated feedlot cattle, which is likely due to vaccine outbreaks [58, 59]. A number of vaccine and virulent field strains were sequenced and important differences identified between the respective strains [60]. Consequently, polymerase chain reaction (PCR) primers are available that allow one to identify MLV strains versus virulent field strains. This knowledge will make it possible to identify vaccine strains, or emerging BoHV-1 strains not protected by existing MLVs that lead to the break.

Killed whole virus vaccines are usually produced by chemical treatments: for example, formaldehyde, β-propiolactone, or binary ethyleneimine. Killed vaccines are safe but typically require more than one injection to achieve acceptable neutralizing antibody levels and do not always induce cellular immune responses. With respect to formaldehyde-inactivated killed vaccines, antigens may also be denatured, which can affect the immunogenicity of vaccine preparations. Killed vaccines also require suitable adjuvant formulations and adjuvants can induce injection-site reactions. Better adjuvants may improve the efficacy while reducing the number of vaccinations necessary to achieve good protection in cattle. In summary, better vaccines that do not cause abortions or reactivate from latency need to be developed.

http://dx.doi.org/10.5772/63750

4. Transition from acute infection to establishment of latency: latency-related gene products promote latency

4.1. Productive infection

Acute infection of calves induces programmed cell death, inflammation, and high levels of virus shedding [1, 2, 32]. Viral gene expression during productive infection occurs in three distinct phases: immediate early (IE), early (E), or late (L). IE transcription unit 1 (IEtu1) encodes two crucial viral regulatory proteins, bICP0 and bICP4, which activate viral gene expression and DNA replication [61–63] (**Figure 1A**). IEtu2 encodes bICP22 [62]. A viral tegument protein, VP16 (also known as bTIF), is a viral structural protein present in the tegument that specifically trans-activates IE promoters. VP16 interacts with two cellular proteins (Oct1 and HCF-1) and this complex binds specific sequences in IE promoters [64, 65]. E genes, in general, encode nonstructural proteins that promote viral DNA replication. L genes encode proteins that comprise infectious virus particles.

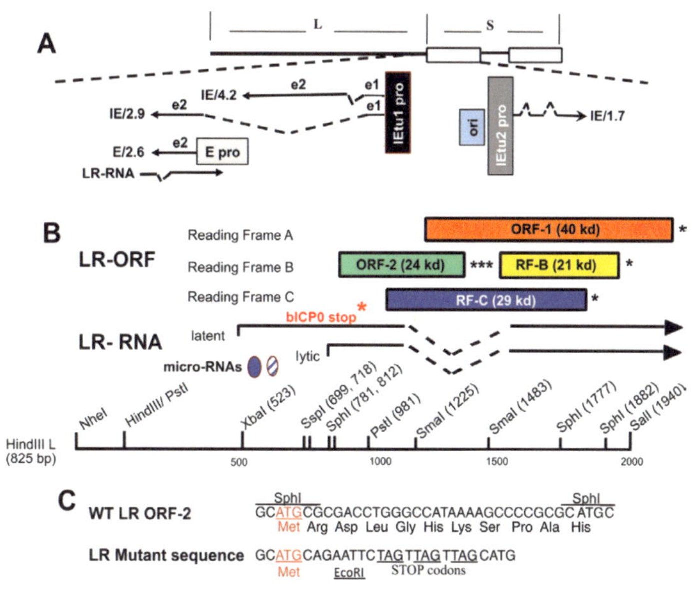

Figure 1. Schematic of BoHV-1 genes encompassing the LR gene. Panel A. Positions of IE transcripts and the LR transcript (LR-RNA) are presented [62, 63, 161]. The bICP4 protein is translated from the IE/4.2 transcript. The bICP0 protein is translated from the IE/2.9 transcript. The IEtu1promoter activates the expression of IE/4.2 and IE/2.9, and is denoted by the black rectangle (IEtu1 pro). The bICP0 protein can also be translated from an early transcript designated as E/2.6 because exon 2 (e2) contains all of the protein-coding sequences. An early promoter (E pro) drives the expression of the E/2.6 transcript. The origin of replication (ORI) separates IEtu1 from IEtu2. The IEtu2 promoter (IEtu2 pro) drives the expression of the bICP22 protein. Solid lines in the transcript position map represent exons (e1, e2, or e3) and dashed lines denote introns. The viral origin of replication (ori) is located near IETu2 promoter. **Panel B**. Partial restriction map of the LR gene. The LR gene contains two open reading frames (ORF-1 and ORF-2) [4]. Reading frame B (RF-B) and RF-C do not contain a methionine at the beginning of the open reading frame. The asterisks denote the position of stop codons that are in frame with the respective open reading frame. **Panel C**. Wild-type sequences near the N-terminus of ORFS compared to that in the LR mutant virus [12, 73].

4.2. Sensory neurons are the primary site for establishing latency

Cell-to-cell viral transmission leads to viral entry into sensory neurons. Following a burst of viral gene expression, lytic cycle viral gene expression is subsequently extinguished. If infection is initiated within the oral, nasal, or ocular cavity, the primary site for latency is sensory neurons in trigeminal ganglia. Lytic cycle viral gene expression [66] and infectious virus [12] are detected in TG from 2 to 6 days after infection. In contrast to infection of mucosal epithelial cells, significant numbers of infected neurons survive and these surviving neurons harbor intact viral genomes. This phase is operationally defined as the establishment of latency. Periodically, reactivation from latency occurs, virus is shed from peripheral sites, and consequently BoHV-1 is widespread in cattle [1, 7, 8, 67]. Other types of neurons may be latently infected; however, this has not been explored. Lymphocytes that reside in the tonsil and circulating blood have been reported to contain viral genomes when collected from latently infected calves [68].

4.3. The BoHV-1 latency-related gene locus is abundantly expressed in infected TG neurons and encodes several products

The LR gene is the only locus in the viral genome abundantly expressed in latently infected neurons [4, 6–8, 67, 69]. LR-RNA has unique start sites in TG and is antisense and overlaps the bICP0 gene, suggesting that it inhibits bICP0 expression [9, 70] (**Figure 1B**). The LR gene has two well-defined open reading frames (ORF1 and ORF2), and two reading frames that lack an initiating methionine (RF-B and RF-C). Two micro-RNAs encoded by the LR gene are abundantly expressed in latently infected neurons and they reduce bICP0 protein expression, but not ICP0 RNA levels in transient transfection studies [11]. The micro-RNAs have different predicted binding sites on bICP0 mRNA suggesting that they cooperate to reduce bICP0 protein levels. A small ORF located downstream from bICP0 (ORF-E) is expressed in latently infected TG neurons [71] and induces neurite formation in mouse neuroblastoma cells [72], suggesting that ORF-E regulates certain aspects of the latency-reactivation cycle.

An LR-mutant virus that contains three stop codons at the N-terminus of ORF2 was constructed and analyzed (see **Figure 1C** for location of stop codons). Following infection of calves, the LR-mutant virus exhibits diminished clinical symptoms during acute infection, and reduced virus shedding from the eye, TG, or tonsils [12, 73, 74]. Although the LR-mutant virus grows like wild-type BoHV-1 and the LR-rescued virus in cultured bovine cells, it expresses LR-RNA earlier than wild-type (wt) virus and stimulates a stronger interferon response in cultured cells and tonsils of acutely infected calves [75]. ORF1 and ORF2 expression are not detected in TG neurons during latency following infection with the LR-mutant virus [10, 76]. Wt BoHV-1, but not the LR-mutant virus, efficiently establishes latency and consistently reactivates from latency following a single injection of the synthetic corticosteroid DEX [12]. Although the LR-mutant virus grow less efficiently compared to wild-type BoHV-1 in TG [73], the LR mutant induces higher levels of apoptosis in TG during establishment of latency [77]. ORF2, in the absence of other viral genes, can inhibit apoptosis in Neuro-2A cells [78] suggesting that ORF2 has important roles during the latency-reactivation cycle.

ORF2 is a 181-amino acid protein that has little or no amino acid similarity to known proteins. The protein localizes to the periphery of the nucleus in transfected Neuro-2A cells and contains a functional nuclear localization signal. When the nuclear localization signal is deleted, ORF2 localizes to the plasma membrane of transfected Neuro-2A cells. Neuro-2A cells were used for these studies because ORF2 protein expression is consistently detected; conversely, other common cell lines that can be readily transfected do not support ORF2 expression. ORF2 preferentially interacts with single-stranded DNA; however, alanine substitution of threonine or serine residues in consensus protein kinase A (PKA) or protein kinase C (PKC) phosphorylation sites generates a protein that preferentially interacts with double-stranded DNA [81]. ORF2 does not appear to specifically bind to DNA sequences or interact with RNA. ORF2 stability is regulated by C-terminal sequences and PKA/PKC phosphorylation sites [79, 82].

ORF2 or an ORF2 isoform interacts with three cellular transcription factors (Notch1, Notch3, and c/EBP-alpha) [83, 84]. Since c/EBP-alpha stimulates IEtu1 promoter activity [85] and Notch 1 can slightly stimulate productive infection and certain viral promoters [83], ORF2 may promote the establishment of latency by interfering with lytic cycle viral gene expression. ORF2 amino acid sequences that interfere with Notch functions do not overlap ORF2 sequences necessary for inhibiting apoptosis [80], suggesting that these functions are separable. The ability of ORF2 to interfere with Notch functions stimulates the differentiation of Neuro-2A cells into differentiated neuronal-like cells, as judged by neurite sprouting [79, 82, 86]. It is well established that Notch family members inhibit differentiation of neural progenitor cells [87–91], suggesting that ORF2 helps infected neurons recover from infection and promotes normal neuronal functions. In summary, ORF2, ORF-E, and two micro-RNAs encoded by the LR gene possess properties that are predicted to enhance the establishment of latency.

5. Maintenance of latency

5.1. LR gene products are likely to promote maintenance of latency

Maintenance of latency lasts for the life of the host. Hallmarks of maintaining latency include the following: (1) infectious virus is not detected by standard virus isolation procedures, (2) abundant expression of lytic cycle viral genes does not occur, and (3) LR gene products are abundantly expressed in latently infected sensory neurons. The most obvious difference between maintenance versus establishment of latency is the initial burst of lytic cycle viral gene expression that occurs following infection of sensory neurons, and is extinguished during the establishment of latency.

Herpes simplex virus 1 latency-associated transcript (LAT), such as the LR gene, is abundantly expressed during latency and was reported to promote the maintenance of latency, reviewed in [7, 67, 92]. A recent study concluded that LAT maintains a pool of latently infected neurons that have the potential to reactivate from latency [93]. A cellular micro-RNA that interferes with the expression of the HSV-1 regulatory protein (ICP0) [94] and a cellular transcription factor (ATF3) [95] that enhances LAT expression are proposed to support the maintenance of latency. LR gene products, in particular the ability of both micro-RNAs to inhibit bICP0 expression, are candidates to suppress lytic cycle viral gene expression during maintenance of latency. The ability of ORF2 and ORF-E to stimulate neurite formation may help latently infected neurons retain their differentiated phenotype and normal functions.

5.2. Potential roles of cellular genes during maintenance of latency

Our recent studies demonstrated that a cellular transcription factor, β-catenin, is readily detected in latently infected TG neurons, but not in TG neurons from uninfected calves. Nearly all β-catenin+ neurons are also ORF2+; however, β-catenin+ neurons do not express the lytic cycle viral regulatory protein (bICP0) suggesting that ORF2 regulates β-catenin expression. During the course of reactivation from latency, the number of β-catenin+ neurons decreases significantly, which correlates with the induction of two Wnt antagonists, dickkopf-1 (DKK-1) and secreted frizzled-related protein 2 (SFRP2).

Wnt is a family of secreted glycoproteins that interacts with frizzled and the coreceptor LRP5/LRP6, reviewed in [96]. In the absence of the Wnt ligand or when a Wnt antagonist is expressed at high levels, a β-catenin destruction complex forms in the cytoplasm (**Figure 2A**). This complex (axin, adenomatous polyposis gene (APC), GSK3β, and CKIα) hyper-phosphorylates β-catenin: consequently, β-catenin is polyubiquitinated and degraded by the proteasome.

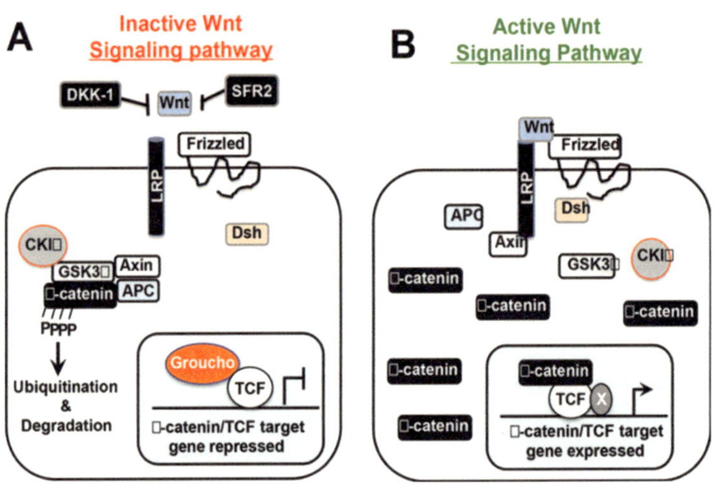

Figure 2. Schematic of canonical Wnt signaling pathway. Panel A: Key regulators of inactive Wnt pathway. In the absence of Wnt ligand, a β-catenin destruction complex, Axin, APC (adenomatous polyposis gene), GSK3β, and CKIa hyper-phosphorylate β-catenin, which leads to ubiqutination and degradation. Soluble frizzled-like proteins (DKK-1 and FRP2) prevent Wnt binding to its true receptors. In the absence of active Wnt signaling, TCF bound to DNA interacts with transcriptional repressors and transcription is repressed. **Panel B: Key regulators of active Wnt pathway**. Binding of Wnt to LRP and frizzled family members disrupts the β-catenin destruction complex and hypo-phosphorylated β-catenin accumulates in the nucleus. Nuclear β-catenin binds TCF family members, displaces repressors of TCF-dependent transcription, and recruits additional transcriptional regulators (denoted by X) resulting in transcriptional activation.

http://dx.doi.org/10.5772/63750

Wnt binding to its receptor disrupts the β-catenin destruction complex (**Figure 2B**). Consequently, the transcription factor β-catenin is stabilized, enters the nucleus, and interacts with TCF (T-cell factor) family members bound to the consensus site AGATCAAGG. β-catenin binding to TCF displaces bound corepressors (e.g., Groucho) and recruits coactivators (denoted as X) to activate Wnt target genes.

β-catenin activation regulates navigation of axons to their synaptic targets and stimulates axonal growth, reviewed in [97–101]. Several lines of evidence have concluded that disrupting the Wnt signaling pathway stimulates neurodegeneration, reviewed in [97, 98, 102]. Wnt signaling via β-catenin activation also inhibits apoptosis in several cell types [103–105], including neurons [106]. Chronic stress or increased corticosteroids induce a secreted Wnt antagonist, dickkopf-1 (DKK-1), which stimulates neuronal damage in the hippocampus [107], and ischemic neuronal death [108]. DKK-1 also mediates glucocorticoid-induced changes in human neuronal progenitor cell growth and differentiation [109]. Secreted frizzled-related protein 2 SFRP2 may also stimulate neuronal survival because it induces cell death in the developing hindbrain [110]. The ability of LR gene products, ORF2, for example, to stabilize β-catenin protein levels may promote maintenance of latency [103].

6. Reactivation from latency

6.1. Activation of viral gene expression during reactivation from latency

BoHV-1 reactivation from latency is consistently initiated by the synthetic corticosteroid DEX [6–8, 12, 67, 111], suggesting that DEX flips a molecular switch that disrupts the maintenance of latency (see **Figure 3** for schematic of putative steps leading to reactivation from latency). Within 6 h after DEX treatment, LR gene products are nearly undetectable in TG [6, 11, 82], lytic cycle viral RNA expression is detected in TG neurons of latently infected calves [68, 112], and apoptosis of T cells persisting in TG can be detected [112]. CD8+ T cells also persist in TG of humans or mice latently infected with HSV-1 [113–119] and have been reported to promote maintenance of latency [120, 121–124]. CD8α dendritic cells have also been reported to regulate the HSV-1 latency-reactivation cycle using mouse models of infection [125]. CD8+ T cells and/or CD8α dendritic cells may be important regulators of the BoHV-1 latency-reactivation cycle.

Two viral regulatory proteins, bICP0 and VP16, are expressed in the same neuron within 90 min after DEX treatment of latently infected calves; conversely, two other late proteins (gC and gD) are not readily detected until 6 h after DEX treatment [105, 126]. Fewer neurons express gC or gD relative to bICP0 or VP16. The fact that VP16 is a late gene implies that a novel mechanism induces VP16 expression very soon after DEX administration. However, the VP16 promoter is not activated by DEX or any of the DEX-induced transcription in transient transfection assays [127, 128]. With respect to HSV-1, VP16 has been proposed to be an important factor during initial stages of reactivation [129, 130]. Nearly all bICP0+ and VP16+ neurons express the glucocorticoid receptor (GR) suggesting that GR+ latently infected neurons are more likely to reactivate. The IEtu1 promoter that drives bICP0 and bICP4 (two crucial viral transcriptional regulators; **Figure 1A**) expression is stimulated by DEX and contains a consensus GR-binding site bound by the activated GR [128]. Inspection of the BoHV-1 genome revealed that more than 100 GR-binding sites are present, suggesting that additional viral promoters are stimulated by corticosteroids during reactivation from latency.

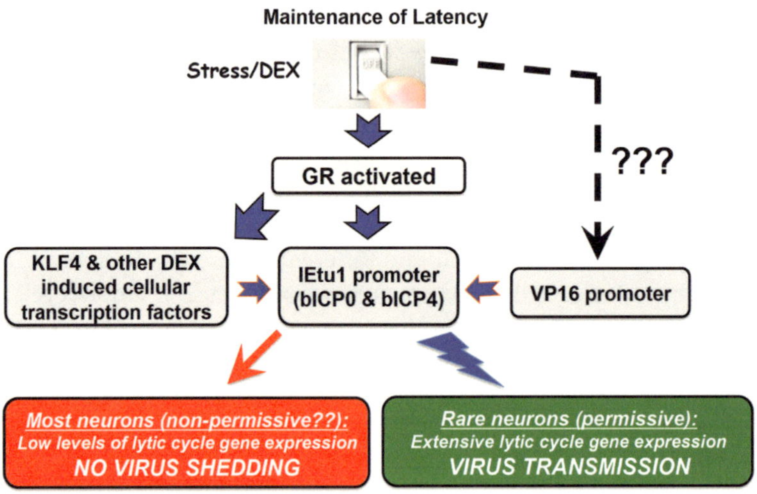

Figure 3. Putative steps leading to reactivation from latency. Stress, as mimicked by the synthetic corticosteroid dexamethasone (DEX), is a molecular switch that is predicted to stimulate viral gene expression via activation of the GR- and DEX-induced transcription factors. The IEtu1 is a crucial promoter that appears to be stimulated during the early stages of reactivation from latency. The mechanism by which VP16 expression is stimulated is not known. Many latently infected neurons lack cellular factors and are unable to support virus production and consequently reestablish latency. A small subset of latently infected neurons possesses the necessary factors to support extensive lytic cycle viral gene and production of infectious virus. The fate of these neurons is unclear.

6.2. Regulation of cellular gene expression in TG neurons during early phases of DEX-induced reactivation from latency

Within 3 h after DEX treatment, Pentraxin 3, a regulator of innate immunity and neurodegeneration [131], and two cellular transcription factors, promyelocytic leukemia zinc finger (PLZF) and Slug, are induced at least 15-fold in TG [127]. Additional DEX-induced cellular transcription factors were also identified in TG: Sam-pointed domain Ets transcription factor (SPDEF) and three Kruppel-like transcription factors (KLF), KLF4, KLF6, and KLF15. Immunohistochemistry studies confirmed that these cellular transcription factors are expressed in TG neurons during early stages of DEX-induced reactivation from latency. In general, overexpression of a DEX-induced cellular transcription factor stimulated productive infection and certain viral promoters, including IEtu1and the bICP0 early promoter.

The finding that four KLF family members (KLF4, KLF6, KLF15, and PLZF) are stimulated during DEX-induced reactivation from latency is significant because KLF family members resemble the SP1 transcription factor family and both families of transcription factors interact with GC-rich motifs, reviewed in [132, 133]. In general, genomes of Alphaherpesvirinae

http://dx.doi.org/10.5772/63750

subfamily members, including BoHV-1 and HSV-1, are GC rich and many viral promoters contain Sp1 consensus-binding sites and additional GC-rich motifs [132]. KLF15 stimulates HSV-1 ICP0 promoter activity more than 400-fold, but not the HSV-1 VP16 and ICP4 promoters [134]. KLF4, SPDEF, and Slug also stimulate ICP0 promoter activity at least 100-fold. These transcription factors are induced in mouse TG neurons following explant and addition of DEX generally enhanced their expression. These studies provide evidence that KLF transcription factors stimulate BoHV-1 and HSV-1 transcription, which may consequently enhance productive infection and reactivation from latency.

Lytic cycle viral gene expression is not readily detected during the maintenance of latency because HSV-1 and presumably BoHV-1 genome exist as "silent" chromatin during latency, reviewed by [135–137]. In contrast to many transcription factors, the activated GR can specifically bind silent chromatin [138–140], generate a nuclease-hypersensitive site, and then promote initiation of transcription [141–142]. Activated GR only binds a subset of GREs in silent chromatin [143–144] and thus fits the criteria for being a "pioneer transcription factor," reviewed in [145, 146]. Purified KLF4, a DEX-induced transcription factor in TG neurons [127, 134], is also a pioneer transcription factor [145, 146] that can bind nucleosomes in vitro and preferentially targets silent sites enriched for nucleosomes in vivo [147]. We suggest that these two pioneer transcription factors (GR and KLF4) have the potential to convert a silent BoHV-1 genome into a transcriptionally active genome that subsequently expresses abundant levels of lytic cycle viral genes and produces infectious viral particles.

There appears to be a bottleneck with respect to completion of successful reactivation (production of an infectious virus particle). Many latently infected neurons apparently do not support extensive lytic cycle viral transcription and/or cellular factors necessary to produce an infectious viral particle that are missing or not expressed in sufficient quantities. These neurons are operationally defined as nonpermissive. Evidence for the existence of nonpermissive neurons comes from three studies: (1) few neurons express late proteins (gC and gD) relative to neurons that express VP16 and bICP0 [126], (2) only a small subset of latently infected sensory neurons produce infectious viral particles [6], and (3) the LR mutant does not reactivate from latency following DEX treatment even though the viral genome and LR-RNA are detected in TG during latency [12]. Many nonpermissive neurons are predicted to survive a stressful stimulus and reestablish latency. It is unclear whether a permissive neuron that reactivates from latency and sheds infectious virus can survive and reestablish latency. In a mouse model of HSV-1, neurons that support reactivation in vivo do not appear to survive [148].

7. Conclusions and unresolved questions

The latency-reactivation cycle of Alphaherpesvirinae subfamily members, including BoHV-1, is regulated by a complex series of virus-host interactions. Furthermore, BoHV-1 and cattle have evolved with each other making it difficult to model the latency-reactivation cycle in small animal models or cultured neurons. The HSV-1 LAT and BoHV-1 LR gene encode at least three common functions crucial for the latency-reactivation cycle: (1) inhibit apoptosis [78, 149–152], (2) interfere with productive infection [11, 152, 153], and (3) promote sprouting of neurites in mouse neuroblastoma cells [79, 82, 154], which is predicted to promote neuronal repair and restore normal neuronal functions following infection. Although the LR gene restores wt levels of reactivation to an HSV-1 LAT null mutant [155] and ORF2 plays a role in this process [156], LAT does not appear to encode a protein. Thus, LAT-encoded microRNAs and other small noncoding RNAs are proposed to regulate the latency-related cycle.

A brief discussion of several unresolved questions is presented as follows:

- Is it necessary for viral DNA replication to occur in a latently infected sensory neuron that produces an infectious virus particle? Although it is clear that viral DNA replication must occur at peripheral sites for virus transmission or recurrent disease to occur during a reactivation episode, published reports that have directly tested whether viral DNA replication occurs in neurons during reactivation from latency are lacking. From a minimalist's standpoint, it would seem to be advantageous for the viral genome to merely express sufficient levels of viral proteins necessary to package the viral genome such that cell-to-cell transmission will occur. Considering that sensory neurons do not enter the cell cycle and replicate their chromosomes, there must be ingrained epigenetic signals that prevent the expression of cellular proteins necessary for DNA replication.

- What is the threshold of stress that leads to successful reactivation from latency? Mammals face stressful stimuli everyday but reactivation from latency (at least episodes that lead to virus shedding) does not occur every day. For successful reactivation episodes (one that leads to virus shedding from peripheral sites), there must be a relatively intense stimulus or a prolonged stimulus.

- Do neurons that produce infectious virus particles survive and reestablish a latent infection? As mentioned above, latently infected neurons yielding infectious virus particles probably do not survive in a mouse model of HSV-1 infection [148]. However, this study needs to be confirmed.

- Do other Alphaherpesvirinae subfamily members utilize similar pathways for regulating the latency-reactivation cycle as BoHV-1? HSV-1 does not reactivate as consistently as BoHV-1 following DEX treatment, suggesting that the GR is not as important. However, it should be noted that increased "stress" correlates with a higher incidence of reactivation from latency in humans [157–159]. DEX also stimulates reactivation from latency in TG neuronal cultures prepared from latently infected mice [114] and TG organ cultures latently infected with HSV-1 [160]. Although the exact mechanism is not likely the same, common pathways may flip a switch that initiates reactivation from latency.

Acknowledgements

This research was supported by a grant from the USDA-NIFA Competitive Grants Program (13-01041), funds derived from the Sitlington endowment, and support from the Oklahoma

http://dx.doi.org/10.5772/63750

Center for Respiratory and Infectious Diseases (National Institutes of Health Centers for Biomedical Research Excellence Grant # P20GM103648).

Author details

Clinton Jones

Address all correspondence to: clint.jones10@okstate.edu

Department of Veterinary Pathobiology, Center for Veterinary Health Sciences, Oklahoma State University, Stillwater, Oklahoma, USA

References

[1] Jones C. Regulation of innate immune responses by bovine herpesvirus 1 and infected cell protein 0. Viruses. 2009;1:255–75.

[2] Jones C and S. Chowdhury. A review of the biology of bovine herpesvirus type 1 (BHV-1), its role as a cofactor in the bovine respiratory disease complex, and development of improved vaccines. Adv Anim Health. 2007;8:187–205.

[3] Jones, C., L.F. da Silva, and D. Sinani (2011). Regulation of the latency-reactivation cycle by products encoded by the bovine herpesvirus 1 (BHV-1) latency-related gene. J Neurovirol 17: 535-545.

[4] Kutish G, T. Mainprize, and D. Rock. Characterization of the latency-related transcriptionally active region of the bovine herpesvirus 1 genome. J Virol. 1990;64(12):5730–7.

[5] Rock DL, A.B. Nesburn, H. Ghiasi, J. Ong, T.L. Lewis, J.R. Lokensgard, et al. Detection of latency-related viral RNAs in trigeminal ganglia of rabbits latently infected with herpes simplex virus type 1. J Virol. 1987;61(12):3820–6.

[6] Rock D, J. Lokensgard, T. Lewis, and G. Kutish. Characterization of dexamethasone-induced reactivation of latent bovine herpesvirus 1. J Virol. 1992;66(4):2484–90.

[7] Jones C. Herpes simplex virus type 1 and bovine herpesvirus 1 latency. Clin Microbiol Rev. 2003;16(1):79–95.

[8] Jones C, V. Geiser, G. Henderson, Y. Jiang, F. Meyer, S. Perez, et al. Functional analysis of bovine herpesvirus 1 (BHV-1) genes expressed during latency. Vet Microbiol. 2006;113(3–4):199–210.

[9] Hossain A, L.M. Schang, and C. Jones. Identification of gene products encoded by the latency-related gene of bovine herpesvirus 1. J Virol. 1995;69(9):5345–52.

[10] Jiang Y, M. Inman, Y. Zhang, N.A. Posadas, and C. Jones. A mutation in the latency related gene of bovine herpesvirus 1 (BHV-1) inhibits protein expression of a protein from open reading frame 2 (ORF-2) and an adjacent reading frame during productive infection. J Virol. 2004;78:3184–9.

[11] Jaber T, A. Workman, and C. Jones. Small noncoding RNAs encoded within the bovine herpesvirus 1 latency-related gene can reduce steady-state levels of infected cell protein 0 (bICP0). J Virol. 2010;84(13):6297–307.

[12] Inman M, L. Lovato, A. Doster, and C. Jones. A mutation in the latency-related gene of bovine herpesvirus 1 disrupts the latency reactivation cycle in calves. J Virol. 2002;76(13):6771–9.

[13] Metzler AE, H. Matile, U. Gasman, M. Engels, and R. Wyler. European isolates of bovine herpesvirus 1: a comparison of restriction endonuclease sites, polypeptides and reactivity with monoclonal antibodies. Arch Virol. 1985;85:57–69.

[14] Oirschot JT van. Bovine herpesvirus in semen of bulls and the risk of transmission: a brief overview. Vet Q. 1995;17:29–33.

[15] Edwards S, H. White, and P. Nixon. A study of the predominant genotypes of bovine herpesvirus 1 isolated in the U.K. Vet Microbiol. 1990;22:213–23.

[16] D'Arce RCF, R.S. Almedia, T.C. Silva, A.C. Spilki, P.M. Roehe, and C.W. Ams. Restriction endonucleases and monoclonal antibody analysis of Brazilian isolates of bovine herpesvirus 1 and 5. Vet Microbiol. 2002;88:315–34.

[17] Yates WDG. A review of infectious bovine rhinotracheitis, shipping fever pneumonia, and viral-bacterial synergism in respiratory diesease of cattle. Can J Comp Med. 1982;46:225–63.

[18] Hodgson PD, P. Aich, A. Manuja, K. Hokamp, F.M. Roche, F.S.L. Brinkman, et al. Effect of stress on viral-bacterial synergy in bovine respiratoryt disease: novel mechanisms to regulate inflammation. Comp Funct Genom. 2005;6:244–50.

[19] Jones C and S. Chowdhury. Bovine herpesvirus type 1 (BHV-1) is an important cofactor in the bovine respiratory disease complex. In: Broderson VLCaB, editor. Veterinary Clinics of North America, Food Animal Practice, Bovine Respiratory Disease, vol. 26. New York, NY: Elsevier; 2010. pp. 303–21.

[20] Carter JJ, A.D. Weinberg, A. Pollard, R. Reeves, J.A. Magnuson, N.S. Magnuson. Inhibition of T-lymphocyte mitogenic responses and effects on cell functions by bovine herpesvirus 1. J Virol. 1989;63(4):1525–30.

[21] Griebel P, H.B. Ohmann, M.J. Lawman, and L.A. Babiuk. The interaction between bovine herpesvirus type 1 and activated bovine T lymphocytes. J Gen Virol. 1990;71(Pt 2):369–77.

[22] Griebel P, L. Qualtiere, W.C. Davis, A. Gee, H. Bielefeldt Ohmann, M.J. Lawman, et al. T lymphocyte population dynamics and function following a primary bovine herpesvirus type-1 infection. Viral Immunol. 1987;1(4):287–304.

[23] Griebel PJ, L. Qualtiere, W.C. Davis, M.J. Lawman, and L.A. Babiuk. Bovine peripheral blood leukocyte subpopulation dynamics following a primary bovine herpesvirus-1 infection. Viral Immunol. 1987;1(4):267–86.

[24] Highlander SK, N.D. Fedorova, D.M. Dusek, R. Panciera, L.E. Alvarez, and C. Renehart. Inactivation of *Pasteurella (Mannheimia) haemolytica* leukotoxin causes partial attenuation of virulence in a calf challenge model. Infect Immun. 2000;68:3916–22.

[25] Highlander SK. Molecular genetic analysis of virulence in *Mannheimia (Pasteurella) haemolytica*. Front Biosci. 2001(1):D1128–50.

[26] Zecchinon L. T. Fett, and D. Desmecht. How *Mannheimia haemolytica* defeats host defense through a kiss of death mechanism. Vet Res. 2005;36:133–56.

[27] Rivera-Rivas JJ, D. Kisiela, and C.J. Czuprynski. Bovine herpesvirus type 1 infection of bovine bronchial epithelial cells increases neutrophil adhesion and activation. Vet Immunol Immunopathol. 2009;131:167–76.

[28] Songer JG and K.W. Post. The genera *Mannheimia* and *Pasteurella*. In: Bacterial and Fungal Agents of Animal Disease. L. Duncan St Louis, MO: Elsevier Saunders; 2005.

[29] Frank GH. Bacteria as etiologic agents in bovine respiratory disease. In: Bovine Respiratory Disease. College Station, R.W. Loan. TX: Texas A&M University Press; 1984.

[30] Rice JA, LC-M, D.C. Hodgins, and P.E. Shewen. *Mannheimia haemolytica* and bovine respiratory disease. Animal Health Research Reviews. 2008;8:117–28.

[31] Hodgins DC and P.E. Shewen. Pneumonic pasteurellosis of cattle. In: Infectious Disease of Livestock, 2nd ed. Cape Town, South Africa: Oxford University Press; 2004.

[32] Wang J, J. Alexander, M. Wiebe, and C. Jones. Bovine herpesvirus 1 productive infection stimulates inflammasome formation and caspase 1 activity. Virus Res. 2014;185:72–6.

[33] Nataraj C, S. Eidmann, M.J. Hariharan, J.H. Sur, G.A. Perry, and S. Srikumaran. Bovine herpesvirus 1 downregulates the expression of bovine MHC class I molecules. Viral Immunol. 1997;10(1):21–34.

[34] Hariharan MJ, C. Nataraj, and S. Srikumaran. Down regulation of murine MHC class I expression by bovine herpesvirus 1. Viral Immunol. 1993;6(4):273–84.

[35] Hinkley S, A.B. Hill, and S. Srikumaran. Bovine herpesvirus-1 infection affects the peptide transport activity in bovine cells. Virus Res. 1998;53(1):91–6.

[36] Koppers-Lalic D, E.A.J. Reits, M.E. Ressing, A.D. Lipinska, R. Abele, J. Koch, et al. Varicelloviruses avoid T cell recognition by UL49.5-mediated inactivation of the transporter associated with antigen processing. Proc Natl Acad Sci. 2005;102:5144–9.

[37] Lipińska AD, D. Koppers-Lalic, M. Rychlowski, P. Admiraal, F.A.M. Rijsewijk, K., Bieńkowska-Szewczyk, et al.. Bovine herpesvirus 1 UL49.5 protein inhibits the transporter associated with antigen processing despite complex formation with glycoprotein M. J Virol. 2006;81:5822–32.

[38] King P and S. Goodbourn. The beta-interferon promoter responds to priming through multiple independent regulatory elements. J Biol Chem. 1994;269:30609–15.

[39] Goodbourn S, K. Zinn, and T. Maniatis. Human beta-interferon gene expression is regulated by an inducible enhancer element. Cell. 1985;41:509–20.

[40] Munshi N, M. Merika, J. Yie, K. Senger, G. Chen, and D. Thanos. Acetylation of HMG I(Y) by CBP turns off IFN beta expression by disrupting the enhanceosome. Mol Cell. 1998;2(4):457–67.

[41] Yoneyama M, W. Suhara, M. Fukuhara, M. Fukuda, E. Nishida, and T. Fujita. Direct triggering of the type 1 interferon system by virus infection: activation of a transcription factors containing IRF-3 and CBP/p300. EMBO J. 1998;17:1087–95.

[42] Sharma S, B.R. tenOever, N. Grandvaux, G.-P. Zhou, R. Lin, and J. Hiscott. Trigerring the interferon antiviral response through and IKK-related pathway. Science. 2003;300:1148–51.

[43] Au WC, P.A. Moore, W. Lowther, Y.T. Juang, and P.M. Pitha. Identification of a member of the interferon regulatory factor family that binds to the interferon-stimulated response element and activates expression of interferon-induced genes. Proc Natl Acad Sci U S A. 1995;92:11657–61.

[44] Wilson V, A.J. Jeffreys, and P.A. Barrie. A comparison of vertebrate interferon gene families deteced by hybridization with human interferon DNA. J Mol Biol. 1983;166:457–75.

[45] Valarcher J-F, J. Furze, S. Wyld, R. Cook, K.-K. Conzelman, and G. Taylor. Role of alpha/beta interferons in the attenuation and immunogenecity of recombinant bovine respiratory syncitial viruses lacking NS proteins. J Virol. 2003;77:8426–39.

[46] da Silva LF and C. Jones. Infection of cultured bovine cells with bovine herpesvirus 1 (BHV-1) or Sendai virus induces different beta interferon subtypes. Virus Res. 2011;157(1):54–60.

[47] Saira K, Y. Zhou, and C. Jones. The infected cell protein 0 encoded by bovine herpesvirus 1 (bICP0) induces degradation of interferon response factor 3 (IRF3), and consequently inhibits beta interferon promoter activity. J Virol. 2007;81:3077–86.

[48] Saira K. Functional analysis of the bovine herpesvirus-1 gene encoding bICP0, a promiscuous trans-activator, that stimulates productive infection and interferon signaling pathways (PhD thesis). Lincoln: University of Nebraska; 2008.

[49] Saira K and C. Jones. The infected cell protein 0 encoded by bovine herpesvirus 1 (bICP0) associates with interferon regulatory factor 7 (IRF7), and consequently inhibits beta interferon promoter activity. J Virol. 2009;83:3977–81.

[50] da Silva LF and C. Jones. The ICP27 protein encoded by bovine herpesvirus type 1 (bICP27) interferes with promoter activity of the bovine genes encoding beta interferon 1 (IFN-β1) and IFN-β3. Virus Res. 2012(169):162–8.

[51] Gaudreault N and C. Jones. Regulation of promyelocytic leukemia (PML) protein levels and cell morphology by bovine herpesvirus 1 infected cell protein 0 (bICP0) and mutant bICP0 proteins that do not localize to the nucleus. Virus Res. 2011;156:17–24.

[52] Everett RD, W.C. Earnshaw, J. Findlay, and P. Lomonte. Specific destruction of kinetochore protein CENP-C and disruption of cell division by herpes simplex virus immediate-early protein Vmw110. EMBO J. 1999;18(6):1526–38.

[53] Everett RD, P. Lomonte, T. Sternsdorf, R. van Driel R, and A. Orr. Cell cycle regulation of PML modification and ND10 composition. J Cell Sci. 1999;112(Pt 24):4581–8.

[54] Parkinson J and R.D. Everett. Alphaherpesvirus proteins related to herpes simplex virus type 1 ICP0 affect cellular structures and proteins. J Virol. 2000;74(21):10006–17.

[55] Van Drunen Littel-van den Hurk S. Rationale and perspectives on the success of vaccination against bovine herpesvirus-1. Vet Microbiol. 2005;113:275–82.

[56] O'Toole D and H. Van Campen. Abortifacient vaccines and bovine herpesvirus-1. J Am Vet Med Assoc. 2010;237:259–60.

[57] O'Toole D, M.M. Miller, J.L. Cavender, and T.E. Cornish. Pathology in Practice. Vet Med Today. 2012;241:189–91.

[58] Ellis J, C. Waldner, C. Rhodes, and V. Ricketts. Longevity of protective immunity to experimental bovine herpesvirus-1 infection following inoculation with a combination modified-live virus vaccine in beef calves. J Am Vet Med Assoc. 2005;227:123–8.

[59] Van Drunen Littel-van den Hurk S, D. Myers, P.A. Doig, B. Karvonen, M. Habermehl, L.A. Babiuk, et al. Identification of a mutant bovine herpesvirus-1 (BHV-1) in post-arrival outbreaks of IBR in feedlot calves and protection with conventional vaccination. Can J Vet Res. 2001;65:81–8.

[60] Fulton RW, J.M. d'Offay, and R. Eberle. Bovien herpesvirus-1: comparison and differentiation of vaccine and field strains based on genomic sequence variation. Vaccine. 2013;31:1471–9.

[61] Fraefel C, J. Zeng, Y. Choffat, M. Engels, M. Schwyzer, and M. Ackermann. Identification and zinc dependence of the bovine herpesvirus 1 transactivator protein BICP0. J Virol. 1994;68(5):3154–62.

[62] Wirth UV, B. Vogt, and M. Schwyzer. The three major immediate-early transcripts of bovine herpesvirus 1 arise from two divergent and spliced transcription units. J Virol. 1991;65(1):195–205.

[63] Wirth UV, C. Fraefel, B. Vogt, C. Vlcek, V. Paces, and M. Schwyzer. Immediate-early RNA 2.9 and early RNA 2.6 of bovine herpesvirus 1 are 3′ coterminal and encode a putative zinc finger transactivator protein. J Virol. 1992;66(5):2763–72.

[64] Misra V, A.C. Bratanich, D. Carpenter, and P. O'Hare. Protein and DNA elements involved in transactivation of the promoter of the bovine herpesvirus (BHV) 1 IE-1 transcription unit by the BHV alpha gene trans-inducing factor. J Virol. 1994;68(8):4898–909.

[65] Misra V, S. Walker, S. Hayes, and P. O'Hare. The bovine herpesvirus alpha gene trans-inducing factor activates transcription by mechanisms different from those of its herpes simplex virus type 1 counterpart VP16. J Virol. 1995;69(9):5209–16.

[66] Schang L and C. Jones. Analysis of bovine herpesvirus 1 transcripts during a primary infection of trigeminal ganglia of cattle. J Virol. 1997;71(9):6786–95.

[67] Jones C. Alphaherpesvirus latency: its role in disease and survival of the virus in nature. Adv Virus Res. 1998;51:81–133.

[68] Winkler MTC, A. Doster, and C. Jones. Persistence and reactivation of bovine herpesvirus 1 in the tonsil of latently infected calves. J Virol. 2000;74:5337–46.

[69] Rock DL, S.L. Beam, and J.E. Mayfield. Mapping bovine herpesvirus type 1 latency-related RNA in trigeminal ganglia of latently infected rabbits. J Virol. 1987;61(12):3827–31.

[70] Bratanich AC, N.D. Hanson, and C. Jones. The latency-related gene of bovine herpesvirus 1 inhibits the activity of immediate-early transcription unit 1. Virology. 1992;191(2):988–91.

[71] Inman M, J. Zhou, H. Webb, and C. Jones. Identification of a novel transcript containing a small open reading frame that is expressed during latency, and is antisense to the latency related gene of bovine herpes virus 1 (BHV-1). J Virol. 2004;78:5438–47.

[72] Perez S, F. Meyer, G. Henderson, Y. Jiang, S. Sherman, A. Doster, et al. A protein encoded by the bovine herpesvirus 1 ORF E gene induces neurite-like morphological changes in mouse neuroblastoma cells and is expressed in trigeminal ganglionic neurons. J Neurovirol. 2007;13:139–49.

[73] Inman M, L. Lovato, A. Doster, and C. Jones. A mutation in the latency-related gene of bovine herpesvirus 1 leads to impaired ocular shedding in acutely infected calves. J Virol. 2001;75:8507–15.

[74] Perez S, M. Inman, A. Doster, and C. Jones. Latency-related gene encoded by bovine herpesvirus 1 promotes virus growth and reactivation from latency in tonsils of infected calves. J Clin Micro. 2005;43:393–401.

[75] Perez S, F. Meyer, K. Saira, A. Doster, and C. Jones. Premature expression of the latency-related RNA encoded by bovine herpesvirus type 1 correlates with higher levels of beta interferon RNA expression in productively infected cells. J Gen Virol. 2008;89(Pt 6): 1338–45.

[76] Meyer F, S. Perez, Y. Jiang, Y. Zhou, G. Henderson, and C. Jones. Identification of a novel protein encoded by the latency-related gene of bovine herpesvirus 1. J Neurovirol. 2007;13:569–78.

[77] Lovato L, M. Inman, G. Henderson, A. Doster, and C. Jones. Infection of cattle with a bovine herpesvirus 1 (BHV-1) strain that contains a mutation in the latency related gene leads to increased apoptosis in trigeminal ganglia during the transition from acute infection to latency. J Virol. 2003;77:4848–57.

[78] Shen W and C. Jones. Open reading frame 2, encoded by the latency-related gene of bovine herpesvirus 1, has antiapoptotic activity in transiently transfected neuroblastoma cells. J Virol. 2008;82(21):10940–5.

[79] Sinani D, Y. Liu, and C. Jones. Analysis of a bovine herpesvirus 1 protein encoded by an alternatively spliced latency related (LR) RNA that is abundantly expressed in latently infected neurons. Virology. 2014;464–465:244–52.

[80] Sinani D and C. Jones. Localization of sequences in a protein encoded by the latency related gene of bovine herpesvirus 1 (ORF2) that inhibits apoptosis and interferes with Notch1 mediated trans-activation of the bICP0 promoter. J Virol. 2011;85:12124–33.

[81] Pittayakhajonwut D, D. Sinani, and C. Jones. A protein (ORF2) encoded by the latency related gene of bovine herpesvirus 1 interacts with DNA. J Virol. 2013;87:5493–501.

[82] Sinani D, L. Frizzo da Silva, and C. Jones. A bovine herpesvirus 1 protein expressed in latently infected neurons (ORF2) promotes neurite sprouting in the presence of activated Notch1 or Notch3. J Virol. 2013(87):1183–92.

[83] Workman A, D. Sinani, D. Pittayakhajonwut, and C. Jones. A protein (ORF2) encoded by the latency related gene of bovine herpesvirus 1 interacts with Notch1 and Notch3. J Virol. 2011;85:2536–46.

[84] Meyer F, S. Perez, V. Geiser, M. Sintek, M. Inman, and C. Jones A protein encoded by the bovine herpes virus 1 (BHV-1) latency related gene interacts with specific cellular regulatory proteins, including the CCAAT enhancer binding protein alpha (C/EBP-a). J Virol. 2007;81:59–67.

[85] Meyer F and C. Jones. The cellular transcription factor, CCAAT enhancer-binding protein alpa (C/EBP-a) has the potential to activate the bovine herpesvirus 1 immediate early transcription unit 1 promoter. J Neurovirol. 2009;15:1–8.

[86] Liu L and C. Jones. Regulation of Notch-mediated transcription by a bovine herpesvirus 1 encoded protein (ORF2) that is expressed in latently infected sensory neurons. J Neurovirol. 2016 (in press).

[87] Berezovska O, P. McLean, R. Knowles, M. Frosh, F.M. Lu, S.E. Lux, et al. Notch1 inhibits neurite outgrowth in postmitotic primary neurons. Neuroscience. 1999;93:433–9.

[88] El Bejjani R and M. Hammerlund. Notch signaling inhibits axon regeneration. Neuron. 2012;73:268–78.

[89] Hitoshi S, T. Alexson, V. Tropepe, D. Donoviel, A. Elia, J. Nye, et al. Notch pathway molecules are essential for the maintenance, but not the generation, of mammalian neural stem cells. Genes Dev. 2002;16:846–58.

[90] Lassiter RN, M.K. Ball, J.S. Adams, B.T. Wright, and M.R. Stark. Sensory neuron differentiation is regulated by notch signaling in the trigeminal placode. Dev Biol. 2010;344:836–48.

[91] Levy, O.A., J.J. Lah, and A.I. Levey. Notch signaling inhibits PC12 cell neurite outgrowth via RBP-J-dependent and -independent mechanisms. Dev Neurosci. 2002;24:79–88.

[92] Perng G-C and C. Jones. Towards an understanding of the Herpes Simplex Virus Type 1 latency-reactivation cycle. Interdisciplinary Perspect Infect Dis. 2010;2010:1–18.

[93] Thompson RL and N.M. Sawtell. The herpes simplex virus type 1 latency associated transcript locus is required for the maintenance of reactivation competent latent infections. J Neurovirol. 2011;17:552–8.

[94] Pan D, O. Flores, J.L. Umbach, J.M. Pesola, P. Bentley, P.C. Rosato, et al. A neuron-specific host micrRNA targets herpes simplex virus-1 ICP0 expression and promotes latency. Cell Host Microbe. 2014;15:446–56.

[95] Shu M, T. Du, G. Zhou, and B. Roizman. Role of activating transcription factor 3 in the synthesis of latency-associated transcript and maintenance of herpes simplex virus 1 in latent state in ganglia. Proc Natl Acad Sci U S A. 2015;39:E5420–E6.

[96] Clevers H and R. Nusse. Wnt/B-catenin signaling and disease. Cell. 2012;149:1192–205.

[97] Salinas PC. Wnt signaling in the vertebrate central nervous system: from axon guidance to synaptic function. Cold Spring Harb Perpect Biol. 2012;4:a008003.

[98] Purro SA, S. Galli, and P.C. Salinas. Dysfunction of Wnt signaling and synaptic disassembly in neurodegenerative diseases. J Mol Cell Biol. 6(6):75–80.

[99] Bhardwaji D, M. Nager, J. Camats, M. David, A. Benguira, A. dopazo, et al. Chemokines induce axon outgrowth downstream of hepatocyte growth factor and TCF/beta-catenin signaling. Front Cell Neurosci. 2013;7:1–10.

[100] Murase S, E. Mosser, and E.M. Schuman. Depolarization drives beta-catenin into neuronal spines promoting changes in synaptic structure and function. Neuron. 2002;35:91–105.

[101] Bamji SX, B. Rico, N. Kimes, and L.F. Reichardt. BDNF mobilizes synaptic vesicles and enhances synaptic vesicles and enhances synapse formation by disrupting cadherin-beta-catenin interactions. J Cell Biol. 2006;174:289–99.

[102] Grigoryan T, P. Ward, A. Klaus, and W. Birchmeir. Deciphering the function of canonical Wnt signals in development and disease: conditional loss-and gain-of-function mutations of beta-catenin in mice. Gene Dev. 2015;22:2308–41.

[103] Liu Y, M. Hancok, A. Workman, A. Doster, and C. Jones. B-catenin, a transcription factor activated by canonical Wnt signaling, is expressed in sensory neurons of calves latently infected with bovine herpesvirus 1. J Virol. 2016;90(6):3148–59.

[104] Kalamvoki M, T. Du, and B. Roizman. Cells infected with herpes simplex virus 1 export to uninfected cells exosomes containing STING, viral mRNAs, and microRNAs. Proc Natl Acad Sci U S A. 2014;111:E4991–E6.

[105] Kook I, A. Doster, and C. Jones. Bovine herpesvirus 1 regulatory proteins are detected in trigeminal ganglionic neurons during the early stages of stress-induced escape from latency. J Neurovirol. 2015;21:585–91.

[106] Zhao S, J. Fu, X. Liu, T. Wang, J. Zhang, and Y. Zhao. Activation of Akt/GSK-3beta/beta-catenin signaling pathway is invovlved in survival of neurons after traumatic brain injury in rats. Neurol Res. 2012;34:400–7.

[107] Matrisciano F, C.L. Buscetti, D. Bucci, R. Orlando, A. Caruso, G. Molinaro, et al. Induction of the Wnt antagonist Dickkopf-1 is involved in stress-induced hippocampal damage. PLoS One. 2011;6:e16447.

[108] Mastroiacovo F, C.L. Busceti, F. Biagioni, S.G. Moyanova, M.H. Meisler, et al. Induction of the Wnt antagonist, Dickopf-1, contributes to the development of neuronal death in models of brain focal ischemia. J Cereb Blood Flow Metabol. 2009;29:264–76.

[109] Moors M, R. Bose, K. Johansson-Haque, K. Edoff, S. Okret, and S. Ceccatelli. Dickkopf mediates glucocorticoid-induced changes in human neural progenitor cell proliferation and differentiation. Toxicol Sci. 2012;125:488–95.

[110] Ellies DL, V. Church, P. Francis-West, and A. Lumsden. The Wnt antagonist cSFRP2 modulates programmed cell death in teh developing hindbrain. Development. 2000;127:5285–95.

[111] Jones C, T.J. Newby, T. Holt, A. Doster, M. Stone, J. Ciacci-Zanella, et al. Analysis of latency in cattle after inoculation with a temperature sensitive mutant of bovine herpesvirus 1 (RLB106). Vaccine. 2000;18(27):3185–95.

[112] Winkler MT, A. Doster, J.H. Sur, and C. Jones. Analysis of bovine trigeminal ganglia following infection with bovine herpesvirus 1. Vet Microbiol. 2002;86(1–2):139–55.

[113] Cantin EM, D.R. Hinton, J. Chen, and H. Openshaw. Gamma interferon expression during acute and latent nervous system infection by herpes simplex virus type 1. J Virol. 1995;69(8):4898–905.

[114] Halford WP, B.M. Gebhardt, and D.J. Carr. Persistent cytokine expression in trigeminal ganglion latently infected with herpes simplex virus type 1. J Immunol. 1996;157(8): 3542–9.

[115] Liu T, Q. Tang, and R.L. Hendricks. Inflammatory infiltration of the trigeminal ganglion after herpes simplex virus type 1 corneal infection. J Virol. 1996;70(1):264–71.

[116] Shimeld C, J.L. Whiteland, N.A. Williams, D.L. Easty, and T.J. Hill. Reactivation of herpes simplex virus type 1 in the mouse trigeminal ganglion: an in vivo study of virus antigen and immune cell infiltration. J Gen Virol. 1996;77(Pt 10):2583–90.

[117] Shimeld C, J.L. Whiteland, N.A. Williams, D.L. Easty, and T.J. Hill. Cytokine production in the nervous system of mice during acute and latent infection with herpes simplex virus type 1. J Gen Virol. 1997;78(Pt 12):3317–25.

[118] Shimeld C, J.L. Whiteland, S.M. Nicholls, E. Grinfeld, D.L. Easty, H. Gao, et al. Immune cell infiltration and persistence in the mouse trigeminal ganglion after infection of the cornea with herpes simplex virus type 1. J Neuroimmunol. 1995;61(1):7–16.

[119] Theil D, T. Derfuss, I. Paripovic, S. Herberger, E. Meinl, O. Schueler, et al. Latent herpesvirus infection in human trigeminal ganglia causes chronic immune response. Am J Pathol. 2003;163:2179–84.

[120] Liu T, K.M. Khanna, X. Chen, D.J. Fink, and R.L. Hendricks. CD8(+) T cells can block herpes simplex virus type 1 (HSV-1) reactivation from latency in sensory neurons [In Process Citation]. J Exp Med. 2000;191(9):1459–66.

[121] Liu T, K.M. Khanna, B.N. Carriere, and R.L. Hendricks. Gamma interferon can prevent herpes simplex virus type 1 reactivation from latency in sensory neurons. J Virol. 2001;75(22):11178–84.

[122] Khanna KM, R.H. Bonneau, P.R. Kinchington, and R.L. Hendricks. Herpes simplex virus-specific memory CD8+ T cells are selectively activated and retained in latently infected sensory ganglia. Immunity. 2003;18:593–603.

[123] Prbhakaran K, B.S. Sheridan, P.R. Kinchington, K.M. Khanna, V. Decman, K. Lathrop, et al. Sensory neurons regulate the effector functions of CD8+ T cells in controlling HSV-1 latency ex vivo. Immunity. 2005;23:515–23.

[124] Knickelbein JE, K.M. Khanna, M.B. Yee, C.J. Baty, P.R. Kinchington, et al. Noncytotoxic lytic granule-mediated CD8+ T cell inhibition of HSV-1 reactivation from neuronal latency. Science. 2008;322:268–72.

[125] Mott KR, S.J. Allen, M. Zandian, B. Konda, B.G. Sharifi, C. Jones, et al. CD8a dendritic cells drive establishment of HSV-1 latency. PLoS One. 9(4).

[126] Frizzo da Silva L, I. Kook, A. Doster, and C. Jones. Bovine herpesvirus 1 regulatory proteins, bICP0 and VP16, are readily detected in trigeminal ganglionic neurons expressing the glucocorticoid receptor during the early stages of reactivation from latency. J Virol. 2013;87:11214–22.

[127] Workman A, J. Eudy, L. Smith, L. Frizzo da Silva, D. Sinani, H. Bricker, et al. Cellular transcription factors induced in trigeminal ganglia during dexamethasone-induced reactivation from latency stimulate bovine herpesvirus 1 productive infection and certain viral promoters. J Virol. 2012;86:2459–73.

[128] Kook I, C. Henley, F. Meyer, F. Hoffmann, and C. Jones. Bovine herpesvirus 1 productive ifnection and the immediate early transcription unit 1 are stimulated by the synthetic corticosteroid dexamethasone. Virology. 2015;484:377–85.

[129] Thompson RL, C.M. Preston, and N.M. Sawtell. De novo synthesis of VP16 corrdinates the exit form HSV latency in vivo. PLoS Pathog. 2009;5:1–12.

[130] Kim JY, A. Mandarino, M.V. Chao, I Mohr, and A.C. Wilson. Transient reversal of episome silencing precedes VP16-dependent transcription during reactivation of HSV-1 in neurons. PLoS Pathog. 2012;8:e1002540.

[131] Garlanda C, B. Bottazzi, A. Bastone, and A. Mantovani. Pentraxins at the crossroads between innate immunity, inflammation, matrix deposition, and female fertility. Annu Rev Immunol. 2005;23:337–66.

[132] Kaczynski J, T. Cook, and R. Urrutia. Sp1- and Kruppel-like transcription factors. Genome Biol. 2003;4:206.1–8.

[133] Bieker JJ. Kruppel-like factors: three fingers in many pies. J Biol Chem. 2001;276:34355–8.

[134] Sinani D, E. Cordes, A. Workman, P. Thunuguntia, and C. Jones. Stress induced cellular transcription factors expressed in trigeminal ganglionic neurons stimulate the herpes simplex virus type 1 (HSV-1) infected cell protein 0 (ICP0) promoter. J Virol. 2013;87:1183–92.

[135] Deshmane SL and N.W. Fraser. During latency, herpes simplex virus type 1 DNA is associated with nucleosomes in a chromatin structure. J Virol. 1989;63:943–7.

[136] Kubat N, R.K. Tran, P. McAnanny, and D.C. Bloom. Specific histone tail modification and not DNA methylation is a determinant of HSV-1 latent gene expression. J Virol. 2004(78):1139–49.

[137] Knipe DM and A. Cliffe. Chromatin control of herpes simplex virus lytic and latent infection. Nat Rev Microbiol. 2008;6:211–21.

[138] Perlman T. Glucocorticoid receptor DNA-binding specificity is increased by the organization of DNA in nucleosomes. Proc Natl Acad Sci U S A. 1992;89:3884–8.

[139] Perlman TaOW. Specific glucocorticoid receptor binding to DNA reconstituted in nucleosome. EMBO J. 1988;7:3073–9.

[140] Lin QaOW. Translational positioning of a nucleosome: glucocorticoid response element moulates glucocorticoid receptor affinity. Genes Dev. 1993;7:2471–82.

[141] Foy RaWH. Sequence-specific positioning of nucleosomes over the steroid-inducible MMTV promoter. EMBO J. 2003;6:2321–8.

[142] Zaret KSaKRY. Reversible and presistent changes in chromatin structure accompany activation of a glucocorticoid-dependent enhancer element. Cell. 1984;258:1780–4.

[143] John S, P.J. Sabo, R.E. Thurman, M.H. Sung, S.C. Biddie, T.A. Johnson, G.L. Hager, and J.A. Stamatoyannopoulos. Cromatin accessibility pre-determined glucocorticoid receptor binding patterns. Nat Genet. 2011(43):264–8.

[144] Voss TC, R.L. Schiltz, M.H. Sung, P.M. Yen, J.A. Stamatoyannopoulos, S.C. Biddie, et al.. Dynamic exchange at regulatory elements during chromatin remodeling underlies assisted loading mechanism. Cell. 2011;146:544–54.

[145] Zaret KS and J.S. Carrol. Pioneer transcription factors: establishing competence for gene expression. Genes Dev. 2011;25:2227–41.

[146] Iwafuchi-Doi M and K.S. Zaret. Pioneer transcription factors in cell reprogramming. Genes Dev. 2014;28:2679–92.

[147] Soufi A, M.F. Garcia, A. Jaroszewcz, N. Osman, M. Pellegrini, and K.S. Zaret. Pioneer transcription factors target partial DNA motifs on nucleosomes to initiate reprogramming. Cell. 2015;161:555–68.

[148] Shimeld C, D.L. Easty, and T.J. Hill. Reactivation of herpes simplex virus type 1 in the mouse trigeminal ganglion: an in vivo study of virus antigen and cytokines. J Virol. 1999;73(3):1767–73.

[149] Inman M, G.-C. Perng, G. Henderson, H. Ghiasi, A.B. Nesburn, S.L. Wechsler a, et al. Region of herpes simplex virus type 1 latency-associated transcript sufficient for wild-type spontaneous reactivation promotes cell survival in tissue culture. J Virol. 2001;75(8):3636–46.

[150] Perng G-C, C. Jones, J. Ciacci-Zanella, M. Stone, G. Henderson, A. Yukht, et al. Virus-induced neuronal apoptosis blocked by the herpes simplex virus latency-associated transcript (LAT). Science. 2000;287:1500–3.

[151] Ciacci-Zanella J, M. Stone, G. Henderson, and C. Jones. The latency-related gene of bovine herpesvirus 1 inhibits programmed cell death. J Virol. 1999;73(12):9734–40.

[152] Shen W, M.S.e. Silva., T. Jaber, O. Vitvitskaia, S. Li, G. Henderson, et al. Two small RNAs encoded within the first 1.5 kb of the herpes simplex virus type 1 (HSV-1) latency-associated transcript (LAT) can inhibit productive infection, and cooperate to inhibit apoptosis. J Virol. 2009;90:9131–9.

[153] Umbach JL, M.F. Kramer, I. Jurak, H.W. Karnowski, D.M. Coen, and B.R. Cullen. MicroRNAs expressed by herpes simplex virus 1 during latent infection regulate viral mRNAs. Nature. 2008;454:780–5.

[154] Li S, D. Carpenter, C. Hsiang, S.L. Wechsler, and C. Jones. The herpes simplex virus type 1 latency-associated transcript (LAT) locus inhibits apoptosis and promotes neurite sprouting in neuroblastoma cells following serum starvation by maintaining active AKT (protein kinase B). J Gen Virol. 2010;91:858–66.

[155] Perng G-C, B. Maguen, L. Jin, K.R. Mott, N. Osorio, S.M. Slanina, et al. A gene capable of blocking apoptosis can substitute for the herpes simplex virus type 1 latency-associated transcript gene and restore wild-type reactivation levels. J Virol. 2002;76:1224–35.

[156] Mott K, N. Osorio, L. Jin, D. Brick, J. Naito, J. Cooper, et al. The bovine herpesvirus 1 LR ORF2 is crucial for this gene's ability to restore the high reactivation phenotype to a Herpes simplex virus-1 LAT null mutant. J Gen Virol. 2003;84:2975–85.

[157] Cassidy L, J. Meadows, J. Catalan, and S. Barton. Are stress and coping style associated with frequent recurrence of genital hereps? Genitourin Med. 1997;73:263–6.

[158] Glaser R, J.K. Kiecolt-Glaser, C.E. Speicher, and J.E. Holliday. Stress, loneliness, and changes in herpesvirus latency. J Behav Med. 1985;8:249–60.

[159] Padgett DA, J.F. Sherida, J. Dorne, G.G. Berntson, J. Candelora, and R. Glaser. Social stress and the reactivation of latent herpes simplex virus type 1. Proc Natl Acad Sci U S A. 1998;95:7231–5.

[160] Du T, G. Zhou, and B. Roizman. Induction of apoptosis accelerates reactivation from latent HSV-1 in ganglionic organ cultures and replication in cell cultures. Proc Natl Acad Sci U S A. 2012;109:14616–21.

[161] Wirth UV, K. Gunkel, M. Engels, and M. Schwyzer. Spatial and temporal distribution of bovine herpesvirus 1 transcripts. J Virol. 1989;63(11):4882–9.